Functional Movement Development
Across the Life Span

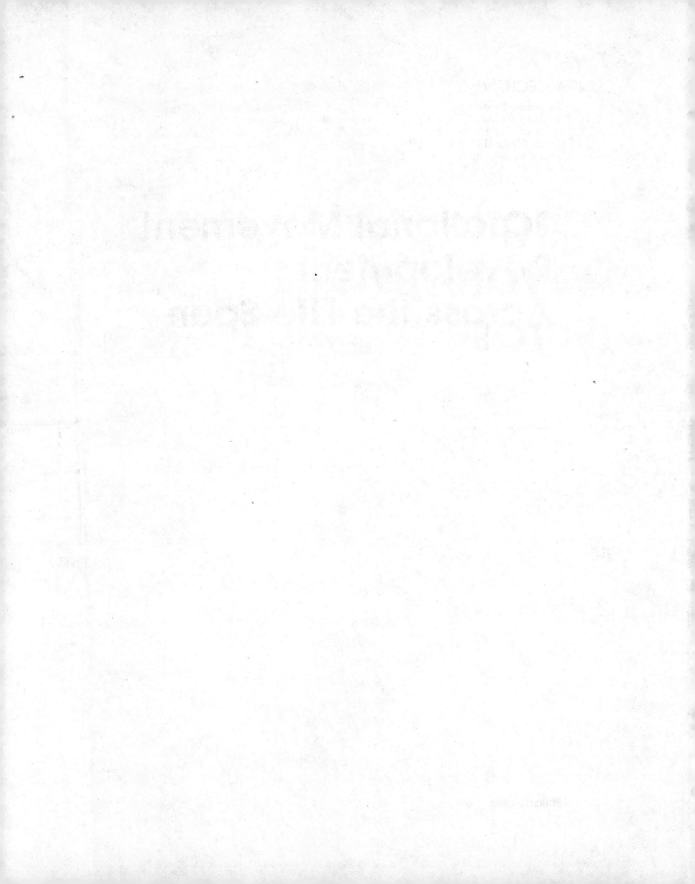

whereas others may not be able to do the things they need to do. The terms "disability" and "handicap" are frequently used when daily tasks cannot be performed. In general, the term "disability" refers to an individual's diminished functional capacity (Jette, 1985). "Handicap" is a frame of reference defined by society. When an individual is no longer viewed as being able to perform the tasks society would expect of him or her, he or she is considered handicapped. It must be emphasized that loss of functional ability does not necessarily result in disability or handicap.

HEALTH STATUS MODELS

Several models have been proposed to analyze the spectrum of status from functional independence to disability. By using these models, health care providers can more easily categorize their patients according to functional status. This categorization is helpful in identifying appropriate services and planning treatment programs. The two most popular models are the International Classification of Impairments, Disabilities, and Handicaps (ICIDH) proposed by the World Health Organization (WHO, 1980) and the model of health status proposed by sociologist Saad Nagi (Nagi, 1991). These two models are compared in Figure 1–1.

The ICIDH defines impairment as any limitation or abnormality in anatomic, physiologic, or psychologic processes. Disability refers to a deficit in the performance of daily activities. Handicap is related to an individual's inability to perform expected social roles, leading to a diminished quality of life. This model does provide basic categories for classifying a patient's functional outcome status. Not all patients can easily and neatly fit into the categories.

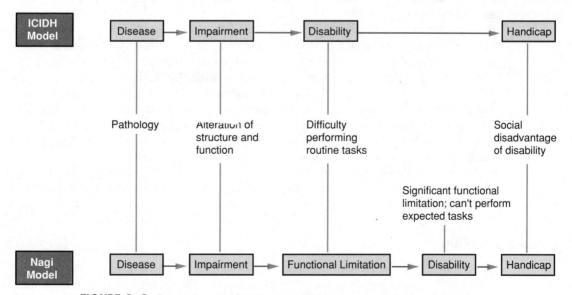

FIGURE 1–1. Comparison of ICIDH and Nagi Classification Systems of Health Status.

Some people can have impairments that do not automatically mean they are disabled in their performance of daily activities. Others may have the ability to perform a task such as dressing, but choose not to perform this task independently if it takes too much time or is too exhausting. They may draw upon the assistance of others, use assistive devices, or adjust the environment to make the task easier. Do they then have a disability? (Guccione, 1991; Haley et al, 1992).

The model proposed by Nagi, although similar in its definition of impairment to the ICIDH, introduces another category into the classification scheme. The category of *functional limitation* is included to describe deficits occurring because of an impairment and affecting a person's ability to perform his or her usual activities. Within the Nagi model, the presence of disease and impairment does not necessarily result in functional limitations. Consider a patient with an impairment of elbow range of motion who cannot fully extend the elbow. This impairment will cause more of a functional limitation for a baseball pitcher than it would for a pianist. The term "disability" is also used differently in the Nagi model. Disability refers to patterns of behavior that emerge when functional limitations are too great to allow successful completion of a task. The Nagi classification system supports the identification of limitations in functional tasks appropriate and important for the person. By using this approach, health care providers are aided in identifying the most appropriate focus for their interventions (Guccione, 1993; Haley et al, 1992).

In assessing health status of individuals, health care providers need to understand and differentiate among the issues of impairment, functional limitation, and disability. This knowledge will allow the provider to focus on the issues most important to the patient and to consider if interventions can effect change in an impairment, minimize a functional limitation, or diminish a disability.

In working with patients of different ages, it is also important to understand if limitations reflect presence of disability or development. Is the 3-year-old who cannot tie his shoe disabled? Of course not. Developmentally it is normal for a child to require adult assistance with this task. By 8 years of age, usually the child no longer needs adult assistance because the child has developed skills in this area. If an older adult with severe arthritis cannot put on her shoe because of mobility limitations in hip flexion or finger mobility, is she disabled? Again, not necessarily. If that adult uses a long-handled shoehorn, she may be quite good at completing the task. Developmental issues, social expectations, family attitudes, and adaptability of the environment are all issues that help determine whether limitations or disabilities are present (Guccione, 1993; Haley et al, 1992).

Functional Skills

Functional skills have been defined as the variety of skills that are frequently demanded in natural domestic, vocational, and community environments, allowing an individual to perform as independently as possible in all settings

(Brown et al, 1979). Functional skills and activities not only support an individual's physical and psychologic well being, but also allow that individual to incorporate what is important to him or her into meaningful, everyday life (Guccione et al, 1988). From early infancy to late adulthood, individuals must develop or adapt functional skills to best access the environment they live in and meet their own needs as independently as possible. Performance of functional activities not only depends on one's physical abilities, but is also affected by emotional status, cognitive ability, and social/cultural expectations. These factors together define an individual's functional performance (Fig. 1–2).

In general, certain categories of functional activities, such as eating, maintaining personal hygiene, dressing, ambulating, and grasping, are common to everyone. Other tasks related to one's job or recreation vary from one person to the next. Within the health care model, personal care activities such as ambulating, feeding, bathing, dressing, grooming, maintaining continence, and toileting are referred to as *basic activities of daily living (BADL)*. Other important activities relate to how well one can manage within the home setting and in the community. These activities are referred to as *instrumental activities of daily living (IADL)* and include tasks such as cooking, cleaning, handling finances, shopping, working, and using personal or public transportation. As discussed in Chapter 5, the health care provider often assesses BADL

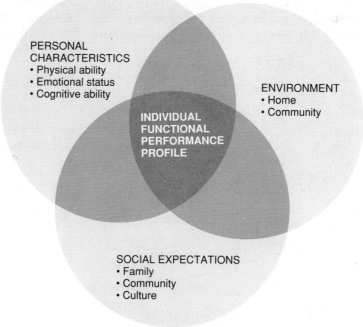

FIGURE 1–2. Factors defining an individual's functional performance.

and IADL to define patient status and develop appropriate intervention programs.

Function from a Life Span Perspective

Function defines mastery and competency over the environment (Guccione, 1993). Throughout the life span, from conception until old age, the individual demonstrates varying abilities and levels of mastery over the environment in which he or she lives. Initially, an individual is concerned with being able to survive and masters a level of function concerned with self-need. Next the individual learns to function well within the home environment, and finally the individual learns to function within the community (Fig. 1–3). For example, to ensure survival, the infant learns to cry for food or when in discomfort. He can also turn his head to keep his airway clear and coordinate important tasks such as breathing and swallowing. The toddler learns to function safely within her home: avoiding electric outlets, climbing stairs, feeding herself, using the toilet. Finally, the school-age child learns to safely cross the street on the way to school. These same levels of mastery are mirrored at all life stages, as functional expectations change. The adult masters self-care tasks such as eating by shopping and cooking or dining out. He provides himself with shelter and keeps that shelter clean and warm. Finally, the adult masters functioning in a larger community including the workplace.

From these examples, it is obvious that an individual's functional ability is in part defined by his or her age. As children get older they are expected to gain independence in a wide variety of functional tasks and in an expanding environment. The 5-year-old must meet the challenges of becoming competent within the new environment of school. Many 16-year-olds assume the respon-

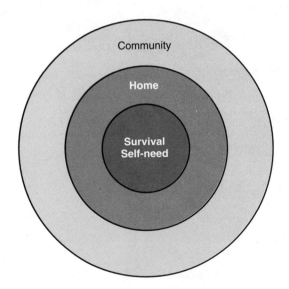

FIGURE 1–3. Acquisition of function: Levels of mastery over the environment.

sibilities of safely driving a car and functioning within their community. The functional expectations of adults expand as they have children and assume job responsibilities. Older adults may appear to be faced with fewer functional expectations as they retire and their children become independent. They may also be faced with challenges related to maintaining functional independence of even basic needs as they adapt to fixed incomes and declining physical abilities. It is clear that the definition of function and functional independence changes across the life span as a person's abilities change and society's expectations vary.

PHYSICAL GROWTH AND FUNCTION

In many ways a person's functional abilities depend on his or her physical abilities. Physical development not only impacts on the ability to perform physical activity, but also affects a person's ability to interact with his or her environment. Movement has been related to cognitive development, social activity, and communication. Across the life span, the physical capacity of the individual changes and helps to define functional capacity.

Within the embryologic development of the individual, the first 7 to 8 weeks after conception are devoted to growth of the individual. Functional systems, although being formed, have not yet begun to work at their tasks. In the fetal period (8 weeks after conception until birth) the organ systems begin to function and the developing person becomes competent within the protective environment of the womb. Once born, the baby must accommodate to another environment, governed by the force of gravity. Babies attain functional skills in this new environment and systematically continue growing. The 1-year-old may be very proud and excited about his ability to walk. The 2- to 3-year-old adds important functional skills such as feeding and dressing herself. The balance between body growth and functional mastery continues until physical maturity is attained in young adulthood. Adults strive to attain and maintain functionally active lifestyles. The wear and tear that sometimes results from their functional activities can frequently be balanced by growth and the repair abilities of the body. By the time an adult reaches old age, growth and repair functions may be insufficient to maintain the optimal functional state of the body. As performance of functional skills becomes inefficient, the older adult may be less able to participate in activities that are important to him, diminishing his ability to function and maintain a level of mastery over his environment (Guccione, 1993; Sinclair, 1985).

RELATIONSHIP BETWEEN DEVELOPMENT AND FUNCTION

As is emphasized in this book, an individual develops throughout the life span. Development occurs not only as a result of physical changes within the body, but also because of environmental influences. As the individual interacts within family, community, social, and cultural contexts, his or her development is shaped and functional roles or tasks are defined. From this perspec-

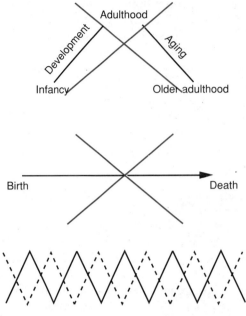

FIGURE 1-4. Interaction of life span and functional development.

Key: ———— = life span; - - - - = functional development

tive, development and function are intertwined throughout the life span, much like a cloth is woven.

Development of function does not refer just to the growth process related to youth or to the decline often associated with aging. Similarly, it cannot necessarily be reflected linearly. Growth and development imply change, either positive or negative, which can be observed at any point within the life span. If the life span and functional development are considered two separate continuums, pleated back on one another to resemble the bellows of an accordian, their impact on one another is obvious (Fig. 1-4). As adolescents experience growth spurts, attaining new height, they also experience losses in flexibility because muscle growth does not keep up with bone growth. Adults may achieve new levels of productivity in the workplace, but at the cost of family or social interactions. The life span approach to development and function appreciates all of the changes seen in an individual's abilities at any point in the life cycle, whether the changes reflect progression, regression, or reorganization (Hultsch & Deutsch, 1981; Van Sant, 1990).

Domains of Function

Functional activities with similar outcomes can be grouped together into categories or domains. Within this text, three domains of function are defined: physical function, psychologic function, and social function (Fig. 1-5). Physical functions are those sensorimotor skills needed to perform activities of daily living such as dressing, ambulating, maintaining hygiene, and cooking. Psy-

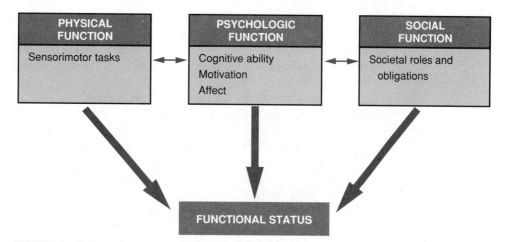

FIGURE 1–5. Domains of function.

chologic function reflects intellectual activities. Motivation, concentration, problem solving, and judgment are all factors contributing to psychologic function. Also included within the domain of psychologic function is affective function, which allows a person to cope with everyday stresses. It also influences how a person perceives his or her ability to function. Factors such as anxiety, depression, emotional well-being, and self-esteem influence affective function (Guccione, 1993). Social function reflects the ability to interact with other people and successfully complete social roles and obligations. Cultural norms or expectations help define social function.

These domains of function parallel domains of development discussed in Chapter 2, reinforcing the interrelationship of function and development. No one domain of function stands alone. All three are interrelated and interdependent in meeting everyday challenges. Many social functions depend on one's mobility and ability to physically manipulate objects. Likewise, a person's physical level of function can easily be influenced by emotional status, intellectual ability, or motivation.

Although all three domains of function are important, only the domain of physical function will be discussed in depth in this chapter. The domains of psychologic and social function are generally discussed within the context of human development and developmental psychology courses and textbooks. This text focuses on physical function because it is in this arena that physical and occupational therapists focus their interventions.

PHYSICAL FUNCTION

Physical function can also be thought of as goal-directed movement. Function is the link between the physical actions we call movement and the environmental context in which they take place. For the act of reaching to be meaningful and therefore functional, it must take place when there is an object to reach for. Walking is functional because it is a means of moving from one place to another. People use movement every day as they interact with their environment. Goal-directed movement is important for an individual to survive, to adapt, and to learn within the environment. When an individual is less able to move, he or she may be less able to meet day-to-day needs. The young athlete with a broken leg suddenly must depend on crutches, making simple tasks such as walking to the bathroom or opening the door a challenge. As movement becomes less efficient, an individual may be faced with diminished functional independence. The individual with arthritis may not be able to quickly and efficiently button clothes. He or she may also have difficulty picking up coins when paying for purchases in a store. As physical function becomes impaired, individuals frequently turn to health professionals for assistance.

Physical and occupational therapy intervention generally focus on improving physical function. Improved physical functioning may also impact positively on psychologic and social functioning. Therapists must first identify their patient's functional difficulties by performing a functional assessment. Additional assessment of sensory, cardiopulmonary, neurologic, or musculoskeletal systems may then identify impairments that interfere with overall function. Impairments may include anatomic or physiologic changes such as limited range of motion or diminished strength. Therapeutic programs can then be devised to improve function by impacting on the identified impairments. The measure of success of these therapeutic programs is the functional change demonstrated by the patient, not isolated changes in range of motion or strength impairments.

It is important for therapists to have an understanding of how physical function changes over time, the relationship of physical function to other domains of function, and the components of physical function that contribute to quality and efficiency of movement. With this foundation, the therapist can most effectively create intervention programs to meet the individual needs of each person.

Development

How does physical function develop? What factors influence its development? Age, environment, and social expectations all contribute to defining normal physical functioning for an individual. Age not only defines size and biologic capacity for movement but also reflects expectations about lifestyle.

During infancy and childhood, body size and the maturity of the body systems involved in movement will limit and define functional abilities. For example, toddlers are able to walk, but because of their short legs, they have trouble keeping up with their parents. It is frequently more efficient and functional for them to be carried or pushed in a stroller. Young children may have trouble sitting at the table without fidgeting at a meal, perhaps because their feet do not reach the floor and they cannot easily sit in the large chair provided for them. Functional limitations in these examples are closely related to the immaturity of the child's skeletal system, but the neuromuscular and cardiopulmonary systems are also undergoing rapid development during this timeframe and impact on the child's physical abilities. Fundamental motor skills such as postural control, locomotion, and prehension develop rapidly during childhood.

Functional expectations of the infant and child also impact on their development of functional skills. Young infants' abilities are basically survival oriented. They can lift and turn their heads; coordinate suck, swallow, and breathing; cry to indicate needs; and socially interact with their caregivers to ensure that they are well taken care of. As the infant begins to control his or her movement, the major "job" or "task" is to explore the environment. Through play, infants learn about the world around them. As the toddler and young child associate some of their play with functional activities, such as eating and dressing, caregivers begin to have higher expectations for functional independence.

Through childhood and adolescence, social roles and expectations continue to undergo constant change. Body growth and maturation of the body systems also continues. Once maturity is attained in adolescence or young adulthood, the systems of the body contributing to motor performance have completed their development. At this point these body systems are ready to operate at peak efficiency. Practice and motivation to excel contribute to the person's ability to learn and refine new motor tasks. Skills are refined as the child/adolescent tries to improve performance in recreational activities such as baseball, ballet, and gymnastics.

Societal roles and lifestyle changes accompanying adulthood again redefine physical function and may result in decreased physical activity levels. Commuting time, combined with a full day at work, may limit time available for physically active recreational pursuits. As activity levels decrease, so does one's level of fitness. Cardiopulmonary functioning and muscle strength may not be supported in their full capacity, resulting in decreased endurance and weakness. Refinement of skills associated with job pursuits continues through adulthood. As the body systems are continually used in day-to-day activities, wear and tear, as well as ongoing developmental changes related to adulthood, are thought to decrease the efficiency of the body in physical functioning.

In the older adult, physical functional ability is thought to further decline because of wear and tear on the body systems, normal development, and lifestyle changes. Retirement from a physically demanding job may result in a less active lifestyle. A common assumption made about the elderly is that they have diminished ability to perform physical activities. When one considers the total population of older adults, however, the majority of them do not have significant functional limitations. They live independently and maintain a relatively active and satisfying lifestyle. Functional ability does decrease with age, but it is in the oldest populations (>85 years old) that physical disability is the greatest. Several functional tasks are required of people who live independently, including basic activities of daily living (self-care and mobility) and instrumental activities of daily living such as cooking, shopping, housekeeping, and transportation. Of these, housekeeping and transportation difficulties are the most often reported by older adults (Jackson & Lang, 1989).

Components

Efficient, effective, graceful, fluid, and smooth are all adjectives frequently associated with movement. Clumsy, awkward, disjointed, and wasted can also describe movement but paint a very different picture than the first set of adjectives. Sports science, physical education, and more recently physical and occupational therapy have tried to define the factors that contribute to efficient, effective movement. Flexibility, balance, coordination, power, and endurance are some dimensions that affect the quality of physical function.

FLEXIBILITY

Most simply, flexibility refers to the capacity to bend. Flexibility can be described for a specific joint, a series of joints, or a specific person. Within human movement, flexibility depends on two different components. The first is the flexibility of the muscles, connective tissue, and skin. These tissues must maintain an appropriate resting length and pliability to allow the joint mobility necessary for completing activities of daily living. The second component of flexibility refers to joint range of motion. The joint structure must be able to move through its entire range, completing the normal range of arthrokinematics and demonstrating adequate laxity of the joint capsule (Kisner & Colby, 1985; Zachazewski, 1989). When a person has good flexibility, the tissues accommodate more easily to stress, which results in efficient, effective movement (Zachazewski, 1989).

Two types of flexibility can be assessed. *Static flexibility* refers to the range of motion available at a joint. *Dynamic flexibility* refers to the resistance offered to active movement of the joint. As resistance increases, dynamic flexibility decreases. When optimal levels of resistance balance the motion around a joint, efficiency of movement is achieved. As flexibility increases, greater force can be exerted in a movement, and speed of performance increases (Northrip et al, 1974).

A person's flexibility is defined by the types of physical activities that are included within his or her day. The flexibility of the baseball pitcher's throwing arm is certainly greater than that of a typist. A gymnast is probably more flexible than a football player. Work and recreational activities of adults certainly impact on their flexibility.

Developmentally, flexibility is fairly stable in boys from age 5 to 8 years, then decreases slightly until 12 to 13 years. After that time it again increases slightly until age 18. In girls flexibility is stable from age 5 to 11 years, then increases until age 14. After that time it plateaus. At all ages, into maturity, females are more flexible than males (Malina & Bouchard, 1991). In older adults, flexibility is thought to decrease because of changes in connective tissue, activity level, muscle strength, and joints. Active older adults maintain greater levels of flexibility than their more sedentary peers.

BALANCE

Balance refers to a state of equilibrium and is an important component of skilled movement. Balance is achieved when one can maintain one's center of gravity over one's base of support, thereby maintaining equilibrium. Several factors contribute to the ability to balance, including efficient function of the nervous system, musculoskeletal system, and sensory systems. Balance is necessary during static activities such as standing still *(static balance)* and during movement *(dynamic balance)*.

During childhood, balance improves with age. Girls appear to do better than boys on balance activities. In adolescence, both groups plateau in balance skills. Boys may perform slightly better than girls in this age group (Malina & Bouchard, 1991). In older adulthood, poor balance is frequently reported as a problem and may be related to impairments in the body systems contributing to balance.

COORDINATION

Coordination implies that various muscles are working together to produce a movement. Smooth, efficient movement results when the right muscles work at the right time with the right intensity (Kisner & Colby, 1985). Coordination is needed to successfully crawl, skip, run to catch a bus, make a bed, or put on a pair of pants in the morning. Another way of looking at coordination is to consider it as the function that constrains the body's limitless movement possibilities into one efficient, functional unit (Crutchfield et al, 1989).

POWER

Power refers to the rate at which work is done. Related to movement, it is the rate at which a muscle can develop tension and produce a force, moving a body part through a range of motion (Mangine et al, 1989). Power is then related to both strength and speed. In childhood, power depends on size and maturity of the neurologic and musculoskeletal systems. In older adults, as strength and speed decrease, power also decreases (Brown, 1987).

ENDURANCE

Endurance refers to the ability to continue performing work over an extended period. Children, for example, can play actively for hours. Endurance is necessary for an individual to perform repetitive activities of daily living, such as stirring food while cooking, using a blow dryer to dry his or her hair, and walking up steps. Recreational and job-related tasks also often require a high level of endurance.

Endurance can be related to an individual muscle, a muscle group, or the total body. Total body endurance usually refers to cardiopulmonary endurance, reflecting the heart's ability to deliver a steady supply of oxygen to working muscle. Muscle endurance is related to muscle strength. Developmentally, muscle endurance has been shown to increase linearly in boys between 5 and 13 years of age, at which point a spurt is seen. In girls a steady linear increase is seen (Malina & Bouchard, 1991).

SUMMARY

This chapter has attempted to define that elusive entity, human function, from a life span perspective. Function has been discussed in relationship to the broader context of health. Models of health status are presented to help differentiate between function and dysfunction (disability). The interactions and interdependence of the domains of physical, psychologic, and social function are what define a person's ability to function. The domain of physical function is looked at in more depth, because this is the area which physical and occupational therapists hope to impact when working with their patients. An attempt is made to define the components that make movement efficient, effective, and most importantly, functional. From this base, therapists can assess how their clients are functioning and successfully meet their goals of improved function.

References

Brown L, Branston MB, Hamre-Mietupski S, Pumpian I, Certo N, Gruenewald L. A strategy for developing chronological age appropriate and functional curricular content for severely handicapped adolescents and young adults. *J Spec Ed* 13:81–89, 1979.

Brown MA. Selected physical performance changes with aging. *Top Geriatr Rehabil* 2:68–76, 1987.

Crutchfield C, Shumway-Cook A, Horak F. Balance and coordination training. In Scully RM, Barnes MR (eds). *Physical Therapy.* Philadelphia: JB Lippincott, 1989, pp 825–843.

Guccione AA, Physical therapy diagnosis and the relationship between impairments and function. *Phys Ther* 71:499–504, 1991.

Guccione AA, Health status: A conceptual framework and terminology for assessment. In Guccione AA (ed). *Geriatric Physical Therapy.* St. Louis: Mosby, 1993, pp 101–111.

Guccione AA, Cullen KE, O'Sullivan SB. Functional assessment. In O'Sullivan S, Schmitz TJ (eds). *Physical Rehabilitation: Assessment and Treatment,* 2nd ed. Philadelphia: FA Davis, 1988, pp 219–235.

Haley SM, Coster WJ, Ludlow LH, Haltiwanger JT, Andrellos PJ. *Pediatric Evaluation of Disability Inventory (PEDI).* Boston: New England Medical Center Hosp., Inc., and PEDI Research Group, 1992.

Hultsch DF, Deutsch F. *Adult Development and Aging: A Lifespan Perspective.* New York: McGraw-Hill, 1981.

Jackson OL, Lang RH. Comprehensive functional assessment of the elderly. In Jackson OL (ed). *Physical Therapy of the Geriatric Patient,* 2nd ed. New York: Churchill Livingston, 1989, pp 239–277.

Jette AM. State of the art in functional status assessment. In Rothstein J (ed). *Measurement in Physical Therapy.* New York: Churchill Livingston, 1985, pp 137–168.

Kisner C, Colby LA. *Therapeutic Exercise: Foundations and Techniques.* Philadelphia: FA Davis, 1985.

Malina RM, Bouchard C. *Growth, Maturation, and Physical Activity.* Springfield, IL: Human Kinetics Press, 1991.

Mangine R, Heckman TP, Eldridge VL. Improving strength, endurance and power. In Scully RM, Barnes MR (eds). *Physical Therapy.* Philadelphia: JB Lippincott, 1989, pp 739–762.

Nagi SZ. Disability concepts revisited: Implications for prevention. In Pope AM, Tarlov AR (eds). *Disability in America: Toward a National Agenda for Prevention.* Washington, DC: National Academy Press, 1991, pp 309–327.

Northrip JW, Logan GA, McKinney WC. *Introduction to Biomechanic Analysis of Sport.* Dubuque, IA: Wm C. Brown, 1974.

Sinclair D. *Human Growth After Birth,* 4th ed. London: Oxford University Press, 1985.

Van Sant AF. Life-span development in functional tasks. *Phys Ther* 70:788–798, 1990.

Webster's New 20th Century Unabridged Dictionary, 2nd ed. New York: Simon & Schuster, 1983, p. 741.

World Health Organization. *The First Ten Years of the World Health Organization.* Geneva: WHO, 1958.

World Health Organization. *International Classification of Impairments, Disabilities, and Handicaps.* Geneva: WHO, 1980.

Zachazewski JE: Improving flexibility. In Scully RM, Barnes MR (eds). *Physical Therapy.* Philadelphia: JB Lippincott, 1989, pp 698–738.

Chapter 2

Theories Affecting Development

Objectives

AFTER STUDYING THIS CHAPTER, THE READER WILL BE ABLE TO:

1   Define and differentiate development, growth, maturation, adaptation, and learning.
2   Discuss representative physical, psychologic, and social theories and theorists.
3   Discuss theories unique to different ages.
4   Relate developmental theories to functional movement.

Development is a topic covered in many professional education programs including education, psychology, and health sciences programs. Each program focuses on aspects of development unique to its profession, with vast bodies of knowledge existing in developmental psychology, physiology, biology, and sociology. A person does not develop in only one arena at a time. In normal human development, interaction among physical, psychologic, and social factors shapes the individual.

This chapter provides a general overview of physical, psychologic, and social theories. From this general introduction, it should become apparent how different arenas and disciplines are inexorably involved in the study of the development of functional movement skills. For example, a child in the United States learns to eat with a fork within the 1st or 2nd year of life. This social skill cannot develop until physical development is sufficiently advanced to allow fine controlled movements of the arm and hand. The child must cognitively understand the relationship among food, the fork, hunger, and the action taken to satisfy that hunger. Social customs shape how the child performs the skill. In fact, an Asian child will be meeting the same functional need at about the same age, but will be using chopsticks.

DEVELOPMENT

Human development refers to changes that occur in a person's life from conception to death. Changes can occur on many levels. Changes in body systems over time can be progressive, reorganizational, or regressive. In muscle, for example, where tissue increases during growth, fiber types differentiate or atrophy because of use or loss of innervation and nutrition. Development can be thought of generally as a change in form and function (Higgins, 1985), such as a sapling's growing into an oak tree or a caterpillar's turning into a butterfly. The form a movement takes is shaped by the function it is intended to carry out. Because functional demands are different at different ages, the movement forms that emerge during development change. Human behavior is the outward manifestation of development and changes through four processes: growth, maturation, adaptation, and learning.

Growth refers to the changes in physical dimensions of the body. A child grows taller and limb lengths increase until skeletal maturity is reached. Head circumference, height, and weight are all examples of dimensions that can be used to assess growth and can be plotted on growth charts. Changes in growth can be used to assess development. The ponderal index (PI) is a growth measure that compares height and weight (weight $\times 100/\text{length}^3$). Body composition manifests age-related increases over time, with the relative amounts of muscle, fat, and bone sometimes contributing to discrepancies between height and weight. Healthy children exhibit stable trends in growth throughout the developmental stages of life.

Maturation contributes to development by producing physical changes that cause organs and body systems to reach their adult form and function (Valadian & Porter, 1977). Many of these processes, such as the appearance of primary and secondary ossification centers in the bones of the skeletal system, are on a genetically controlled timetable. The release of hormones related to growth and development is controlled by the hypothalamus and the endocrine system. Reflexes and reactions emerge sequentially in response to maturation of the nervous system. Myelination is one hallmark of nervous system maturation, whereas puberty is a hallmark of endocrine system maturation. The genetic substrate of behavior does not simply imprint its code on the environment; rather, the genetic base allows the individual to adapt to the environment. An example of the environment altering maturation is seen in the younger onset of puberty that occurs in western societies because of a richer diet. An example of a negative effect the environment can have is shown by delayed motor behavior of understimulated institutionalized infants in the 1940s.

Adaptation and learning are sometimes difficult to separate from maturation. Some structures and functions of organ systems are adaptations to the internal or external environment. Exposure to some type of stimulus that may or may not be a stressor, such as the pull of primitive muscles, can induce change. Development of joints in the embryo requires primitive muscles to pull on bone to produce a joint cavity. If the muscles fail to produce movement, as in arthrogryposis, joint deformities occur in utero. Postnatally, bone remodeling with growth is another example of adaptation. The production of antibodies following exposure to chicken pox is another example of adaptation seen in the immune system. Adaptation is the body's accommodation to the immediate environment. Adaptation, like development, can produce positive or negative changes. Although individuals may adapt differently, all individuals mature in the same manner but at different rates.

Experience plays a crucial role in mastering abilities that are not innate. For example, roller skating is an adaptation to having wheels on your shoes. Hilgard and Marquis (1961, p. 2) define learning as "a relatively permanent change in behavior as a result of practice"; therefore, learning can be considered a form of adaptation. Many motor abilities such as riding a bike, playing soccer, reading, writing, and speaking are learned, but we do not know if there is an optimal time for learning these tasks.

The concept of life span development is relatively new. Baltes et al (1980) defined life span developmental psychology as being "concerned with the description, explanation, and modification (optimization) of developmental processes in the human life course from conception to death" (p. 66). Of all the psychologic theorists, Erikson is the only one who completely addresses the life span (see Table 2–4). Erikson's eight stages embrace the four crucial assumptions that make a theory life span in scope: development (1) is depicted as a lifelong process, (2) is an expression of ontogenetic and evolutionary principles, (3) is multicausal and interactive, based on age-related, history-related, and non-normative life events, and (4) occurs in context.

Geriatrics and gerontology were established as fields of human service and research in the 1950s (Levinson, 1986). Although gerontology has not yet embraced the life span approach, it has fostered an explosion of information on aging. Present population demographics document that the population continues to age. By the year 2050, 22.9 per cent of the total population, or 68.5 million people, will be older than age 65 (Atchley, 1991). Aging is a natural continuation of development and can therefore be considered developmental. However, there is no universally accepted theory of aging, nor do aging theories incorporate early development.

Factors Affecting Development

The process of development is strongly influenced by four factors: genetics, maturation, environment, and culture. None of these influences alone can account for all the changes that occur throughout the life span. The interaction between maturation and experience within specific physical, psychologic, and social environments is thought to account for individual developmental differences. Two children grow up in poverty: one makes it out of the ghetto, the other joins the welfare rolls. What makes the difference? The values and life goals inherited from one's family, society, and culture are just as real as one's biologic heritage.

Genetics and maturation contribute to and control our body's internal environment or internal milieu. The internal milieu includes the body's electrolytes, hormones, autonomic nervous system, and immune system, which control physiologic homeostasis. The body's internal chemistry must be balanced to support growth, development, and functional activities such as movement. Hormones not only play a major role in controlling physical growth and initiating puberty, but also regulate the body's metabolism and ability to utilize chemical sources of energy for growth, maturation, adaptations, and learning. Nutrition is part of the internal and external environments and contributes to the production of a healthy body.

Adequate nutrition supplies fuel for efficient energy production and tissue development. For example, adequate nutrition is critical for the development and function of the nervous system, enabling the execution and control of movement. A person's external environment (surroundings) and culture contribute to the definition of personal nutrition. How much and what type of food is available? There is a vast nutritional difference between having rice and fish as dietary mainstays and having red meat and potatoes. These different diets have been associated with Asian and Western cultures, respectively, and have also been linked to lower or higher incidence of illnesses such as heart disease and cancer (Helsing, 1984). Effects of inadequate nutrition are painfully obvious in areas of the world that have a food shortage. From a more subtle perspective, poor nutrition has been associated with intrauterine growth retardation, a significant cause of developmental disability in the low-birth-weight population (Lin & Evans, 1984). Infants who fail to thrive also have poorer motor skills than their adequately nourished peers. Effects of deprivation on brain development are well documented (Dobbing, 1964). Physical size correlates with strength and motor performance (Malina & Bouchard, 1991). Children in the 95th percentile for height and weight appear to perform better motorically (personal observation). Children do not learn well on empty stomachs.

Development balances the need for the organism to survive, organize, and adapt to environmental surroundings. Development, as a process of change, reflects the transactional nature of the person's interaction with the environment. The child changes and so do the people and things with which the child interacts. Each experience is different. The variables within the physical, psychologic, and social environment have to be considered in the development of functional skills. This interaction is not to be envisioned as a robot-like series of actions, but as one in which variation occurs to produce an adaptive response. The environment includes people, places, and things. Through psychologic interaction with the environment a person develops a sense of identity. Motor learning also occurs as a function of the interactions between the physical body and the environmental task demands.

Periods of Development

The life span is most often divided into age-related segments. The periods referred to throughout the book are listed in Table 2–1 and are depicted in Figure 2–1. Although variations in the age ranges for developmental periods exist, Valadian and Porter's (1977) universally applicable terminology will be

Table 2-1. PERIODS OF DEVELOPMENT

Period	Time Span
Prenatal period	Conception–Birth
Infancy	Birth–2 years
Childhood	2 years–10 years (females)
	2 years–12 years (males)
Adolescence	10 years–18 years (females)
	12 years–20 years (males)
Early adulthood	17 years–45 years
Middle adulthood	40 years–65 years
Older adulthood	60 years–Death

used to describe the early periods of development (conception to adolescence), and Levinson's (1986) terminology will be used to describe adult development.

The *prenatal period* averages 40 weeks in length, beginning with conception and culminating in birth. It is divided into three stages: the *embryonic period,* when all major organ systems form, the *middle fetal period,* when organ systems differentiate, and the *late fetal period,* when rapid body growth occurs. The lengthy *postnatal period* is usually broken down into the categories of infancy, childhood, adolescence, adulthood, and older adulthood. *Infancy* spans the first 2 years of life, from birth to the second birthday, and is divided into three stages, as depicted in Figure 2–1. *Childhood* begins at 2 years of age for both girls and boys but lasts longer for boys because of the time difference in the onset of puberty.

Adolescence lasts 8 to 10 years, beginning at approximately 10 years of age for girls and 12 years of age for boys. As with the prenatal period and infancy, it is divided into three stages. *Prepubescence* consists of the 2 years prior to the adolescent growth spurt and hormonal changes that signal puberty. *Pubescence* refers to the 4 years in which the hormones produce the secondary sexual characteristics and the gonads attain their adult form and function. *Postpubescence* is the final 2 years of adolescence in which the final maturity of adulthood is reached.

Levinson's (1986) periods, as seen in Figure 2–1, describe the stages of *adulthood.* As drawn, there is overlap in these ages because he believes that there are transition stages between adolescence and adulthood and between the eras of *early, middle,* and *late adulthood.* These transition stages are part of the eras they bridge; for example, the mid-life transition comes at the end of early adulthood and the beginning of middle adulthood. In order to more closely study aging, gerontologists subdivide *senescence,* or *late adulthood,* into three stages: *young-old, middle-old,* and *old-old.* The older the adult, the less like other adults he becomes, unlike in early development, which seems to be

24

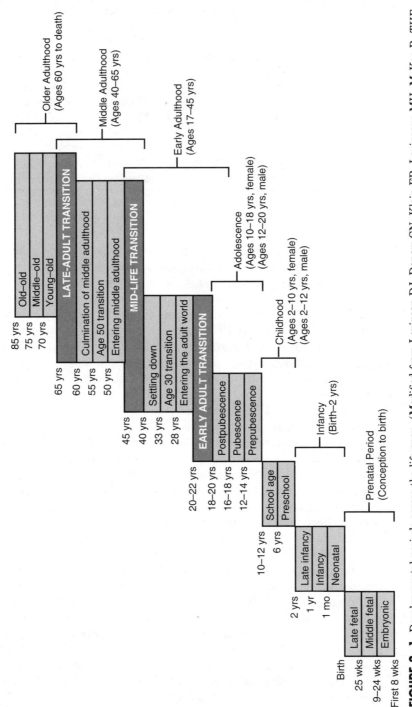

FIGURE 2–1. Developmental periods across the life span. (Modified from Levinson DJ, Danow CN, Klein EB, Levinsons MH, McKee B. *THE SEASONS OF A MAN'S LIFE.* Copyright © 1978 by Daniel J. Levinson. Modified by permission of Alfred A. Knopf, Inc., 1978.)

relatively homogeneous in outward appearance of milestones and development of personality. There is nothing more heterogeneous than an older population whose members have had their own unique life courses. *Life course* (Levinson, 1986) is a descriptive term referring to the concrete character of a life from the beginning to the end.

Development continues throughout adulthood. Structural and functional changes are a normal part of healthy aging. As we journey through the life span and look at those changes that occur and impact on physical function, be aware that there are psychologic and social changes that may either enhance or precipitate loss of function. Aging is a continuation of the developmental process that can have positive and negative outcomes, depending on your perspective. Like other phases of development, aging is not a single process but many processes. Age-related changes produced in a person's organ systems and personal identity result from a lifetime of interactions between the individual, the internal environment, the culture, and society.

"Life span" is defined as *the maximum survival potential for a particular species* (Atchley, 1991). The maximum human life span has not changed appreciably in the last three centuries and remains between 112 and 115 (Timiras, 1972; Cutler, 1985). It is helpful to divide the human life course into three segments: maturation, adulthood, and aging. These broad divisions of life correspond to the age periods in the following way: *maturation* = prenatal, infancy, childhood, and adolescence; *maturity* = adulthood; and *aging* = senescence. The two ends of the spectrum, maturation and senescence, have received the most research attention.

Domains of Function

The processes of growth, development, adaptation, and learning operate at the same time in three different domains: physical, psychologic, and social. Physical growth and development are accompanied by the acquisition of motor skills, intellectual development, and social development. For example, intellectually an infant may be unable to communicate or even understand his or her own physical actions. When the parent supplies meaning to the gestures, looks, or early sound production, the infant's actions are shaped to the parents' expectations of motor performance or communication. The parent interprets a random swipe as a reach, a "ma" as recognition of mother.

Development occurs in more than one domain at the same time. The infant develops perceptual awareness concurrently with motor control, beginning cognition, and attachment. A social smile is evident in most 2-month-olds, although it usually takes several more months before the infant demonstrates sufficient head control to focus attention on caregivers or objects and to be able to direct reaching. The process of human development is interactive, with each domain exerting a positive or negative impact on the other domains. The temperament of a baby can effect the quality of interaction with the caregiver and therapist and thereby affect the attachment process. The physi-

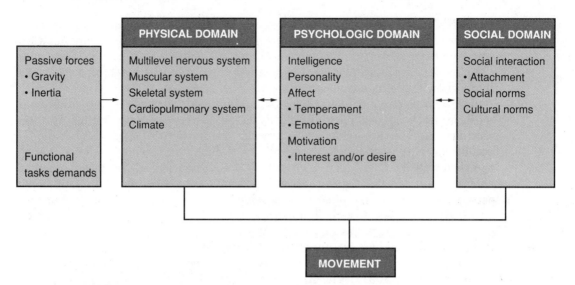

FIGURE 2–2. Domains of development. (Modified from Shephard K. Theory: Criteria, importance and impact. In Lister MF [ed]. *Contemporary Management of Motor Control Problems.* Proceedings of the II Step Conference. Foundation for Physical Therapy, APTA, 1991. Reprinted with permission of the Foundation for Physical Therapy, Inc.)

cal, psychologic, and social selves interact to produce a unique individual. There will never be two people exactly alike.

Each domain—physical, psychologic, and social—contributes to our understanding of motor development. An individual is a biologic organism developing within a psychologic and social environment, a particular culture, and society. This relationship is schematically represented in Figure 2–2. Even though our primary therapeutic emphasis is on the person's ability to move, the therapist must take into account the cognitive and psychosocial status of that person as well as the familial, cultural, and societal movement and life expectations for that person. Each person's own movement behavior will reflect his or her age, ability, level of maturation, experience, and cultural bias.

THEORETICAL ASSUMPTIONS

Theory

Theory, as defined by Shepard (1991), is *an abstract idea or collection of ideas used to explain physical or social phenomena.* It is a reasonable explanation for why things happen and can be applied to many different phenomena. Theories are based on past experiences and observations. They are general beliefs, not always proven by scientific data or supported by documentation. Therefore, theories change as more is learned about the phenomenon being explained.

Theories about motor behavior or psychologic development cannot be directly tested in a laboratory experiment and require a definition of the population to which the theory is applicable. A theory about the behavior of a flightless waterfowl, such as a penguin, does not apply to dogs. A hypothesis or question is posed to test a part of the larger theory. Evidence is gathered that can either support or refute the theory, and knowledge is gained about the conditions or circumstances in which the theory can be applied and in which the theory is accurate. If we hypothesize that flightless waterfowl waddle when they walk on uneven terrain, we can design an experiment to test our hypothesis. The situation is defined by the use of operational definitions that answer questions such as *What is a flightless waterfowl?* and *What do we mean by uneven terrain?* After defining all the variables, data are collected and analyzed, and the hypothesis is proved or unproved.

Related to development is the theory that the child is a miniature adult. In some parts of the skeletal system, where bones are formed in miniature in cartilage first and then replaced by bone, it might appear that the theory is true. However, differential growth occurs in the bones of the face during puberty, so that the adolescent looks much different from the child. Also, many other body systems do not function on an adult level in the child. Because there are more instances in which the theory does not hold true, it is considered a false theory. This chapter presents theories of development that reflect what we currently know about development and provide a basis for our clinical problem solving. If the development of functional movement is based solely on neuromaturation, our therapeutic intervention must follow the developmental sequence. If, however, motor learning occurs during motor development, our therapeutic intervention must also incorporate knowledge of results and practice at solving movement problems. Because what we are presenting are theories, they are changeable, and none of them is totally correct. Theories provide only a starting point from which to understand the complex process of development.

Each of function's three domains (physical, psychologic, and social) represents different disciplines and some domains represent many different disciplines. For instance, both physical and occupational therapists are concerned about physical function, but their approaches to evaluation and treatment of movement dysfunction can be quite dissimilar. Both physical and occupational therapists recognize the value of understanding the whole person and how psychologic and social development affect functional movement.

General Theories of Development

The approach used to describe development provides the framework for discussing reasons for change and allows us to test our hypotheses regarding the ability of a theory to predict future development. The major assumptions about development center around the role of maturation and learning and the nature of developmental changes over time. Theories and theorists differ in the way in which they view the origin of behavior. Is behavior innate or is it the product of our experience? Maturationists argue that our genetic blueprint produces commonalities in our growth and development. Behaviorists take the stand that experience plays a strong role in our personal and social development.

The maturation-experience debate is just another version of the older nature-nurture controversy. It is generally accepted that development of human behavior is strongly influenced by both maturation and experience. Maturation provides a physical base (the body) on which the individual can build a sense of identity and wholeness psychologically (the mind) through experiences within the social environment (family, culture, society). The interplay of maturation and experience is unique for each individual.

The theorists we will be discussing have tried to explain the nature of developmental change over time (Table 2–2). All theorists agree that orderly, sequential changes from simple to complex behavior occur in all domains of function. The theorists debate whether these changes occur in a smooth, continuous manner (continuity or nonstage development) or whether they occur with abrupt stops and starts (discontinuity or stage development).

Continuity implies dependence of later development on what came before. If development is continuous, earlier skills lead to the development of later skills. Continuity appears to be functioning in psychologic development, as exemplified by the statement "the child is the psychological father of the man" (Gottlieb, 1983). In Erikson's theory (1968), successful resolution of each psychologic dilemma is required to proceed to the next level. Development of cognition can be thought of as a continuous line from start to finish.

Stage theory can be thought of quantitatively as a stair-step arrangement with different motor skills such as head control and sitting on each step. Stage theory also postulates that there are qualitative changes that occur throughout development. At each successively higher level of development, or next step, a new characteristic appears that was not previously present. Stage development (discontinuity) is more prevalent than continuity in motor development (Gottlieb, 1983). For example, sitting and standing are sufficiently different to be considered stages in motor development. The major motor milestones—head control, rolling, sitting, creeping, and walking—are considered stages in motor development.

Theories, regardless of the domain focused on, attempt to explain why changes can and do occur over time. However, the time span that is covered by the developmental theory varies greatly. For example, Piaget's theory of intelligence begins at birth and ends in adolescence. Levinson's theory deals exclusively with adult development, a much less understood phenomenon than early or later development. Erikson's theory of personality development is the only true life span approach because his theory accounts for changes that occur from birth to senescence. Theories and theorists selected for discussion present either a perspective unique to an age period or a life span view.

Table 2-2. THEORIES OF HUMAN DEVELOPMENT	
Theorist	**Theory**
Bandura	Social learning —modeling shapes behavior
Bjorksten	Crosslinkage —crosslinkages cause aging
Bronfenbrenner	Ecologic system —environment affects development
Cumming	Disengagement —social disengagement occurs with aging
Erikson	Psychosocial development —psychosocial crises affect personality
Gesell	Developmental schedules —maturation causes development
Harman	Free radical —free radical accumulation causes aging
Hayflick	Hayflick limit —cell replication limits cell age
Maslow	Motivation —hierarchy of needs
McGraw	Biologic maturation —maturation causes development
Neugarten	Activity —activity positively affects aging
Orgel	Error —errors in DNA cause aging
Piaget	Cognitive development —four stages of intelligence
Sears	Social learning —children learn social behavior
Selye	Stress —wear and tear causes aging
Skinner	Behaviorism —behavior is learned and can be conditioned
Walford	Immune —immune system decline causes aging

Theories of Physical Development

MATURATIONISTS

Gesell. The primary proponents of a biologic maturation theory of development are Gesell and McGraw. The maturationists attributed developmental change to genetics and tended to ignore the role of experience. Gesell (1974) studied motor development as a means to understand mental development and in the process became the father of developmental testing. Gesell viewed motor development as the physical entity that allowed functional behavior. As a believer in structure, he defined stages of motor development that he thought governed behavior during each age period. Gesell did recognize the role of individual differences in temperament as a variable during development of stability and change in motor patterns.

McGraw. McGraw (1963) described in exquisite detail movement sequences in infants. She too was interested in the relationship between structure and function in generating developmental change, and she related movement acquisition to biologic maturation (Barnes et al, 1990). Also, like Gesell, she sought answers in the changing activity of the central nervous system (CNS). For example, she tried to correlate changes in an infant's patterns of movement in the prone position (prone progression) with CNS maturation.

The maturationists' view of motor development seeks to correlate all movement acquisition with the onset of changes in the nervous system relative to onset and integration of reflexes/reactions, hierarchy of control, and a timetable of myelination. As biologists, they might consider the possibility that the maturation of other tissues, such as muscle or bone, could contribute to movement production.

AGING THEORIES

Theorists addressing the later aspect of the life span also hypothesize that aging occurs because of physical or biologic changes in the human body. "Aging can be defined as the sum of all the changes that normally occur in an organism with the passage of time" (Matteson, 1988, p. 140). The biologic theories are usually subdivided into genetic and nongenetic theories. The genetic theories are based on the premise that somehow aging is programmed in the cell nucleus. The nongenetic theories assume that changes occur because of influences outside of the cell nucleus and involve some maladaptive response to cell, tissue, or system damage. The damage may be from external, environmental sources or from internal sources.

Another useful classification of aging theories can be made by dividing them into stochastic theories and developmental-genetic theories. *Stochastic theories* state that events occur at random and represent environmental insults to the human body. These events eventually reach a level that is no longer compatible with life. *Developmental-genetic theories* comprise the rest of the aging theories. This class of theories views the process of aging as being on the same continuum as the process of development, with both processes being genetically controlled, and probably programmed, but subject to environmental influence.

"One way to envision the organism's aging scenario is that each cell and tissue type has its own aging trajectory (time course). Death occurs when homeostasis in one or more rapidly aging components of the organism fails beyond the point necessary to maintain the organism. This causes death and terminates the aging trajectory of other, larger-level subsets of cells within the organism" (Cristofalo, 1988, p. 126). Cristofalo makes a case for separating aging in a culture medium and aging of the individual. Aging of cells in a culture medium (in vivo) occurs without any tissue and cell type interaction. What implication does this have on what actually happens in the body? Is there a master timekeeper in the form of a system, or are all individual cells' biologic clocks ticking away independently?

Most gerontologists would agree that an individual's life span is species-specific and therefore intrinsically regulated (Cristofalo, 1988). Theoretically, according to Shock (1977), the maximum length of life that is biologically possible for a human is 120 years. Numerous social and environmental factors such as war, famine, radiation, and toxic chemicals, can negatively impact this figure. Although catastrophic disease is often thought to dramatically shorten many individuals' life spans, if cancer and atherosclerosis were eradicated, it would add only 10 years to our life expectancy (Cristofalo, 1988).

GENETIC THEORIES

The two best known genetic theories are the biologic programming theory (Hayflick, 1983) and error theory. Hayflick and Moorehead (1961) made a profound observation while studying human tumor viruses. When growing human cells in tissue culture, they observed a waxing and waning of cellular proliferation, followed by senescence and eventually death of the cultures. Prior to this time, tissue cultures had been reported to be immortal (Carrel, 1912). Hayflick and Moorehead interpreted their findings to mean that aging was a cellular as well as an organismic phenomenon, and therefore changed the way we view aging and aging research (Hayflick, 1965).

Hayflick (1965) subsequently described, in the *Hayflick limit theory,* the number of cell replications (population doubling potential) possible in the life span to be about 50. Martin et al (1970) linked the replicative life span of specific tissue types in culture to the age of their donor cells. The younger the donor cells, the greater their life span; the older the donor cells, the shorter their life span. Rohme (1981) proved that this holds true for the species from which the cells are derived. In individuals with premature aging, called progeria, the donor cells show a lower Hayflick limit (Fries & Crapo, 1981).

Error theory was originally proposed by Orgel in 1963 as the "error catastrophe" theory. He thought that damage to protein synthesis could occur from a mis-specified enzyme, which would produce a cascade of faulty molecules and lead to an accumulation of malfunctioning systems. Tice and Setlow (1985) postulated that this process resulted from changes in the coding of DNA or the reading of RNA. By passing on incorrect information from the cell's nucleus by mutation, cells would be less able to function normally, and thus organs would become inefficient and senescent. The error theory is the primary example of a stochastic theory of aging.

More recently, other considerations have been suggested to impact on the genetic theories, such as the rate of development, damage relative to longevity, and the rate of repair. Hart and Setlow (1974) suggest that there is a direct correlation between longevity of cell cultures and their ability to repair DNA damage from ultraviolet (UV) radiation. The ability to repair DNA damage appears to slow with maturation (Treton & Courtois, 1981). Data have not substantiated this theory and in fact have demonstrated that aging is *not* accelerated when mis-specified amino acids are introduced—nor do the mis-specified molecules accumulate significantly in aged cells (Sharma & Rothstein, 1980; Hayflick, 1983; Rothstein, 1984).

NONGENETIC THEORIES

Four of the six major aging theories are nongenetic. They include the cross-linkage theory, free radical theory, immunity theory, and neuroendocrine theory. Although considered nongenetic theories, all of the theories could be considered developmental in that they represent change over time and focus on wear and tear on the body. The first two theories have to do with chemical reactions that occur on the cellular level, the latter two with control systems. Bjorksten (1974, 1976) first related the idea of crosslinkage of protein molecules to aging in the 1940s. According to the *crosslinkage theory,* a crosslinking agent attaches itself to two large molecules as a result of a chemical reaction. If the crosslink attaches to only one strand of DNA, it can be repaired. However, if two strands of DNA are crosslinked, the strands are unable to part normally. With aging, the body's ability to repair crosslinkages is thought to decline, causing an increase in cell death related to incomplete division. In looking at collagen, elastin, and DNA molecules, Bjorksten recognized that the occurrence of crosslinkages between compounds might be responsible for the secondary and tertiary signs of aging. One obvious example is seen in the skin. Tanning of the skin produces crosslinkages between collagen and elastin, which leads to a loss of tissue elasticity. Over time, these crosslinking compounds build up and interfere with cell function by impeding cell-to-cell transport. Although age-related changes in collagen, such as loss of flexibility, have been documented (Rockstein & Sussman, 1979), the negative relationship between flexibility and age can be partially compensated for by diet and exercise (Leslie & Frekaney, 1975).

Harmon (1956) originally described the *free radical theory* of aging in 1955. Free radicals are highly charged ions with an orbiting unpaired electron. The separated electron with its high energy level is thought to attack neighboring molecules. The radicals have an affinity for lipid molecules, which are found in abundance in mitochondrial and microsomal membranes. The free radicals then damage cell membranes in a chemical process called lipid peroxidation, which leads to structural changes and malfunctions in the cell. One of the results of the oxidative reactions within the cells is the deposition of lipofuscin, an aging pigment. Lipofuscin accumulates in many organs with aging, particularly in postmitotic (those no longer dividing) organs such as the heart, skeletal muscle, and CNS. Some researchers believe that accumulation of lipofuscin interferes with cell metabolism and information sharing (Pryor, 1983). Others (Meier, 1984; Rowaltt & Franks, 1978; Moss, 1986) do not think the case has been made to support lipofuscin's causative role in cell decline with age. It may be that an excessive accumulation may cause problems while, in general, the presence of lipofuscin is an aging characteristic of some cells. This is certainly true about neurons.

More recently, Pryor (1987) modified Harmon's theory to reflect the role free radicals play in the etiology and development of life-limiting chronic diseases. The diseases having a free radical component are (1) emphysema, (2) atherosclerosis, (3) cancer, (4) arthritis, (5) cirrhosis, and (6) diabetes. There are more free radicals present in individuals with these diseases; emphysema has been linked to deactivating lung enzymes, and atherosclerosis has been linked to damaging low-density lipoproteins (LDLs). Pryor further concludes that although the experimental results do not totally support the free radical theory as originally postulated, there appears to be a strong connection between life-limiting diseases and the oxidative stress to which an organism is subjected. The stress influences the age at which the life-limiting diseases begin to have effect.

The immune system consists of the bone marrow, the thymus gland, the spleen, and the lymph nodes. The first two are primary organs of immunity; the latter two are considered peripherally or secondarily responsible for developing immunity. The bone marrow and thymus are the two organs most affected by the aging process (Makinodan & Kay, 1980). The thymus gets smaller with age; after young adulthood, its ability to produce differentiated T cells needed for cell-mediated immune response declines. As the bone marrow becomes less efficient, the rate of infections, autoimmunity, and cancer rises (Walford, 1980; Felser & Raff, 1983). Walford (1969) first postulated the *immunity theory* based on these facts.

Later, Walford (1980) and Russel (1978) expanded the immunity theory by looking for a genetic origin of immune senescence. They thought that a site on chromosome 6 regulated immunity and aging. Despite the lack of universal application, the fact that the gene locus for the production of enzymes that protect against free radicals occurs at the same site does lend some credence to a connection between immunity and aging. However, there are probably over 100 genes involved in the natural process of longevity (Schneider, 1987), so that it is too simple to think that a single gene could trigger senescence.

Several aging theories implicate the endocrine system as the culprit in the aging process. The maintenance of a stable internal environment is the purview of the endocrine system and the autonomic division of the CNS. With aging, the hormones produced by the endocrine system appear to be intact and potent, although their effective interaction with target body cells is decreased. Put another way, the body's tissues are less responsive. The hypothalamic-pituitary interconnections act as a system to control the body functions of growth, reproduction, and metabolism. This hypothalamic-pituitary axis has been postulated as the master time-keeper for the body because the pituitary gland controls the thyroid gland, which through secretion of thyroxine controls the metabolic rate of the body. A major question regarding aging is whether the body slows down the rate at which it burns calories.

Finch (1987) discusses *neuroendocrine theories* in relationship to the effects of losing hormones, such as estrogen, on bone loss in postmenopausal women. Whitbourne (1985) concludes that the age effects on the neuroendocrine control system seem to occur secondarily to the age effects on the body's tissues. Again, this theory has limited universal application because not all organisms that age have advanced endocrine systems. Secondly, as with the immune theory, observed changes may be a result of aging rather than a cause.

Aging theories would explain the decline in movement performance, both in form and utility of function, as related to a decline in either the individual cells or the various systems of the body. The nervous system's ability to process information and to execute motor programs would be suspected. The raw material to fuel or support movement from the cellular level to the organ level to the systems level would be depleted or would wear out.

Theories of Psychologic Development

INTELLIGENCE

Piaget (1952), a well-known developmental psychologist, identified four stages of cognitive development: sensorimotor, preoperational, concrete operational, and formal operational. Each stage is characterized by different ways of interacting with the environment, as identified in Table 2–3. His theory explains how humans acquire and process information and learn about the world. According to Flavell (1977), Piaget believes that the individual's ultimate goal is to master the environment. Piaget (1952) identified two basic functions of all organisms that make this mastery possible. The first is the individual's ability to organize, which he called *assimilation,* and the second is the ability to adapt, which he called *accommodation.* These two processes allow individuals to learn about and adapt to the world around them.

Assimilation is interpretation of external objects and events in terms of one's own preferred way of thinking about them. Accommodation is a form of

Table 2-3. PIAGET'S STAGES OF COGNITIVE DEVELOPMENT		
Life-Span Period	**Stage**	**Characteristics**
Infancy	Sensorimotor	Pairing of sensory and motor reflexes leads to purposeful activity
Preschool	Preoperational	Unidimensional awareness of environment Begins use of symbols
School age	Concrete operational	Solves problems with real objects Classification, conservation
Pubescence	Formal operational	Solves abstract problems Induction, deduction

From Piaget J. *Origins of Intelligence.* New York: International Press, 1952.

adaptation that involves noticing and taking into account the real properties and relationships of objects and events in the environment (environmental data). Eating is an example of assimilation in which the food is incorporated into the body's structure after the oral-motor system has accommodated to the structure of the food (hard or soft, smooth or lumpy). An example of accommodation is bone remodeling, where the structure of long bones is changed in order to adapt to changes in growth.

The first 2 years of life are seen as a blending of sensory and motor experiences in which the infant uses sensory information (assimilation) to cue movement, and uses movement (accommodation) to explore the environment. The child's sensorimotor system interacts with the environment and, by means of repeated interactions, undergoes developmental change and cognitive growth. Because the developmental therapist is concerned with the impact of maturation and experience on the motor development of infants and children with disabilities, a child's sensory and motor abilities are assessed, and treatment is designed to maximize potential.

The next few years of life are dedicated to acquiring verbal expression as well as using symbols, words or objects to represent things that are not present. The child labels all forms of transportation as "ride" or all four-footed animals as "dog" or "cat," depending on his own frame of reference. Behavior is self-centered, and reasoning is always in relation to the self. "To the right" means to her right. Objects are as alive as people, and they always have a purpose. Toward the end of this stage, most children begin to have some understanding of time, which eventually translates into learning how to wait.

In the concrete operations period, children develop the ability to classify objects according to their characteristics. They can solve concrete problems — that is, those in which the objects are physically present, as in *Which cup is bigger?* or *Which string is longer?* Most of Piaget's famous conservation experiments were carried out to demonstrate the child's ability to transform objects from one set of circumstances to another while preserving the idea that the objects were unchanged. For example, two cups hold equal amounts of water. One cup *(B)* is poured into several other containers *(A)* and the child is asked whether the amount of water poured from cup *B* is the same as what is in *A*. If the child says yes, he demonstrates conservation.

Piaget and Inhelder (1958) describe the highest level of cognitive development as formal operations in which early adolescents are able to deal with hypothetical as well as real situations. A person capable of abstract thought could grasp the experiments with the cups of water described above without having to physically see them. Being able to generate a hypothesis, engage in deductive reasoning, and check solutions are all characteristics of logical decision making. Not all adolescents and adults apply this type of thinking to all aspects of life. They may tend to selectively use this ability only in particular personal or professional situations.

By using biologic terminology, Piaget introduced the concept of a cognitive system developing in parallel with other bodily systems. Furthermore,

Piaget used the model of assimilation and accommodation to describe cognition as another form of ontogenetic adaptation. Ontogenetic adaptation refers to the structural, physiologic, or behavioral characteristics unique to an organism, in this case humans, that increase the survivability of the organism (Oppenheim, 1984).

PERSONALITY

Erikson. Erikson (1968) transformed Freud's psychoanalytical theory into a psychosocial view of human development. Erikson combined biologic needs with cultural expectations and produced the most widely applicable theory of human development for present-day society by replacing Freud's sexual focus with traits of social interaction. Erickson also addresses the entire life span in his eight stages of psychosocial development, as outlined in Table 2–4. These incorporate more than one domain, and each is needed for growth as an individual. Each stage revolves around a psychosocial conflict that the person has to resolve in order to advance in the developmental process. Interestingly, as Erikson himself has aged, his latest works deal more and more with adult stages and aging. He and others (1986) are looking at generational differences and the role of expectations in aging.

The infant's first psychosocial conflict, according to Erikson, is whether to *trust or mistrust* the people within the world. Through physical contact and caregiving, the infant forms positive attachments that are mutually reinforcing. If this does not occur, negative attachments—mistrust of others, of the environment, and even of self—result. The basis of trust is seen in the establishment of positive contact with the environment and the people in it, including touch and the meeting of the infant's needs.

Table 2-4. ERIKSON'S EIGHT STAGES OF DEVELOPMENT

Life-Span Period	Stage	Characteristics
Infancy	Trust vs. mistrust	Self-trust, attachment
Late infancy	Autonomy vs. shame or doubt	Independence, self-control
Childhood (preschool)	Initiative vs. guilt	Initiates own activity
School age	Industry vs. inferiority	Works on projects for recognition
Adolescence	Identity vs. role confusion	Sense of self; physically, socially, sexually
Early adulthood	Intimacy vs. isolation	Relationship with significant other
Middle adulthood	Generativity vs. stagnation	Guiding the next generation
Late adulthood	Ego integrity vs. despair	Sense of wholeness, vitality, and wisdom

From Erikson EH. *Identity, Youth, and Crisis.* New York: WW Norton, 1986.

In toddlers, the basic trust learned in infancy is enhanced by resolving the next psychosocial conflict. The toddler expresses *new-found independence,* both motorically and socially, with the ever-popular statement "me do it." It is important during this stage that the toddler be allowed to be as independent as possible to prevent feelings of doubt concerning emerging abilities. Learning to control one's own movements and those of people and objects within the environment is very important in early development. However, with the assertion of this new-found independence can come conflict between the child's wants and parental boundaries, producing the so-called terrible twos.

Self-regulation develops slowly in the third stage as the child learns the boundaries of appropriate social behavior. Just as an infant learns the rules of moving, the child experiments with social behavior. A growing sense of identity plus parental guidance allows for the development of self-regulation, whether that means becoming toilet trained, learning to share, or learning to take turns. By 3 to 5 years, the preschooler has learned to master many tasks and feels free to initiate his or her own activities. By teaching the child which behaviors are acceptable under which circumstances, the parents encourage the child's confidence in his or her own planning without fear of a negative result or the burden of guilt. During this time, the parents' most important task is to encourage self-regulation of behavior. When children begin to regulate their own behavior, they begin to rely on internalized value and reward systems.

The school-age child deals with the conflict between *industry* and *inferiority.* The initiative developed in the previous stage is applied to learning how to work hard on a project and enjoy the satisfaction of a job well done. With achievement comes a positive self-image. Without success, the child may learn to be helpless, which in turn can produce a negative self-image. The initial self-image formed between 2 and 3 years of age is expanded during middle childhood's struggle with success or failure in school. As the student increases awareness of her own values, goals, and strategies, she becomes more sensitive to the needs and expectations of others. It is during this time that tasks are often undertaken to gain the approval of a favorite teacher.

Adolescence produces one of the most trying psychosocial dilemmas, *identity versus role confusion.* An adolescent's identity is a unique blend of what he or she was in childhood and what he or she will become in adulthood. Identity formation is affected by social and sexual experiences, cognitive abilities, and self-knowledge. To be able to ponder the philosophic question of "Who am I?", the adolescent must be capable of the highest level of cognition. The adolescent spends a great deal of time wondering what he or she would do if "such and such" happened, almost as if the person were trying to play out every possible life scenario before it actually transpired. Self-knowledge is gleaned from past life experiences. This knowledge includes physical information gained from the five senses as well as knowledge of bodily functions. Emotionally, self-knowledge includes self-esteem and self-image. The self is very important to the adolescent, so much so that the self-centeredness (egocentrism) lends itself to feeling like one is "performing on stage." Although emotions are part of adolescent development, they play only one role in the development of a stable identity. Socially, the adolescent is expected to develop appropriate behavior toward his or her own and the opposite sex. One's own sexual identity is established in adolescence, as are a philosophy and a moral ideology to guide socially responsible behavior. Adolescents are expected to achieve emotional independence from their parents and other adults. The end result of a successful adolescence is a unique and stable view of oneself, a life philosophy, and a career path. The pursuit of a career or vocation allows the adolescent to move away from his previous egocentrism (Erikson, 1968). *Role confusion* is the term used by Erikson to describe the failure to form an identity during adolescence. Role confusion may result if adequate support systems are not available (Dennis & Hassol, 1983). Without an identity, a person will be confused about his role in society, have difficulty formulating a life philosophy, and be unable to forge a career or have a family.

Once an identity has been established, the young adult must deal with the conflict of *intimacy versus isolation.* Forming an intimate relationship with a significant other involves sharing the values, hopes, goals, and fears found during the search for identity. Schuster (1986) states that a person learns to share love in many different forms—parental love, spousal love, child love, friend love, and spiritual love. The negative result from losing the battle for intimacy is to become self-absorbed and unable to relate openly with other people. Social and emotional isolation may lead to an overly developed sense of righteousness and outward prejudice toward those with whom one disagrees.

Generativity is an unconscious desire to guide and assist the next generation. The traditional way that this assistance is given is through parenting, but it can also be expressed through an occupation such as teaching or an avocation such as Big Brothers or Big Sisters. At the age of 80, Erikson (1986) stated that making creative contributions to the world and caring for other people's children could substitute for having your own children. The common denominator in this stage is fostering another's well-being. In order to help others, the person must be productive and creative (Dennis & Hassol, 1983). Stagnation is the alternative to generativity, the "is that all there is?" attitude toward life.

The last hurdle to be faced in Erikson's stages of development is conflict between *integrity and despair*—not ethical integrity, but *ego* integrity, a sense of wholeness of self in perspective of the life already lived and the life yet to be experienced. There is a sense of vitality, expectation, and wisdom that comes from the life cycle being reflected back on itself (Erikson et al, 1986). If the older adult does not achieve ego integrity, despair replaces vitality. Erikson attributes the failure to a lack of having built-up inner resources from successful handling of previous psychosocial dilemmas.

Realistically, we can understand that not all determinants of late life satisfaction are under an individual's control. The body ages physically as well as psychologically. The physical self and the life situation (including socioeconomic status, activity level, and availability of transportation) have been shown to have an impact on successful aging (Dennis & Hassol, 1983, p. 268). There is a complex relationship between internal and external factors that shape the end result of a process that includes our past achievements and how we reacted to them. The task of coming to grips with how one led one's life, the choices made and paths not taken, is not easy. The challenge is best met with a strong sense of self-respect and a good sense of humor, remembering that "no one gets through this life alive."

Levinson. If a phenomenon occurs often enough it will become the subject of study. Such is the case of the so-called mid-life crisis. Levinson (1986) and colleagues' initial findings from studying men aged 35 to 45 led to a new view of adult development that extended Erikson's original work by identifying four eras: preadulthood, early adulthood, middle adulthood, and late adulthood (see Fig. 2-1). These are frequently referred to as the Seasons of a Man's Life.

The theory includes the elements of a life course and life cycle, individual life structure, and a conception of adult development. *Life structure,* as defined by Levinson, is a pattern of relationships between the self and the world. This relationship has inner psychologic aspects such as feelings and outer social aspects such as ways of relating to people. He further identifies periods during the adult years in which structure building is most prevalent, and other periods in which structure changing is more prevalent. The structure-changing periods are seen as transitions between the more stable structure-building periods. His research supports the notion that the character of living changes considerably between early and middle adulthood and is associated with age-related periods (Levinson, 1986).

MOTIVATION

Maslow (1954) generated a theory to counteract the seemingly nonhumanistic approach of the psychoanalysts and the behaviorists. His theory of motivation is based on a needs hierarchy, depicted in Figure 2-3, in which each life stage is seen from the perspective of fulfilling a certain need. Every individual has an innate drive to survive, grow, and find meaning to life. The sequence of needs progresses from the physiologic ones related to survival and safety to needing love, self-esteem, and ultimately self-actualization. The last stage occurs when the individual has become all that it is possible for that person to be, and it cannot be achieved unless all other needs have been met.

Maslow might define *movement* as a basic physiologic need to assist with survival of the individual. Other psychologic theorists might view movement as a means to explore and learn about themselves and the environment. Piaget defines early cognition as the combining of sensory and motor actions. What implication does this have on a severely motorically impaired infants' ability to develop intellectually?

Theories of Social Development

BEHAVIORIST

Probably the most famous behaviorist is B. F. Skinner (1938), the father of stimulus-response (S-R) psychology, whose experiments with rats and mazes clearly showed that certain behavior can be conditioned. He applied the prin-

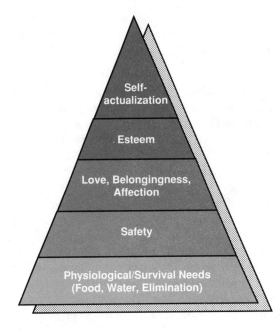

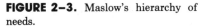

FIGURE 2–3. Maslow's hierarchy of needs.

ciples of operant conditioning to the development of human behavior and believed that the environment was the most influential factor in determining behavioral outcomes. Skinner was even able to condition a fear response in a child. Although the value of reinforcement is universally accepted and behavior modification is a legitimate form of therapeutic intervention, classic conditioning will not be discussed as a formative aspect of development. Behaviorists do not represent a life span view of human development because they focus on development in childhood and adolescence, but they do represent the opposing side to the nature-nurture debate. According to behaviorists, all behavior is learned by observation and imitation and can be conditioned or shaped through reinforcement.

SOCIAL LEARNING THEORY

Robert Sears (1965) attempted to explain the early behavior of the child according to observable social interactions—that is, overt behavior. Although Sears used the Skinnerian S-R cycle, his theory became known as social learning theory and is predicated on identifying the common reinforcers used to produce social behavior. The theory states that behavioral development is learned with the parents as the first teachers, followed by the extended family and, finally, the social group. Sears' theory is outlined in Table 2–5.

Table 2-5. SEARS' PHASES OF SOCIAL LEARNING		
Life-Span Period	**Phase**	**Description**
Infancy	I. Rudimentary behavior: initial behavioral learning	Basic need requirements met within intimate parental environment Positive reinforcement is primary socializing agent
Toddlerhood/preschool	II. Secondary motivational systems: family-centered learning	Socialization within larger family environment Negative reinforcement introduced as socializing agent
School age/adulthood	III. Secondary motivational systems: extrafamilial learning	Social penetration into neighborhood and beyond Controls universally defined and strictly enforced

From Sahler OJZ, McAnarney ER. *The Child from Three to Eighteen.* St. Louis: CV Mosby, 1981.

COGNITIVE SOCIAL LEARNING

Bandura's (1986) social learning theory is mentioned because it explains observational learning. As such, it is more relevant to understanding the abstract learning that occurs from adolescence through adulthood. An essential process in Bandura's cognitive social learning theory is that of modeling. *Modeling* is described as a type of cognitive patterning. Some skills are taught directly by modeling the behavior being taught, such as having a child watch an adult sweep the floor. More complicated behaviors, such as learning values and developing problem solving approaches, are transmitted more subtly. Adults are always amazed at what behaviors children "pick up."

Social theory teaches us that experience is invaluable. An individual registers personal experience with reference to his or her own level of biologic and psychologic maturity. A parent's raising her voice to a toddler may stop the child from an unwanted activity, but verbal warnings can go unnoticed by a teenager. Experience by itself is only an occurrence in time; experience paired with memory connotes learning. The pairing is possible because of the interaction among behavior, cognition, and the environment. Each area is able to influence another; cognition can influence the environment and the environment can influence behavior. For example, teaching children not to play with matches does not preclude them from learning how to safely light a campfire.

Observational learning is used in the socialization process of becoming a professional. Expectations play a large role in structuring or motivating performance. The clinical instructor expects a certain level of performance from a student therapist, and that expectation motivates the student to perform. The reality that is observed in the clinic is more highly valued than the laboratory simulation. Learning is not the result of a single event but of many events within a context of interpersonal relationships.

ECOLOGIC SYSTEMS APPROACH

Bronfenbrenner's (1979) ecologic systems approach is the application of the biologic concept of studying organisms in their natural habitat or ecosystem to human development. A biologist would study trout in a trout stream, not a saltwater marsh. The model in Figure 2–4 represents Bronfenbrenner's perception of the family, community, and culture as interacting systems of society. Each system is named for its relationship to the child and encompasses an

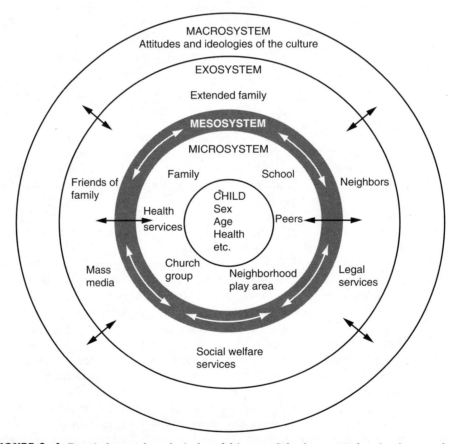

FIGURE 2–4. Bronfenbrenner's ecological model is one of the few comprehensive frameworks for understanding the environment's role in the child's development. (From Garbarino J. from Kopp/ Krakow, *The Child*, © 1982 by Addison-Wesley Publishing Company, Inc. Reprinted with permission of the publisher.)

ever-widening sphere of influence. The child interacts with the members of the family, community, and culture, and they in turn act on the child. Research to date has primarily focused on the effects of the microsystem on attachment, parenting, peer relationships, and school experiences.

SOCIAL THEORIES OF AGING

Age may be the only thing a group of seniors has in common. Life histories and experiences are only a few of the variables present in the life course of individuals. Two divergent social theories have emerged in the last 30 years. The first is the disengagement theory, and the second is the activity theory.

Cumming and Henry (1961) proposed the *disengagement theory,* suggesting that aging people turned inward as a means of withdrawal from family and society. This served to ease the eventual loss of the elder on the family. They originally thought that this was normal, but after considerable research they found that it was neither normal nor natural for this disengagement to occur, at least not totally (Atchley, 1991). Disengagement may occur partially or completely, but it is usually because of circumstances beyond the individual's control, such as placement in a nursing home some distance from the remaining family, a terminal illness, or Alzheimer's disease.

In sharp contrast to the disengagement theory, the *activity theory,* postulated by Neugarten, Havinghurst, and Tobin (1968), suggested that staying actively involved with friends, family, and society is necessary to be successful at aging. Activity is positively correlated with happiness in old age. Being active allows for adaptation, which has always been part of life and is an even more important part of aging. Depending on life circumstances, people may have to adjust to less income, an increase in dependency, loss or change of a job role, or an inability to participate in leisure activities. Those who can adapt and remain active are most successful in aging.

SUMMARY

. . . .

Growth and development are processes that occur simultaneously and are accompanied by the acquisition of motor skills and intellectual and social development. Growth is usually associated with early development and declines with later development. Although this appears to be a simple dichotomy, it is an erroneous one. The only constant seen throughout development is change. Changes that occur in the domains are age-related and can be positive or negative. Change occurs in the physical, psychologic, and social domains simultaneously and consecutively.

Genetics, maturation, the environment, and culture all affect development. Although it is probably true that just because your father was a concert pianist, it doesn't mean that you will inherit musical talent, an individual's genetic makeup will predispose to certain traits; the environment (physical, psychologic, and social) in which you develop, however, can have an equally potent affect.

Theories are ways to predict what will happen. The more theories on a particular subject, the more in flux the state of the research on the subject. This is true with aging, where there is still much to be learned. Adult development is a new area that is only beginning to be researched. Levinson thinks that as more is known about adult development, our understanding of old age will be enhanced. Gerontology, the study of aging, has lagged behind developmental psychology in utilizing the concept of the life cycle. The study of preadult development continues to determine the universal order and general developmental principles that guide the process by which human beings become more individualized (Levinson, 1986). As more and more developmentalists from divergent disciplines of psychology, physical therapy, motor control, and motor learning focus research on motor development across the life span, the process of the development of functional movement will become clearer.

References

Atchley RC. *Social Forces and Aging,* 6th ed. Belmont, CA: Wadsworth, 1991.

Baltes PB, Reese HW, Lipsett LP. Life-span developmental psychology. *Ann Rev Psychol* 31:65–110, 1980.

Bandura A. *Social Foundations of Thought and Action: A Social Cognitive Theory.* Englewood Cliffs, NJ: Prentice-Hall, 1986.

Barnes MR, Crutchfield CA, Heriza CB, et al. *Reflex and Vestibular Aspects of Motor Control, Motor Development and Motor Learning.* Atlanta: Stokesville, 1990.

Bjorksten J. Crosslinkage and the aging process. In Rockstein M, Sussman ML, Chesky J (eds). *Theoretical Aspects of Aging.* New York: Academic Press, 1974, pp 43–59.

Bjorksten J. The crosslinkage theory of aging: Clinical implications. *Compr Ther* 2:65, 1976.

Bronfenbrenner U. *The Ecology of Human Development. Experiments by Nature and Design.* Cambridge, MA: Harvard University Press, 1979.

Carrel A. On the permanent life of tissues outside the organism. *J Exp Med* 15:516–528, 1912.

Cristofalo VJ. An overview of the theories of biological aging. In Birren JE, Bengtson VL (eds). *Emergent Theories of Aging.* New York: Springer, 1988, pp 118–127.

Cumming E, Henry WE. *Growing Old: The Process of Disengagement.* New York: Basic Books, 1961.

Cutler RG. Evolutionary perspective of human longevity. In Andre R, Bierman EL, Hazzard WR (eds). *Principles of Geriatric Medicine.* New York: McGraw-Hill, 1985, pp 22–29.

Dennis LB, Hassol J. *Introduction to Human Development and Health Issues.* Philadelphia: WB Saunders, 1983.

Dobbing J. The influence of early nutrition on the development and myelination of the brain. *Proc R Soc Lond [Biol]* 159:503–509, 1964.

Erikson EH. *Identity, Youth, and Crisis.* New York: WW Norton, 1968.

Erikson EH, Erikson JM, Kivnick HQ. *Vital Involvement in Old Age.* New York: WW Norton, 1986.

Felser JM, Raff MF. Infectious diseases and aging: Immunologic perspectives. *J Am Geriatr Soc* 31:802–807, 1983.

Finch CE, Landsfield PW. Neuroendocrine and automatic functions in aging mammals. In Finch CE, Schneider EL (eds). *Handbook of the Biology of Aging.* New York: Van Nostrand Reinhold, 1985, pp 567–594.

Fries I, Crapo L. *Vitality and Aging.* San Francisco: WH Freeman, 1981.

Flavell JH. *Cognitive Development.* Englewood Cliffs, NJ: Prentice Hall, 1977.

Gesell A, Ilg FL, Ames LB, et al. *Infant and Child in the Culture of Today,* Revised. New York: Harper & Row, 1974.

Gottlieb B. The psychobiological approach to developmental issues. In Haith MM, Campos JJ (eds). *Infancy and Developmental Psychobiology,* vol 2. New York: Wiley & Sons, 1983, pp 1–26.

Harman D. A theory based on free radical and radiation chemistry. *J Gerontol* 11:298–300, 1956.

Hart RW, Setlow RB. Correlation between DNA excision repair and life span in a number of mammalian species. *Proc Natl Acad Sci USA* 71:2169–2173, 1974.

Hayflick L, Moorehead PS. The serial cultivation of human diploid cell strains. *Exp Cell Res* 25:585–621, 1961.

Hayflick L. The limited in vitro lifetime of human diploid cell strains. *Exp Cell Res* 37:614–636, 1965.

Hayflick L. Theories of aging. In Cape R, Coe R, Rodstein M (eds). *Fundamentals of Geriatric Medicine.* New York: Raven Press, 1983, pp 43–50.

Helsing E. Malnutrition in an affluent society. World Health Organization, October, 1984, pp 14–15.

Higgins S. Movement as an emergent form: Its structural limits. *Hum Movement Sci* 4:119–148, 1985.

Hilgard ER, Marquis DG. *Hilgard & Marquis' Conditioning and Learning,* 2nd ed. Revised by Kimble GA. New York: Appleton-Century-Crofts, 1961, p 2.

Leslie D, Frekaney G. Effects of an exercise program on selected flexibility measurements of senior citizens. *Gerontologist* 15:182, 1975.

Lin CC, Evans MI. *Intrauterine Growth Retardation: Pathophysiology and Clinical Management.* New York: McGraw Hill, 1984.

Levinson DJ. A conception of adult development. *Am Psychol* 41:3–13, 1986.

Makinodan T, Kay MB. Age influence on the immune system. In Kunkel HG, Dixon FJ (eds). *Adv Immunol* 1980, 34:287–330.

Malina RM, Bouchard C. *Growth, Maturation, and Physical Activity.* Springfield, IL: Human Kinetics Press, 1991.

Martin GM, Spargue CA, Epstein CJ. Replication lifespan of cultivated human cells: Effects of damage, tissue, and genotype. *Lab Invest* 23:86—92, 1970.

Maslow A. *Motivation and Personality.* New York: Harper & Row, 1954.

Matteson MA. Biological theories of aging. In Matteson MA, McConnel ES. *Gerontological Nursing.* Philadelphia: WB Saunders, 1988, pp 139–142.

McGraw MB. *The Neuromuscular Maturation of the Human Infant.* New York: Halfner, 1963.

Meier DE. The cell biology of aging. In Cassel CK, Walsh JR (eds). *Geriatric Medicine, vol I: Medical Psychiatric and Pharmacological Topics.* New York: Springer-Verlag, 1984, pp 3–12.

Moss A. Cardiac disease in the elderly. In Calkins E, Davis P, Ford A (eds). *The Practice of Geriatrics.* Philadelphia: WB Saunders, 1986, pp 303–326.

Neugarten BL, Havinghurst RJ, Tobin SS. Personality and patterns of aging. In Neugarten BL (ed). *Middle Age and Aging.* Chicago: University of Chicago Press, 1968, 173–177.

Oppenheim RW. Ontogenetic adaptation in neural development: Toward a more "ecological" developmental psychobiology. In Prechtl HFR (ed). *Continuity of Neural Functions From Prenatal to Postnatal Life.* Philadelphia: JB Lippincott, 1984, pp 16–30.

Orgel LE. The maintenance of the accuracy of protein synthesis and its relevance to aging. *Proc Nat Acad Sci USA* 49:517–521, 1963.

Piaget J. *Origins of Intelligence.* New York: International University Press, 1952.

Piaget J, Inhelder B. *The Child's Concept of Space.* New York: WW Norton, 1956.

Pryor W. The free-radical theory of aging revisited: A critique and a suggested disease-specific theory. In Warner HR, et al (eds). *Modern Biological Theories of Aging.* New York: Raven Press, 1987, pp 89–112.

Pryor W. Free radical and autoxidation in aging. In Armstrong D, et al (eds). *Aging, vol 27: Free Radicals in Molecular Biology, Aging and Disease.* New York: Raven Press, 1983, pp 13–41.

Rockstein M, Sussman M. *Biology of Aging.* Belmont, CA: Wadsworth, 1979.

Rohme D. Evidence for a relationship between longevity of mammalian species and lifespan of normal fibroblasts in vitro and erythrocytes in vivo. *Proc Natl Acad Sci USA* 78:3584–3588, 1981.

Rothstein M. Changes in enzymatic proteins during aging. In Roy AK, Chatterjee B (eds). *Molecular Basis of Aging.* New York: Academic Press, 1984, pp 43–50.

Rowaltt C, Franks LM. Aging in tissues and cells. In Brocklehurst J (ed). *Textbook of Geriatric Medicine and Gerontology.* New York: Churchill Livingstone, 1978, pp 3–17.

Russel ES. Genes and aging. In Behnke JA, Finch CE, Moment GB (eds). *The Biology of Aging.* New York: Plenum Press, 1978, pp 235–245.

Schneider EL. Theories of aging: A perspective. In Warner HR, Butler RN, Sprout RL, Schneider EL (eds). *Modern Biological Theories of Aging.* New York: Raven Press, 1987, pp 1–4.

Schuster CS. Study of the human life span. In Schuster CS, Asburn SS (eds). *The Process of Human Development: A Holistic Approach.* Boston: Little, Brown, 1980.

Sears RR, Rau L, Alpert R. *Identification and Child Rearing.* Stanford, CA: Stanford University Press, 1965.

Selye H. *The Stress of Life.* New York: McGraw-Hill, 1976.

Sharma HK, Rothstein M. Altered enolase in age Turbatrix aceti results from conformational changes in the enzyme. *Proc Natl Acad Sci USA* 77:5865–5868, 1980.

Shepard K. Theory: Criteria, importance and impact. In Lister MF (ed). *Contemporary Management of Motor Control Problems: Proceedings of the II Step Conference.* Alexandria, VA: Foundation for Physical Therapy, APTA, 1991, pp 5–10.

Shock NW. Biological theories of aging. In Birren JE, Schaie KW (eds). *Handbook of the Psychology of Aging.* New York: Van Nostrand Reinhold, 1977, pp 103–115.

Skinner BF. *The Behavior of Organisms: An Experimental Analysis.* New York: Appleton-Century-Crofts, 1938.

Strehler BL. *Time, Cells and Aging,* 2nd ed. New York: Academic Press, 1977.

Tice RR, Setlow RB. DNA repair and replication in aging organisms and cells. In Finch CE, Schneider EL (eds). *Handbook of the Biology of Aging,* 2nd ed. New York: Van Nostrand Reinhold, 1985, pp 173–224.

Timiras PS. *Developmental Physiology and Aging.* New York: Macmillan, 1972.

Treton J, Courtois Y. Evolution of the distribution, proliferation, U-V repair capacity of the rat lens epithelium cells as a function of maturation and aging. *Mech Ageing Dev* 15:251–267, 1981.

Valadian I, Porter D. *Physical Growth and Development from Conception to Maturity.* Boston: Little Brown, 1977.

Walford RL. Immunology and aging. *Am J Clin Pathol* 74:247–253, 1980.

Walford RL. *The Immunological Theory of Aging.* Baltimore: Williams & Wilkins, 1969.

Whitbourne SK. *The Aging Body—Physiological Changes and Psychological Consequences.* New York: Springer-Verlag, 1985.

Chapter 3

Motor Control and Motor Learning

by ANN F. VANSANT

Objectives

AFTER STUDYING THIS CHAPTER, THE READER WILL BE ABLE TO:

1 Define motor control and motor learning.
2 Relate motor control, motor learning, and motor development to appropriate theoretic foundations.
3 Distinguish between hierarchic and systems models of motor control.
4 Delineate the stages of motor learning.
5 Relate theories of motor learning to practice issues.

Motor control and motor learning are two ways of studying motor behavior that are different from, yet related to, the study of motor development. The different approaches of development, control, and learning share a common focus—to promote understanding of motor behavior. They provide therapists with complementary forms of knowledge about human movement. Each of these three areas of study has been influenced by individuals working in allied fields. Motor control theory was influenced by a developmental model of neural function: one that grew from a view of how the nervous system evolved (Taylor, 1958). Similarly, motor development scholars were strongly influenced by studies of reflexes (Wyke, 1975; Peiper, 1963), which have long been considered a fundamental unit of motor control. Currently, motor learning and motor control theory share common themes (Rosenbaum, 1991), and the researchers in these areas share ideas that mutually influence each other's work (Brooks, 1986; Schmidt, 1988). An understanding of the differences between these areas helps one to appreciate the unique contributions of each to our knowledge of motor behavior.

The study of motor control focuses on the control and coordination of posture and movement. The field of motor control grew primarily from the specialized study of neurophysiology. Most of what is known about motor control has been determined for relatively simple movement tasks. For example, the electrical activity of brain cells and the flexor and extensor muscles of the elbow might be monitored during a simple task of elbow flexion and extension. A common postural task that has been studied extensively is standing balance. In studies of postural control, as quiet standing is perturbed, muscle activity and forces generated on supporting footplates help researchers understand how the nervous system contributes to the control of balance.

Motor learning is concerned typically with how "motor skills" are acquired. Because motor learning has been studied most by psychologists and physical education specialists, the term "skill" is used to refer to the highly complex and practiced behaviors often associated with specialized work-related tasks or athletic performance. Motor learning studies often require individuals to move accurately toward a target. The learner is provided with different types of feedback, or the conditions under which practice is conducted are varied.

In contrast, motor development scholars describe changes in motor behavior that are related to age. Like motor learning, the study of motor development has roots in psychology. Typically, researchers in motor development study individuals of different ages performing the same task. They describe "age differences" in performance and often suggest that age-appropriate standards be used to judge the motor performance of infants, children, teens, adults, and the elderly. Motor development studies are less likely to be concerned with changing one's performance than with documenting naturally occurring age-related change.

Another way to distinguish among the control, learning, and developmental perspectives is to focus on the time base that is used to study motor behavior within each area (VanSant, 1991) (Fig. 3–1). Motor development processes transpire across intervals typically referred to as "age." Commonly age is measured in years. Motor control processes occur within very small intervals: typically, fractions of seconds. Motor learning is a process that occurs across hours, days, and weeks. Some of the most useful understanding of motor behavior comes from a blending of these three areas, when a "motor learner" takes a developmental perspective or when a developmentalist begins to study motor control.

This chapter explores the specific contributions of motor control and motor learning to our current understanding of motor behavior. Motor control is addressed first. The issues that most affect how therapists view motor control are highlighted. Concepts that are shared with the sister field of motor learning are introduced. The second part of the chapter focuses on motor learning. Because this is a relatively new formal foundation science for physical therapists, the areas of greatest clinical relevance will be stressed, including the stages of learning, the use of feedback that assists learning, and how to structure practice to achieve the greatest benefit for patients.

MOTOR CONTROL

Motor control is the set of processes that organize and coordinate functional movements. To some, these mechanisms are physiologic; to others, they are

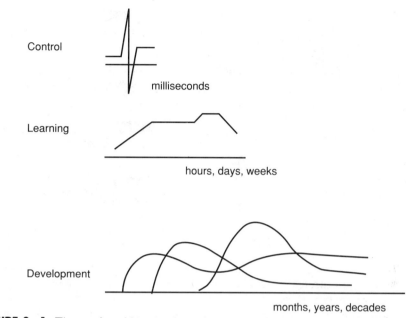

Control
milliseconds

Learning
hours, days, weeks

Development
months, years, decades

FIGURE 3–1. Time scales of interest from a motor control, motor learning, and motor development perspective.

psychologic. The blending of physiologic and psychologic perspectives has greatly enriched the study of how movements are governed. Currently, there are two competing views of how the brain organizes movements: one is a hierarchic view, the other a systems perspective. Each of these will be discussed in turn.

Hierarchic Models of Motor Control

Hierarchic models of motor control are characterized by three main concepts. These traditionally have been reflexes, "levels of function," and volition. Reflexes are stereotypic responses to specific sensory stimuli. Some examples include the flexor withdrawal reflex and the asymmetric tonic neck reflex. To evoke the flexor withdrawal reflex, a noxious stimulus is applied to the sole of the foot. The stereotypic response is flexion of the lower limb at the ankle, knee, and hip. This action withdraws the foot from the potentially harmful stimulus. The asymmetric tonic neck reflex is brought about by positioning the head so that it faces left or right. The response is extension of the upper limb toward which the face is turned, and flexion of the opposite upper limb. The concept of a reflex was developed back in the early 20th century by Sherrington, the father of neurophysiology. His work profoundly influenced many fields of study and practice. As physical therapists, our knowledge of the reflex is rooted in Sherrington's work.

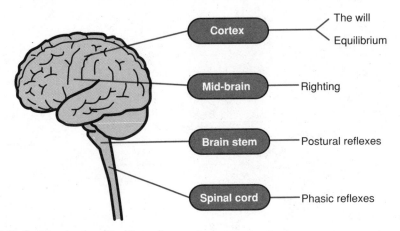

FIGURE 3-2. The classic reflex hierarchy.

A hierarchy of control is composed of levels. These levels traditionally comprise reflex responses, with the highest-level reflexive responses exerting dominance over lower-level reflexive responses. However, in many motor control hierarchies, reflexes are represented only at the lowest levels, with more complex, variable, and volitional functions assigned to higher levels.

In the classic reflexive hierarchy, the levels that have been most commonly included correspond to specific anatomic regions of the nervous system: the spinal cord, the brain stem, the mid-brain, and the motor cortex. Specific reflexes are associated with the distinct functions of each level (Fig. 3-2).

Reflexes mediated in the spinal cord are deemed "phasic" because they are typically of short duration. Spinal reflexes also are characterized by patterns of reciprocal inhibition. According to Sherrington, reciprocal inhibition is a process through which agonistic muscles are facilitated for contraction while their antagonists are inhibited. Concurrent inhibition of the antagonist permits movement as a result of unopposed contraction of the agonist. The monosynaptic stretch reflex, the flexor withdrawal, and the extensor thrust reflexes are examples of phasic reflexes. Each produces movements of short duration.

In contrast to phasic spinal function, reflexes mediated at the brain stem level are characterized as "tonic" because of their long duration. Tonic reflexes such as the tonic neck, tonic labyrinthine, grasp, and positive support reflexes are characterized by co-contraction of agonist and antagonist muscles. Co-contraction patterns enable primitive forms of "posture." The positive support reflex, brought about by pressure on the ball of the foot, turns the lower limb into a rigid pillar of support.

In the hierarchic model of motor control, the motor behaviors of the mid-brain are complex behaviors that align the body with respect to gravity. This function is termed "righting." The righting function is composed of a series of movements that bring the body from recumbency to standing. Righting behaviors believed to be mediated at the mid-brain level are brought about by complex sensory signals arising from a variety of sources including the eyes, the labyrinths of the ears, and the cutaneous and proprioceptive sensory receptors of the body. The stimulus for these reactions is any complex set of sensory signals that indicate discomfort or malalignment of the head or segments of the body. Righting behaviors are quite variable in their form and, as a result, were termed "reactions" rather than "reflexes." The term *reaction* emphasizes their variability when compared to stereotypic reflex responses. Five righting reactions have been identified:

Head or labyrinthine righting reaction: Is responsible for bringing the head into an upright posture.

Head on the body righting reaction: Provides mechanisms for the movements that enable the body to assume a normal alignment with respect to the position of the head.

Body on head righting reaction: Assures that the head is aligned with the body.

Body on body righting reaction: Enables various segments of the axial region to align with respect to each other, so that the shoulder and pelvic girdles may move into alignment with each other.

Optical righting reaction: Allows the head to align with respect to the visual environment.

The highest level of the motor control hierarchy is the cortical level. Two functions are attributed to this level. First, equilibrium or balance reactions are thought to be mediated at this level. The use of the term "reaction" is also quite appropriate to describe balancing activities, for they too vary considerably in form and, like righting reactions, arise from a complex set of sensory signals. Motor behaviors of balance are directed toward preserving the current posture of the body. It is this purpose that differentiates balance reactions from righting reactions. When one rights the body, one assumes a new posture in which the center of mass of the body is higher above the support surface — for example, moving from a prone position to sitting. When one balances, one attempts to preserve and maintain the current posture — for example, maintaining the hands-and-knees posture. Moving the body up against the force of gravity to assume a new posture is righting. Maintaining a posture against the pull of gravity or other perturbing forces is balancing.

In addition to balance reactions, the cortex is also the sight of the "will," or volitional functions that inhibit and control reflexes and initiate purposeful action.

Neurologists have explained motor behavior exhibited by patients with brain injury using this traditional hierarchy (Denny-Brown, 1950; Seyffarth & Denny-Brown, 1948; Twitchell, 1951). According to classic theory, disease or damage to the brain causes "dissolution" of brain function. Dissolution means that neural function regresses to a primitive level characteristic of an earlier phase of nervous system development. After performing a clinical test of reflexes, the behavior of the patient is interpreted to represent a particular level of function. For example, if the patient's behavior is dominated by tonic reflex responses, the behavior is interpreted as representing "brain stem level" function. Classic treatment theories for individuals with brain damage were founded on this view of motor control.

More contemporary motor control hierarchies have been proposed by Gallistel (1980) and Brooks (1986). These theorists incorporate more complex organizational units of motor control into their hierarchies, replacing the reflex as the control mechanism at higher levels. Two of these new elements are oscillators and motor programs.

GALLISTEL'S MODEL

Gallistel (1980) proposed an adaptation of a control hierarchy originally proposed by Paul Weiss (1941), a comparative psychologist and developmentalist. Weiss originally proposed a hierarchy of six functional levels of motor coordination. These were closely tied to anatomic structures and included the following:

Level 1—The level of the neuron represents the simplest form of neuromotor organization: the motor unit. The motor unit is composed of the motor neuron and the muscle fibers innervated by that neuron.

Level 2—The level of the muscle represents orderly graded contraction of a collective of motor units.

Level 3—The level of the muscle group represents the orderly function of several muscles working at a single joint.

Level 4—The level of the organ (or several joints making up a body segment, such as a limb or the trunk) incorporates control of so-called two-joint muscles that span several joints. In Weiss's hierarchy, limb movement requires a higher order of coordination than does movement of a single joint.

Level 5—The level of the organ system represents combinations of movements organized for a purposeful function such as locomotion. One would speak of the locomotor system as the unit of coordination for walking.

Level 6—The level of the organism as a whole places the motor functions in the context of the animal as a whole. At this, the highest level of coordination, sensory systems provide the animal with information concerning the environment, which is coupled with the internal state of the organism, inherited response mechanisms, and past experience to serve the biologic purposes of the organism. According to Weiss, "progression becomes an instrument of preying," and eye movements enable orientation in space.

LEVEL   FUNCTION

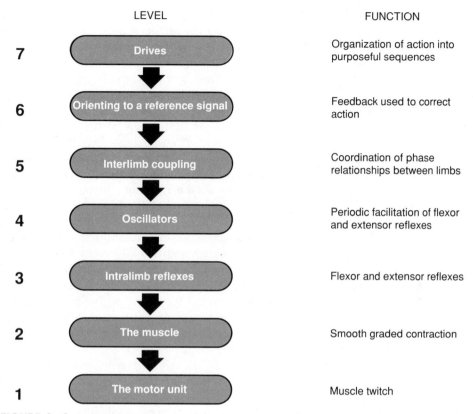

7   Drives   Organization of action into purposeful sequences

6   Orienting to a reference signal   Feedback used to correct action

5   Interlimb coupling   Coordination of phase relationships between limbs

4   Oscillators   Periodic facilitation of flexor and extensor reflexes

3   Intralimb reflexes   Flexor and extensor reflexes

2   The muscle   Smooth graded contraction

1   The motor unit   Muscle twitch

FIGURE 3–3. Gallistel's hierarchy.

Gallistel's hierarchy corresponds to that proposed by Weiss at levels 1 and 2 (Fig. 3–3). At level 3, reflexes involving the entire limb are represented: the flexor reflex and the extensor reflex. At level 4, the mechanism of an oscillator is incorporated. The oscillator periodically facilitates the flexion and extension reflex mechanisms represented at level 3. This enables a stepping action involving alternate flexion and extension of the limb. At level 5, there is control across limbs to allow forward and backward locomotion. This requires that the oscillators controlling the stepping action within limbs be coordinated with the stance and swing phases of stepping in the other limbs. This process is termed "coupling" and follows a relatively well-known set of coordinative principles.

Level 6, the level of acts of the individual as a whole, incorporates the process of orienting toward or away from a reference point. This process is termed "taxis." In Gallistel's model, orienting behavior is enabled through the process of feedback. A set of complex sensory signals provides information regarding the relative condition of the individual with respect to the standard. If the standard is not met, error signals are used to generate behavior to reach the goals or approach the reference standard. For example, the heating systems within our homes use temperature feedback to turn the furnace on and off. If the thermostat is set for 70 degrees F and the temperature is only 65, the 5-degree difference serves as the error signal, and the furnace will be turned on until the temperature reaches 70 degrees. At that point there is no error signal and the furnace will be shut off.

Of course, Gallistel's orienting mechanisms involve motor actions. He discusses as an example phototaxis, the attraction to light common among moths and other insects. For human beings, orienting against the force of gravity is a common motor behavior that could be thought of as an orienting behavior. Given complex sensory information regarding our body position with respect to gravity, motor control signals generate corrective actions that enable us to assume an erect posture against the force of gravity. Earlier in the chapter this same behavior was called a *righting reaction*. Within two different motor control hierarchies, the traditional reflex hierarchy and Gallistel's hierarchy, two different explanations of righting behaviors can be found. Which is correct? It is helpful to think about which explanation might be more useful. If as a therapist you were trying to help a child right the body, it might be useful to think in terms of righting reactions that you could initiate through sensory stimulation. In this example, the traditional reflex hierarchy is useful. On the other hand, if you were trying to understand why a child did not come completely to standing, you might use the concept of faulty feedback to help explain the failure. In the latter instance, Gallistel's concept of an orienting mechanism is useful.

From the previous discussion of righting reactions, you will recall that reactions, unlike reflexes, are quite variable in form. Like the traditional motor control hierarchy, the higher levels of Gallistel's hierarchy produce more variable behaviors directed toward a general goal. The lower levels produce less variable and more constrained behaviors.

Gallistel's hierarchy does not end with level 6. He goes one step further and adds level 7. At the highest level of this motor control model, single acts are organized into behavioral sequences that serve the overall well-being of the individual. Gallistel borrows the concept of drives, which facilitate a set of acts that serve a common purpose. Although in classic literature only one drive can be active at a single time, Gallistel admits that as humans we often operate with mixed motives. Thus, at the highest level in this control hierarchy, the concept of motivation becomes important as an organizing process.

Feedback: An Element of Self-Control. Feedback, the mechanism on which Gallistel's level 6 depends, is a very important feature of motor control. Feedback and error signals are important for two reasons. First, feedback provides a steppingstone toward understanding processes of self-control. Reflexes are initiated and controlled by sensory stimuli from the environment surrounding the individual. Motor behavior generated from feedback is initiated as a result of an error signal produced by a process within the individual. Many motor hierarchies have included at the highest level a volitional, or self-control, function. But there has been very little explanation of how self-control operates. It is as though the will were just a little commander in the brain telling

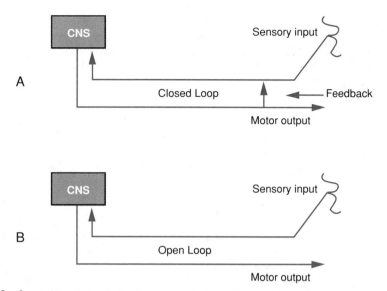

FIGURE 3-4. Models of the feedback process. *A*, Closed loop. *B*, Open loop.

the individual what to do. Having a little commander in the brain controlling movement is not a useful solution, because at some point the question arises, "But how does the little commander control movement?"

Feedback also provides the fundamental process for learning new motor skills. For this reason, feedback is a common element in motor control and motor learning theories. Although the kinds of feedback of concern may vary between these two fields, the common interest in feedback mechanisms is apparent.

Open- and Closed-Loop Control. Feedback is such an important element in current theory that terminology has been created to distinguish between theories that include feedback and those that do not. The terms "open-loop" and "closed-loop" are use to designate these two different types of control. Closed-loop processes are based on feedback. If one were to draw a model of the feedback process as is seen in Figure 3-4*A*, one would say that information regarding a motor action is fed back into the nervous system to assist in planning the next action. A loop between sensory information and motor actions is created. This is a closed loop. An example of a closed-loop action can be seen in many computer games that require guiding a figure or object across a screen.

In contrast, open-loop movements are driven by either a central structure (Schmidt, 1988) or sensory information from the periphery (Smith & Henry, 1967) without benefit of feedback (Fig. 3-4*B*). Motor behavior can be carried out without benefit of feedback. This is particularly true for very fast actions termed "ballistic movements." Some movements occur so fast that they may be completed before feedback loops can provide information that would alter the action. On the other hand, no one can learn without feedback. Whether one relies on a teacher or coach to provide the feedback, or on one's own capacity to gather information about performance, feedback is necessary to correct faulty actions. But movements that have already been learned can proceed without feedback.

Motor Programs. As a result of a debate over the role of sensory information in motor actions, another concept of great importance to current control and learning theories arose (Lashley, 1951). That concept is the "motor program." A motor program is a memory structure that provides instructions for the control of actions. A program is a plan that has been stored for future use. The concept of a motor program is useful because it provides a means by which the nervous system can avoid having to create each action from scratch, and thus can save time when initiating actions. There has been much debate over what is contained in a motor program. Different researchers have proposed a variety of programs. We will discuss a contemporary theory of motor control that uses the motor program concept extensively.

BROOKS' MODEL

Brooks, a well-known motor physiologist, proposed a hierarchy of motor control that comprises three major levels: simply termed, they are the higher, middle, and lower levels (Brooks, 1986). These levels in many ways parallel the functions of the traditional motor control hierarchy outlined above, specifically, in roughly corresponding to anatomic structures. Reflexes are predominantly the function of the lowest level of the spinal cord, and volitional, or intended, movements depend on the sensorimotor cortex. The levels also comprise functional elements termed plans, programs, and subprograms. Brooks views motor plans and programs as communications within the nervous system. They are based on previous experiences and contribute to the creation of intended actions. Plans, programs, and subprograms are learned. Plans are made up of several programs, which in turn are made up of several subprograms. Reflexes, mediated at the lower level of the hierarchy, unlike plans and programs, are an innate rather than a learned functional element.

The nervous system creates and controls motor actions through two fundamental divisions of the nervous system: the sensorimotor system and the limbic system (Brooks, 1986). The sensorimotor system is concerned with sensations, perceptions, and motor actions. The limbic system is composed of a set of cortical structures that connect with "lower centers" of the mid-brain and brain stem that control vital functions. The limbic system is of particular importance in Brooks' model. The limbic system is involved in the control and regulation of emotions and drives related to feeding, reproduction, and other

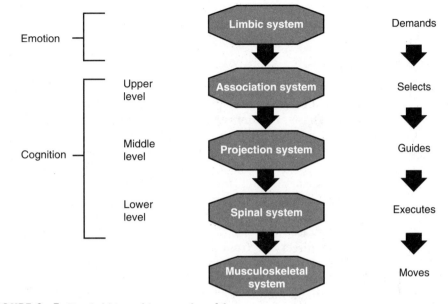

FIGURE 3–5. Brooks' hierarchic control model.

activities that are vital for the preservation of the species. Additionally, the limbic system is involved in the process of learning. The relationship between the limbic system and the sensorimotor system is important because it assists in understanding how goal-directed behavior is initiated. Drives arising through the limbic system are formatted into motor goals through cortical processes carried out in the sensorimotor system. The two systems are described by Brooks as "essential and inseparable partners" (Brooks, 1986, p 22) that function together to produce motor behavior. Figure 3–5 illustrates the command hierarchy beginning at the level of the limbic system, which is superimposed on the sensorimotor hierarchy of plans, programs, and subprograms used in the execution of motor behavior.

The limbic system expresses needs and drives to the highest level of the sensorimotor system, the so-called association system of the association cortex. The association cortex, which is the highest level of Brooks' motor hierarchy, selects the best plan of action and relays that information to the projection system, composed of sensorimotor cortex, cerebellum, basic ganglia, and other subcortical structures. This projection system signals the spinal cord about how and when to direct the musculoskeletal system into action.

Despite an emphasis on plans, programs, and subroutines, all of Brooks' control levels receive feedback and therefore represent a potential for closed-loop motor control and motor learning, but they also suggest that learned movements can be carried out without benefit of feedback through programs and subroutines that have been stored in memory.

Systems Models of Motor Control

Feedback, which provides information flow between elements of the hierarchy, is one of the fundamental characteristics of motor control models that are not hierarchies. These are referred to as "systems models of motor control."

Systems are composed of a set of structural-functional units. They differ from traditional control models in that the units participate collectively in the process of control. Through cooperative and interactive processes among the structural-functional units, the individual is capable of self-regulation and can construct and control behavior.

Four features can be used to distinguish a systems model of control from a traditional hierarchy (Davis, 1976). First, in a hierarchy, information typically flows in one direction: from the top downward. This is not the case in a system. Rather, there is a reciprocal flow of information among units of the system.

Second, in a hierarchy, functions are attributed to specific levels. For example, in the classic hierarchy described earlier in this chapter, phasic reflexes were specifically related to the spinal level of the nervous system, and tonic reflexes were controlled at the brain stem level. In contrast, in a system, a function is a property of the system as a whole. Thus, functions are shared or distributed among the units of the system.

Third, properties of a hierarchy are the properties of each unit within the hierarchy. In contrast, properties of the system emerge though interaction among the elements of the system. For example, a rhythmic repetitive movement may arise through a circular arrangement of neural elements rather than being the property of one neuron (Fig. 3-6).

Fourth, in a hierarchy, the command function is typically the province of the highest level. In a systems model, command is usually an emergent property arising from the cooperation, collaboration, and sharing of information among units of the system.

In contemporary systems models, units other than the central nervous system are given a role in motor control (Gordon, 1987; Horak, 1991; Scholtz, 1990). Other biologic systems such as the musculoskeletal and the cardiopulmonary systems, as well as the physical, psychologic, and social environments in which we function, also contribute to motor control. One of the advantages of a systems model of control is its flexibility. The system can vary its coordinative arrangements depending on the context, or situation in which the individual must operate. Actions are organized to meet specific goals. The process of motor control can be envisioned as a process of solving a problem. Depending on the goal, a variety of structural-functional units have the potential to assume control. Which unit is in command is a function of the specific situation in which the goal must be attained. Information about the situation or context in which the action must be performed is gathered to determine

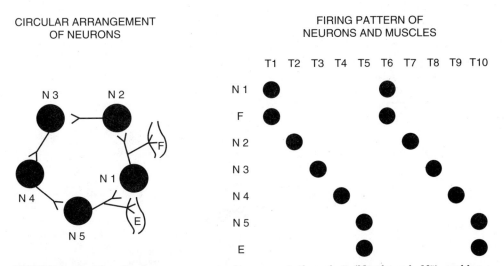

FIGURE 3–6. The circular arrangement of neurons 1 through 5 (N1 through N5) enables a patterned firing of the flexor (F) and extensor (E) muscles. The firing pattern at time one (T1) is characterized by activity of neuron 1 (N1) and the flexor muscle (F). At time 2 (T2), neuron 2 (N2) fires; at time three, neuron 3 fires; at time 4, neuron 4 fires; and at time 5, neuron 5 and the extensor muscle fire. This pattern then repeats beginning at time 6 (T6).

which movement strategy will be used. To understand more fully how such a control system operates, consider the model of postural control developed by Nashner.

NASHNER'S MODEL OF POSTURAL CONTROL

Over the course of some 20 years, Nashner evolved a model for the control of standing balance (Nashner, 1990). This model is currently well known among physical therapists. Nashner's model is a good example of systems theory. Over the years, Nashner has studied the many sensory systems that contribute to the control of standing balance. These include the visual, vestibular, and so-called somatosensory (cutaneous and proprioceptive) systems. In addition, he has described the various strategies or movement patterns that the individual uses to maintain standing balance during external disturbances. Through an ingenious method of varying the surface on which the subject stands and the visual field surrounding the subject, he has been able to identify the contributions of the various sensory systems to the control of standing posture. The role of each system varies according to the specific situation. In some instances, the visual system provides accurate information for the control of standing. But when the visual field moves in concert with the individual's postural sway, the eyes cannot be relied on to provide accurate information for the organization of postural responses. In this instance, the individual must switch control from the visual to the vestibular system. The flexibility of

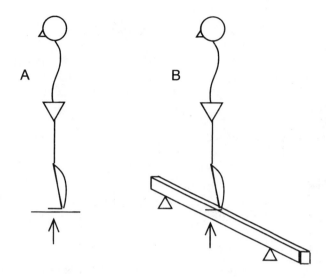

FIGURE 3–7. Sway strategies. *A,* Postural sway about the ankle in quiet standing, foot fully supported. *B,* Postural sway about the hip in standing on a balance beam.

the system is even more clear if one considers the different strategies that can be used to maintain stance.

Three action strategies have been defined: the ankle strategy, the hip strategy, and the stepping strategy. Depending on the characteristics of the support surface, the speed of perturbation, and the degree of displacement, different strategies emerge. Postural sway about the ankle is the norm under conditions of quiet standing in which the foot is fully supported (Fig. 3–7A). This strategy depends on solid contact under the foot to provide a resistive force, enabling the ankle muscles to exert their effect through "reverse action." In the ankle strategy, with the foot fixed on the ground, the plantar flexors and dorsiflexors contract to pull the leg backward and forward with respect to the foot, keeping the body within the limits of stability. When the plantar flexors contract, they produce plantar flexion through reverse action of the muscles: by pulling the leg backward with respect to the foot. For this strategy to be successful, the support surface must extend under the ball of the foot. Similarly, the dorsiflexors operate to pull the leg forward with respect to the foot, producing dorsiflexion through reverse action of the muscles, but only when there is support to provide a reactive force.

If one were to stand crosswise on a narrow balance beam, as shown in Figure 3–7B, the strategy of using ankle musculature to keep the body over the base of support could not be used. This is because there is nothing under the toes and heels to provide a reactive force to the ankle motion. In such instances, the only successful strategy is the so-called hip strategy, in which hip flexion and extension in combination with knee extension and flexion are used to assure balance. Thus, the conditions under which the ankle strategy can be successful are limited. In this example, it is clear that constraints of the physical environment contribute to the control of posture.

Embedded in Nashner's concept of postural control are the concepts of distributed function. Specifically, the control of standing balance is shared among the several sensory systems. Which system assumes control depends on the situation. The flexibility of the system has many ramifications for physical therapy. Postural control is not attributed to a specific set of reflexes, mediated at a specific level of a hierarchy, but is served by a very flexible and dynamic system.

A systems model of motor control provides useful ideas for physical therapists. If one were to take a traditional view of brain dysfunction, damage to higher centers of the brain would result in motor control by lower centers. In the instance of damage to the cerebral cortex, motor behavior would be mediated by the undamaged primitive structures: the mid-brain, brain stem, and spinal levels. Equilibrium or balance reactions typically attributed to the cortical level would be lost. On the other hand, if one ascribes to a systems model, one could assume that damage to one system would not completely eliminate a behavior; rather, remaining systems could be called on to take over for the damaged structural-functional units. Although the balancing function would not be as versatile and flexible, the function would not be lost.

Motor control theories influence strongly how physical therapists view our patients' behaviors and, accordingly, how we evaluate and treat them. If you understand more than one theoretic perspective of motor control, you will have more than one way to view your patients' motor control problems. It is useful to be able to apply a different theory when at first our understanding of a patient's problem leads to treatments that are not totally effective.

DYNAMIC SYSTEMS THEORY

Currently, there is increasing interest among physical therapists in what can be termed "dynamic systems" theories. A dynamic system is any system that demonstrates change over time (Heriza, 1991). Rather than being one cohesive theory, the dynamic systems perspective has several branches that continue to evolve. At the heart of dynamic systems theory is the idea that motor behavior emerges from cooperation among many subsystems within a task-specific context. The nervous system is just one of many components that interact to produce motor behavior.

One of the common issues addressed across this set of theories is how complex patterns of behavior arise out of so many possibilities. This is what has been termed "the degrees of freedom problem." Considering all the neurons, motor units, muscles, joints, and limbs that must be controlled to produce a goal-directed action, how does coordinate behavior arise (VanSant, 1991)? Individuals studying motor behavior from this perspective look for simple ways of capturing or describing complex behavior. These simple descriptors are called "order parameters." An order parameter is a quantitative measure that collectively represents a complex motor function. For example, the phase relationship between the right and left legs during walking is an example of an order parameter. That phase relationship captures the essence of the complex behavior of walking. Other order parameters that have been studied include the spatial relationships between the hip and knee joint angles in stepping, and the relationships between speed of movement and position of the leg while walking.

Order parameters, as expressions of complex relationships within a motor behavior, can be studied to help us understand and predict qualitative changes in the form of movement—for example, the transition from walking to running. Because the quality of motor behavior has long been an interest of physical therapists, newer theories that examine the qualitative changes in movements are particularly appealing.

According to dynamic systems theories, control parameters are those variables that act as catalysts for change in motor behavior. Prior to the evolution of dynamic systems theories, it was believed that qualitative change in motor behavior was brought about either by learning or by a maturation process. Now, changes in motor behavior are being attributed to parameters that previously went unnoticed. For example, therapists are developing a renewed interest in physical growth parameters. It is possible that some qualitative changes in movement patterns are catalyzed by a change in the size of body parts. Women who are in the final 3 months of pregnancy change the movement patterns that they use to rise to standing (Overbaugh, et al, in preparation). Following delivery, they resort to patterns of rising that were more characteristic during the 1st and 2nd trimesters of pregnancy. The new pattern seen during the final trimester of pregnancy is an emergent property of a dynamic or changing system. Dynamic systems theories hold a great deal of promise for advancing our understanding of the changing form of movements that we observe in our patients. Finding descriptors of complex behavior that can be used to study abnormal movements and to study how changes in movement patterns can be fostered is still on the horizon. But therapists look forward to the knowledge this new set of dynamic systems theories will bring to our understanding of motor control.

In summary, the two major theoretic perspectives on motor control are the hierarchic and systems theories. For physical therapists, the hierarchic theory is classic and fundamental to our basic understanding of motor control. Reflexes fulfill a basic role in hierarchic theories as the fundamental unit of behavior. Hierarchies are composed of levels that closely relate to anatomic structures. Volitional movements, which are complex and variable in form, are carried out by the higher levels, whereas more simple, reflexive behaviors are characteristic of lower levels of a motor hierarchy.

Systems theories have been introduced more recently to the physical therapy literature. Systems are structural functional units that have properties of self-organization and sharing of coordination and control among system units. A postural control model advanced by Nashner clearly illustrates the flexibility of a systems perspective of motor control. Newer dynamic systems theories hold promise for physical therapists who are seeking to understand how qualitative change in movements can be described and fostered in patients.

MOTOR LEARNING THEORY AND PRINCIPLES

Motor learning is the process that brings about a relatively permanent change in the capacity for motor performance that is a result of practice or experience. This definition, taken from Schmidt (1988), has several distinct features. First, motor learning, like motor control, is a process. According to Schmidt, motor learning results in a change in the capacity to perform. This is an important feature of the definition because it does not imply that in every instance what has been learned will be apparent. Often, highly skilled individuals have a "bad day." Their performance is less than what they might expect after long hours of training and practice. Yet, we know that on another day they will demonstrate what they have learned. Performance varies from time to time as a result of many temporary factors. Learning, in contrast, results in a relatively permanent change in the capacity of the performer. Another feature of the definition that is important is the fact that learning is defined simply as a change in the capacity to perform. The change may result in either an increase or a decrease in the capacity to perform. Sometimes, as a result of instruction and practice, skill is lessened, although in most cases learning results in an increased ability. Finally, motor learning is a result of practice or experience. This element of the definition is included to distinguish changes resulting from learning from changes that might result from maturational or aging processes (Oxendine, 1984). For example, an older person may gradually lose range of motion or strength as a result of natural physiologic changes in the musculoskeletal system. Motor behavior may be permanently altered in this instance to accommodate the change, but this change is not considered to be learning.

As Gordon (1987) pointed out, until recently, therapists had been concerned with facilitating and inhibiting movement patterns and less concerned with the teaching and learning of motor skills. Therapists were focusing on performance and not on learning as defined by Schmidt (1988). Often the patient was a passive recipient of the therapist's handling and guidance. The therapist controlled the patient's movements by providing inhibitory and facilitative stimuli, to provide the patient with a kinesthetic sense of correct performance. Patients were not encouraged to participate in generating movements not only because their volitional effort might result in abnormal movement patterns, but because automatic rather than volitional movements were the goal of treatment.

This approach to treatment has undergone rapid change over the past several years, and recently Schmidt compared a physical therapy session to a session of motor learning (Schmidt, 1991). Although not a physical therapist, he has come to understand that what therapists do in treatment of patients involves the fundamental characteristics of motor learning. We provide instruction, feedback, opportunities to practice, and encouragement to our patients.

Stages

Fitts (1964) provided a very clear outline of three stages of motor learning that lead from the initial fumbling attempts to mastery of a skill. These stages are the cognitive, associative, and autonomous phases.

COGNITIVE PHASE

The initial phase of motor learning is a time when the learner is gathering information from all possible sources in order to understand the task and develop a plan for performance of the skill. All sensory systems are typically involved in gathering information. Consider teaching a school-age child a sliding board transfer to and from a wheelchair. In the first phase of learning, the patient would benefit from a demonstration or videotape of the activity or from watching another child perform transfers. Verbal instructions that could be used to help the child develop a plan of action would also be important (e.g., pointing out key safety features during the performance and using short phrases that can serve as reminders of the appropriate sequence during learning, such as "First lock the breaks; now remove your foot pedals"). This stage of learning is relatively short. The child is not expected to demonstrate skill or independence, but rather is developing an appreciation of what needs to be done and in what order.

ASSOCIATIVE PHASE

This is the period of practice and feedback. The child will gradually improve performance, making fewer mistakes and becoming relatively smooth in sequencing the components of the skill. In our example of transfer training, there would be relatively little hesitancy as the patient approaches the task. The breaks would be locked quickly and the foot pedals removed in quick succession. Improvements would be noted in speed and dexterity. This phase of motor learning lasts quite a bit longer than the initial cognitive phase. Often, many practice sessions are involved. A therapist would be concerned with keeping the child motivated, providing accurate and appropriate amounts of feedback, and providing the best schedule for practice. You might provide variability within the practice sessions by having the patient try various types of transfers to bed, chair, mat, or car. It is also important that during this phase of learning, children be encouraged to identify and correct their own errors. Asking children to analyze their own performance and determining what they would do to improve is a helpful strategy during this phase of learning.

AUTONOMOUS PHASE

During this most advanced phase of learning, the task is performed efficiently and without conscious attention. Learners are now able to attend to more important details. For example, they would be able to engage in conversation during the transfer without losing a step, or carry an object during the transfer. It is not uncommon for wheelchair-bound children to develop this level of skill.

Theories

There are two theories of motor learning that have generated a great deal of study of how we acquire motor skills. These two theories have provided some important information that can be used for the benefit of our patients. They are Adams' closed-loop theory of motor learning (Adams, 1971) and Schmidt's schema theory (Schmidt, 1975). They differ in the amount of emphasis placed on open-loop processes that can occur without benefit of ongoing feedback (Schmidt, 1988, p 482). Schmidt incorporated many of Adams' original ideas when formulating his schema theory in an attempt to explain acquisition of both slow movements that could be mediated by ongoing feedback and movements that were carried out so fast that feedback could not be used to monitor and correct performance.

ADAMS' CLOSED-LOOP THEORY

The name of Adams' theory emphasizes the crucial role of feedback. The concept of a closed loop from the previous discussion of motor control is one in which sensory information is funneled back to the central nervous system for processing and control of motor behavior.

The basic premise of Adams' theory is that movements are performed by comparing the ongoing movement to an internal reference of correctness that is developed during practice. This internal reference is termed a "perceptual trace." The perceptual trace represents the feedback one would receive if the task were performed correctly. By ongoing comparison of the feedback to the perceptual trace, a limb may be brought into the desired position. The quality of performance is directly related to the quality of the perceptual trace. A perceptual trace, formed as the learner repeatedly performs an action, is made up of a set of intrinsic feedback signals that arise from the learner. Intrinsic feedback here means the sensory information that is generated through performance: for example, the kinesthetic feel of the movement. The perceptual trace becomes stronger with repetition and more accurately represents correct performance as a result of external feedback provided by a teacher or therapist.

In the closed-loop theory, there are two types of feedback: intrinsic feedback arising from the learner, and external feedback arising from the teacher or therapists. External feedback in motor learning is referred to as "knowledge of results (KR)." Rather than just viewing KR as a means of reinforcing correct performance, Adams emphasized the role KR plays in providing information to help the learner solve a motor problem. KR does not produce learning; rather, it helps the learner accomplish the process of learning.

The perceptual trace is a memory of correct performance. Adams was concerned that this memory could not also be the initiator of action. If it were, there would be no way to detect if an error in the selection of the movement occurred. For this reason, he included in his theory what he termed a "memory trace." A memory trace is a limited motor program that contains the specifications to get the movement going, at which point the perceptual trace takes over and guides the movement to an accurate completion.

Adams' theory has been criticized (Schmidt, 1988). A specific limitation of the theory is that it was developed to explain what are known as *slow positioning movements,* such as those used to track slowly moving targets. His theory did not explain how fast movements were controlled and learned.

SCHMIDT'S SCHEMA THEORY

Schema theory was developed in direct response to Adams' closed-loop theory and its limitations. Schema theory is concerned with how movements that can be carried out without feedback are learned, and it relies on an open-loop control element: specifically, the motor program.

The term "schema" refers to an abstract memory that represents a rule, or generalization, about skilled actions. According to schema theory, when an individual produces a movement, four kinds of information are stored for a brief period:

1. The initial conditions under which the performance took place (e.g., the position of the body, the kind of surface on which the individual carried out the action, or the shapes and weights of any objects that were used to carry out the task).
2. The parameters assigned to the motor program (e.g., the force or speed that was specified at the time of initiation of the program).
3. The KR that specified the outcome of the performance.
4. The sensory consequences of the movement (e.g., how it felt to perform the movement, the sounds that were made as a result of the action, or the visual effect of the performance).

These four kinds of information are analyzed to gain insight into the relationships among them and to form two types of schema.

The *recall schema* is an abstract representation of the relationship between the initial conditions surrounding performance, parameters that were specified within the motor program, and the outcome of the performance (KR). The learner, through the analysis of parameters that were specified in the motor program and the outcome, begins to understand the relationship between these two factors. For example, the learner may come to understand how far a wheelchair travels when varying amounts of force are generated to push the chair on a gravel pathway.

The learner stores this schema, and the next time performance on a gravel path is required, the amount of force needed to move the chair a desired distance is estimated and the parameters of the motor program are adjusted accordingly.

The *recognition schema* represents the relationship between the initial conditions, the outcome of performance (KR), and the sensory consequences that are perceived by the learner. Because it is formed in a manner similar to that of the recall schema, once established, the recognition schema is used to produce an estimate of the sensory consequences of the action that will be used as a basis for evaluation of the movement.

One of the limitations of schema theory is its failure to address how motor programs are created. Recall and recognition schemata are used to adjust and evaluate motor performance *given a motor program.* But the formation of the motor program is not explained.

KNOWLEDGE GENERATED BY THESE THEORIES

These competing theories of motor learning are responsible for a great surge of interest and a large increase in the number of research studies carried out to test their predictions. As an example, we can examine the predictions of the two theories related to varying performance during practice.

In Adams' theory the perceptual trace is strengthened by a series of "correct" performances and weakened by performances that stray from the mark. On the other hand, in schema theory, recall and recognition schemata are strengthened by a variety of experiences that allow the learner to extract the general relationship among initial conditions, program parameters, outcomes, and sensory consequences. Thus, schema theory predicts a beneficial effect of variability in practice trials (i.e., varying initial conditions and changing parameters such as force or speed), and the closed-loop theory predicts the opposite.

It has since been shown that variable practice within the confines of a single motor program is beneficial, enabling successful performance in novel situations (Catalano & Kleiner, 1984). Further, Shapiro and Schmidt (1982) have shown that variability in practice is particularly effective for children's formation of schemata. These theories are driving research that furthers our understanding of the process of motor learning.

Recently Schmidt (1991) and Winstein (1991) outlined some of the recent research on practice conditions and provision of feedback to the learner that has a clear relationship to the way therapists can design training sessions for their patients.

Conditions of Practice. As a physical therapist you will have control over how treatment sessions are organized. How much time is spent in practice of each task you are teaching, and the order in which the tasks are practiced, are important. There are two ways to schedule or organize practice: blocked practice and random practice. *Block practice* is characterized by devoting a set of practice trials all to the same task. *Random practice* involves switching among tasks on practice trials. It has been demonstrated that random practice is better for learning than blocked practice (Shea & Morgan, 1989). Thus, if there were several tasks that you were teaching your patient, such as sit-to-stand transfers, and moving from supine to sitting, practicing them in either a random order or in a natural order would promote learning more than would repeated practice of just one of the tasks. A patient could come to sitting and then stand. After performing some other activity the patient could sit and then come to stand, return to lying, sit, and then stand again. According to Winstein (1991), if the critical element of later performance is to recall a skill under different performance conditions, then practice should be structured to enable the patient to practice that kind of processing. Specifically, the patient should recall the skill under a variety of conditions. Often, performance on a practice trial deteriorates when different conditions are presented, but learning is enhanced, and learning is the object of training sessions.

Another feature of practice that is of concern to therapists is embodied in the "whole-part" practice debate. For a long time therapists have assumed that breaking a skill down into component parts would make the process of learning easier. Practice of one part of a task was thought to enhance learning of the whole task. Winstein recently reported her study of a comparison of two methods of gait training for hemiplegic patients (1991). One group received weight transfer training and standard gait training; the other group received just standard gait training. After training, there was no difference between the groups in the gait performance measures. Members of the group that received weight transfer training were more symmetric in their weight distribution during standing, but they did not have an advantage in gait. Winstein proposed that because other studies have shown some advantage to groups who practice parts of a whole task, the issue is how similar the "part" is to its natural occurrence in the context of the whole task. She surmised that standing weight transfer as practiced by her subjects was not analogous to the smooth transfer of weight from one foot to the other that occurs during gait. Therefore, the standing weight transfer task was not a natural subunit of the walking task in this example.

Feedback During Practice. Another practice issue is the kind of feedback that is provided to learners and the scheduling of that feedback. The "relative frequency of KR" is the term used to refer to the proportion of trials for which the learner is provided KR. Generally, therapists have assumed that more feedback is better. And, in fact, to the extent that the feedback is used to correct performance, the learner appears to perform better. But a high relative frequency of KR may be detrimental to learning. In fact, Winstein reported a study conducted with Schmidt in which the effects of KR were compared in two groups: one with KR provided after each trial, and one with KR provided after only half of the trials. The 50% relative frequency group demonstrated poorer performance in trials without feedback but better performance during a later retention trial (Schmidt, 1991), indicating that more learning took place. In studies extending this work, Nicholson and Schmidt (1989) were reported to have examined the schedule, or timing, of feedback. They found that reducing the frequency of KR as the number of trials increases appears to have the best effect on learning. This is termed "fading the feedback."

SUMMARY

In summary, motor learning theory and research provide practical information for therapists designing treatment programs. Physical therapists such as Winstein and Nicholson are now involved in the study of motor learning in patients. Our profession will surely benefit from such research, much as we have benefitted from the involvement of physical therapists such as Horak in research on postural control. These areas of movement science—motor control and motor learning—greatly affect how we practice as physical therapists; and now these areas are beginning to be affected by our professional concerns. As one studies motor development, one should not lose sight of the sister sciences and the vast amount of information they provide to the student of motor development.

References

Adams JA. A closed-loop theory of motor learning. *J Motor Behav* 3:110–150, 1971.

Brooks VB. *The Neural Basis of Motor Control.* New York: Oxford University Press, 1986.

Catalano JF, Kleiner BM. Distant transfer and practice variability. *Percept Mot Skill* 58:851–856, 1984.

Davis WJ. Organizational concepts in the central motor networks of invertebrates. In Herman RL, Grillner S, Stein PSG, et al (eds). *Advances in Behavioral Biology: Neural Control of Locomotion.* New York: Plenum Publishing, 1976, pp 265–292.

Denny-Brown D. Disintegration of motor function resulting from cerebral lesion. *J Nerv Ment Dis* 112:1–45, 1950.

Fitts PM. Perceptual motor skills learning. In Melton AW (ed). *Categories of Human Learning.* New York: Academic Press, 1964, pp 243–285.

Gallistel CR. *The Organization of Action: A New Synthesis.* Hillsdale, NJ: Lawrence Erlbaum, 1980.

Gordon J. Assumptions underlying physical therapy intervention: Theoretical and historical perspectives. In Carr JH, Shepherd RB, Gordon J, et al (eds). *Movement Science: Foundations for Physical Therapy in Rehabilitation.* Rockville, MD: Aspen Publishers, 1987, pp 1–30.

Heriza C. Motor development: Traditional and contemporary theories. In Lister M (ed). Contemporary Management of Motor Control Problems. Proceedings of the II Step Conference. Alexandria, VA: Foundation for Physical Therapy, 1991, pp 99–126.

Horak FB. Assumptions underlying motor control for neurologic rehabilitation. In Lister M (ed). Contemporary Management of Motor Control Problems. Proceedings of the II Step Conference. Alexandria, VA: Foundation for Physical Therapy, 1991, pp 11–27.

Lashley KS. The problem of serial order in behavior. In Jeffress LA (ed). *Cerebral Mechanisms in Behavior.* New York: John Wiley & Sons, 1951, pp 112–136.

Nashner LM. Sensory, neuromuscular and biomechanical contributions to human balance. In

Duncan P (ed). *Balance: Proceedings of the APTA Forum.* Alexandria, VA: American Physical Therapy Association, 1990, pp 5–12.

Nicholson DE, Schmidt RA. Scheduling information feedback: Fading, spacing, and relative frequency of knowledge of results. In Proceedings of the North American Society for the Psychology of sport and physical activity: June 1–4, 1989. Kent, OH: Kent State University, p 47.

Overbaugh D, Widener K, Zapotchny T, VanSant AF. Changing movement patterns during pregnancy. (Work in progress).

Oxendine JB. *Psychology of Motor Learning.* Englewood Cliffs, NJ: Prentice Hall, 1984.

Peiper A. *Cerebral Function in Infancy and Childhood.* New York: Consultants Bureau, 1963.

Rosenbaum DA. *Human Motor Control.* New York: Academic Press, 1991.

Schmidt RA. A schema theory of discrete motor skill learning. *Psychol Rev* 82:225–260, 1975.

Schmidt RA. *Motor Control and Learning,* 2nd ed. Champaign, IL: Human Kinetics, 1988.

Schmidt RA. Motor learning principles for physical therapy. In Lister M (ed). Contemporary Concepts of Motor Control Problems. Proceedings of the II Step Conference. Alexandria, VA: Foundation for Physical Therapy, 1991, pp 49–63.

Scholtz JP. Dynamic pattern theory: Some implications for therapeutics. *Phys Ther* 70:827–843, 1990.

Seyffarth H, Denny-Brown D. The grasp reflex and the instinctive grasp reaction. *Brain* 71:109, 1948.

Shapiro DC, Schmidt RA. The Schema theory: Recent evidence and developmental implications. In Kelso JAS, Clark JE (eds). *The Development of Movement Control and Coordination.* New York: John Wiley & Sons, 1982, pp 113–150.

Shea JB, Morgan RL. Contextual interference effects on the acquisition, retention, and transfer of a motor skill. *J Exp Psychol* 5:179–187, 1989.

Smith KU, Henry JP. Cybernetics of rehabilitation. *Am J Phys Med* 46:379–467, 1967.

Taylor J (ed). *Selected Writings of John Hughlings Jackson.* New York: Basic Books, 1958.

Twitchell TE. The restoration of motor function following hemiplegia in man. *Brain* 74:443–480, 1951.

VanSant AF. Life-span motor development. In Lister M (ed). Contemporary Management of Motor Control Problems. Proceedings of the II Step Conference. Alexandria, VA: Foundation for Physical Therapy, 1991, pp 77–83.

Weiss P. Self-differentiation of the basic patterns of coordination. Comp Psychol Monogr 17(4), 1941.

Winstein DJ. Designing practice for motor learning: Clinical implications. In Lister M (ed). Contemporary Management of Motor Control Problems. Proceedings of the II Step Conference. Alexandria, VA: Foundation for Physical Therapy, 1991, pp 65–76.

Wyke B. The neurological basis for movement: A developmental review. In Holt KS (ed). *Movement and Child Development.* Clin Develop Med 55:19–33, 1975.

Chapter 4

Movement Skills

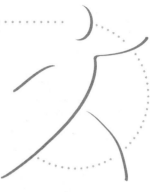

Objectives

AFTER STUDYING THIS CHAPTER, THE READER WILL BE ABLE TO:

1 Differentiate the process of motor development from the achievement of motor skill.
2 List factors that affect movement skill development.
3 Relate developmental theories to motor skill development.
4 Discuss basic concepts related to movement skill development.
5 Describe motor skill development across the life span.

GENERAL DEVELOPMENT

Development is a result of (genetic) maturation, physical growth, and learning (environmental adaptation). Maturation guides development genetically, such as in the physical changes that occur as a result of internal body processes — organ differentiation in the embryo, myelination of nerve fibers, and the appearance of primary and secondary ossification centers. Growth is the process whereby changes in physical size and shape take place — for example, the dramatic changes in facial and body growth that occur during adolescence. Children can be classified as early, average, and late maturers according to the relationship between physiologic growth parameters and chronologic age. Adaptation is how the body changes in response to the environment. For example, a muscle increases bulk with strength training; the immune system produces antibodies when exposed to a pathogen; and bones heal after a fracture. *Ontogeny,* the development of the individual, recapitulates *phylogeny,* the development of the species. One is a reflection of the other. There are similarities in development among species and within individuals of any given species.

MOTOR DEVELOPMENT

Motor development is the change in motor behavior experienced over the life span. Motor development is also the process whereby these changes occur in a sequential manner. The process and the product of motor development are related to age. Central nervous system maturation is one of the primary determinants of early motor behavior. In the infant's nervous system, there is a vertical hierarchy of control, with the infant exhibiting spinal cord reflexes in response to touch or pain. As the nervous system matures, reflexes and reactions that are mediated by the brain stem and mid-brain emerge. Finally, voluntary control from the cortex is seen with purposeful movements such as reaching and walking. There is also a horizontal hierarchy of increasingly complex connectivity within the nervous system. Synaptic connections increase between areas of the cortex, allowing exchange of information. These horizontal connections monitor the timing and execution of motor commands, as well as store movement and perceptual information.

Changes in growth are used as markers for development. Although we routinely use age as the yardstick of motor development, we should think more about relating body size to motor skill achievement. Think of a small 3-year-old being assessed on how he ascends a standard set of stairs. Does he use the railing because of poor motor skills or because the steps are too tall for his short legs? The effects of physical size and body proportion on motor skill acquisition or movement proficiency have been examined in adolescence but are just beginning to be explored in younger age groups. Does the changing weight and proportion of the limb segments constrain the production of movement? Thelen and Fisher's (1982) research appears to support the possibility that infants cease reflex stepping because the limbs get too heavy, not because of any change in the nervous system.

Another factor that affects how a person develops movement is genetic coding. Group differences are reflected in gender and in the culture in which children are raised. Males have an innate ability to develop more muscle and greater strength (Malina & Bouchard, 1991). A child's experience gleaned from various child-rearing practices (including physical handling), sensory and motor feedback, and sensorimotor integration combine with a genetic predisposition to produce movement skills. Why does one person become a triathlete, or another a prima ballerina, while others have difficulty riding a bike, water skiing, or hitting a ball with various sports equipment?

THEORIES

There are two theoretic perspectives that have been most prevalent in motor skill acquisition: the maturation perspective and the perceptual-cognitive perspective. The maturationists, Gesell (1974) and McGraw (1945), predicated motor development and emerging motor behaviors on the neuromaturation of the cerebral cortex. The perceptual-cognitive perspective came from researchers in the field of motor learning and motor control (Clark et al, 1990). They view information processing as a foundation for movement.

The observable changes in motor behavior that occur across the life span are a result of the interaction between biologic factors (maturation, genes) and environmental factors (learning, culture). Together they produce change or adaptation in the individual. Maturation and learning depend on each other because learning does not occur unless the system is ready to learn. The rate of maturation is affected by the amount and type of learning experiences, and the type of learning experiences is affected by the social-cultural environment (Higgins, 1985).

Maturation

Although maturation is only one part of the explanation for motor development, Gesell's theory has provided us with an invaluable concept about movement skill acquisition that is still important. That concept is reciprocal interweaving.

RECIPROCAL INTERWEAVING

Gesell (1974) coined the term reciprocal interweaving to describe the spiral-like development that alternates between periods of equilibrium and disequilibrium. Periods of equilibrium are marked by stable behavior, whereas periods of disequilibrium are marked by instability. The cycles occur frequently in the first year and decrease in frequency with increasing maturity. Gesell applied this concept to all types of behavior—motor, adaptive, linguistic, and personal-social.

The application of reciprocal interweaving can be seen by looking at the pattern of development of head control. Head control in a newborn is relatively good. The newborn is able to hold the head in the mid-line if held upright and is able to lift the head when held at one's shoulder or in prone. At 2 months, the head appears to be more wobbly, but at 4 months control is again excellent in upright and in prone positions. A cycle of stability, instability, and renewed stability is evident in this development of head control.

The development of balance in children is another example of this concept. Schumway-Cook and Woollacott's (1985) study of the growth of stability in standing also reinforces Gesell's concept of reciprocal interweaving. They found that the immature pattern of postural response, the hip strategy, was replaced by the adult pattern, the ankle strategy. Strategies are patterns of muscle activation observed when the supporting surface is moved. Between the two extremes was an intervening period in which highly variable postural responses were seen. This sequence of immature, transitional, and mature motor patterns can be documented throughout development—in fact, throughout the life span.

COMPETITION OF MOTOR PATTERNS

The competition of motor patterns is a concept brought forward by Italian pediatricians Milani-Comparetti and Gidoni (1967). They thought that certain patterns of movement compete for primacy at certain periods during develop-

Table 4-1. REFLEX CORRELATES OF MOTOR BEHAVIOR	
Reflex	**Motor Behavior**
MUST BE PRESENT:	**PRIOR TO:**
1. Labyrinthine righting on head	Prone on elbows Trunk extension in sitting
2. Body righting on body	Rolling to prone
3. Equilibrium reactions in prone	Prone weight bearing on extended arms
4. Parachute (protective extension) sideways	Sitting with hand support
5. Symmetric tonic neck	Quadruped
6. Forward parachute	Quadruped
MUST BE SUPPRESSED:	**PRIOR TO:**
1. Hand grasp	Prone on elbows
2. Immature neck-righting	Body-righting
3. Asymmetric tonic neck	Segmental rolling
4. Moro	All parachute and equilibrium reactions
5. Symmetric tonic neck	Creeping
6. Foot grasp	Walking

Data from Milani-Comparetti A, Gidoni E. Routine developmental examination in normal and retarded children. *Dev Med Child Neurol* 9:631–638, 1967.

ment. The acquisition of certain motor behaviors was correlated with the appearance and suppression of reflexes, as listed in Table 4–1. For example, the asymmetric tonic neck reflex (ATNR) is cued by head turning in the infant. The motor response consists of the face arm extending and the skull arm flexing. Head turning in the infant can also result in the turning of the whole body in the same direction, as in log rolling. This movement is called an immature neck-righting reaction. The ATNR and the neck-righting patterns of movement compete normally during development, with the neck-righting reaction becoming more prevalent as the child matures. Later the log-rolling pattern of the immature neck-righting is replaced by the mature form of the reaction, which causes the body to turn in segments in response to head turning (Barnes et al, 1978). Milani-Comparetti and Gidoni's competition of motor patterns may be only an extension of Gesell's reciprocal interweaving concept.

Perceptual-Cognitive

The perceptual-cognitive perspective provides for the importance of sensory processing and the effect that intellectual abilities have on the acquisition and performance of motor skills. The speed of processing information can significantly impact motor performance. Fitt's Law (1954) is a mathematical calculation that describes the relationship among speed, accuracy, and distance in motor performance. According to the law, it takes longer to touch a small object that is farther away than to touch a large object that is closer. Distance to the target, width of the object or target, and the index of difficulty of the movement are all accounted for when applying Fitt's Law. The movement time increases with the index of difficulty. Children perform in a fashion similar to that of adults but at a lower absolute level of performance.

The role of sensation in movement changes over the life span. First, sensation is paired with movement in the form of reflexes. Sensation is used as feedback to refine movement and as a stimulus for postural responses. Eventually, sensation is fed forward in anticipation of a motor action and is used less in feedback of familiar actions. Sensation can still be used to reinforce or refine new movements, but the speed of processing sensory information declines with age. The decline makes it more difficult for someone to learn a new motor skill such as playing the guitar or piano later in life. There is an interaction between cognition and sensation in learning that also applies to motor skills.

Gibson (1987) recently reviewed the research findings related to infant perception in an attempt to shed some light on the theories involved in human perceptual performance. She discussed eight conclusions that provide another view of the perceptual-cognitive perspective, as related to the relationships between perception and movement:

1. Perception is an active and exploratory process.
2. Perception is externally directed toward distal sources of stimulation.
3. Perception not only uses but depends on information given in motion.
4. Perception is of a three-dimensional world.
5. Perceptual constancy for various object properties such as size and shape exist before reaching, grasping, and handling objects become manifest.
6. Perception is coherent, that is, makes sense.
7. Perception is coordinated between different sensory modalities.
8. Perceptually guided actions are organized and flexible, not reflexive or mechanical stimulus-response sequences.

These conclusions point out the sophistication present in the perceptual abilities of the infant. Movement plays an important role in affording perception. A 4-month-old can distinguish an object's movement from his or her own movement (Kellman et al, 1987). Perceptual information reinforces posture, as when visual information is used to stabilize head posture at 2 months (Butterworth & Pope, 1982, cited in Gibson, 1987) and to stabilize the trunk at 6 months (Butterworth & Hicks, 1977). Just as movement appears to organize behavior, perception may be the ability to detect order and structure in the world, not merely the means to organize sensory information.

ADDITIONAL CONCEPTS AFFECTING MOVEMENT SKILL DEVELOPMENT

Many concepts apply to the acquisition and production of movement across the life span. One major concept of movement skill acquisition is that it is sequential. Other concepts are directional in that they identify the direction in which growth and development, and hence change, occur. Still other concepts relate to the type of movement exhibited during movement skill development, such as the kinesiologic concepts of extension-flexion and mobility-stability. With maturation, movement development proceeds from being a predominately reflexive behavior to a voluntary one. All of these concepts are important to the attainment of mature motor behavior.

Developmental Sequence

One of the most important concepts about movement, and possibly the most universal concept, is that movement skill development is sequential. Movement development in the broadest sense is based on what came before. Each movement learned is used again in a slightly different way to achieve something else. Although the rate of development may vary normally from individual to individual and is referred to by the term "individual differences," the sequence is the same for similar populations and cultures.

The majority of theorists, regardless of their perspective, agree that development occurs sequentially, but they do not agree on whether change occurs continuously or in stages. Continuity in development implies that change occurs continuously with a different end result. Movement patterns change with age, each being quantitatively different yet dependent on what came before. When motor development is viewed as a series of qualitative changes that are stage-like or discontinuous, each higher level of motor development must represent something different that was not there at the lower level, such as head control or rolling.

Movement skill acquisition exhibits continuity and discontinuity. The developmental sequence for the 1st year of life consists of the acquisition of motor milestones. These milestones act as a guide to the progression of movement and are viewed as stages. Within the stages there appears to be continuous change, as in the development of independent sitting (Fishkind & Haley, 1986). Movement patterns continue to change with age even after the last milestone, walking, is achieved.

Development is sequential, but that sequence is not necessarily universal. Although African babies sit and walk earlier than American infants, Oriental and Native American Indian infants normally lag behind their Caucasian counterparts in the acquisition of motor skills. This lag appears only during early development; all of the children eventually exhibit the same skills (Cintas, 1988).

Directional Concepts

CEPHALOCAUDAL

Traditionally, development is said to progress cephalocaudally, that is, from the head to the foot. Head control develops before trunk control. Control of arm movements for reaching develops before control of leg movements for creeping. The first part of the body to develop is the neck. In utero, the neural tube closes first at the level of the fourth cervical vertebra and continues to close in two directions, toward the head (cephalo) and toward the feet (caudal). Development is said to proceed from the neck (cervico) both cephalically and caudally, or cervicocephalocaudally.

PROXIMAL-DISTAL

The second concept of directional development is that development occurs from proximal to distal. In this case proximal refers not only to the proximal parts of the extremities, such as the shoulder or pelvic girdles, but to the mid-line of the body, the neck and trunk, which are referred to as "axial structures." Once again the infant first controls the mid-line of the neck, then the mid-line of the trunk, then the shoulders and pelvis before controlling arms, legs, hands, and feet.

ASYMMETRIC-SYMMETRIC

Newborns begin life asymetrically with the head turned to one side, gazing at one hand, and become more symmetric around the 4th month of life. Mid-line orientation consists of holding the head in the mid-line and discovering the two hands held out in space at the mid-line. Reaching changes from a symmetric bilateral pattern of batting to an asymmetric unilateral swiping pattern.

GROSS MOTOR—FINE MOTOR

The last directional concept involves the direction of overall change in movement skill acquisition, which is from gross, large muscle movements to fine, more discrete movements. Total body movement responses to stimuli are seen before isolated head and trunk movements. Arms and legs thrust in play before single limb reaching occurs. Mass grasp is possible before individual finger movements. However, the infant learns to move and respond on many levels at the same time. Not all gross motor skills come before fine motor skills. The infant reaches for objects before head control is completely established. In general, mass movements occur before more discrete ones.

In reality, the body is a system of linked structures; thus, movement in one area affects the relationship of the structures not only in the moving part but also in the other parts. While the infant is working on perfecting head

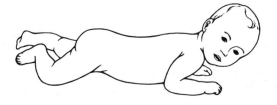

FIGURE 4–1. Head lifting in a new-born.

control, rolling occurs, and while not able to sit alone, the infant can reach for and hold objects. Figure 4–1 shows the newborn trying to lift the head while prone with the extremities flexed. Because of the weight of the head, the task is very difficult. Attempts to lift the head result in movement throughout the body. The head lifts much more easily once the pelvis is flat.

Dissociation. Sensorimotor maturation is characterized by *dissociation,* that is, the breaking up of gross movement patterns, which involve the total body, into finer, more selective patterns, which permit parts of the body to move independently of other parts. An example of dissociation of head from shoulder movements is seen when the child learns to turn the head in all directions without affecting the body as a whole (Connor et al, 1978). Dissociation is also evidenced by the ability to perform neck and trunk rotation. Dissociation, and hence rotation, is necessary to move in and out of most positions. Motor development provides many examples of dissociation. One upper extremity may be dissociated from the trunk for reaching, or the upper and lower extremities may be dissociated from the trunk for creeping. In the latter instance, the upper trunk is also dissociated from the lower trunk and rotated in one direction while the lower trunk is dissociated from the upper trunk and rotated in the opposite direction, providing counter-rotation.

Kinesiologic Concepts

EXTENSION-FLEXION

Development in utero proceeds from a relatively extended posture to one of increasing flexion. At birth, the "fetal position" is synonymous with total body flexion. Flexor tone dominates the newborn's body. In fact, the flexed posture of an infant is used as a measure of gestational age. Physiologic flexion is gradually replaced as gravity acts to change posture and the infant actively initiates extension against gravity. The infant first learns to actively extend the head and neck against gravity and then at 3 months uses neck flexion to hold the head in the mid-line position. After scapular stabilizers and trunk extensors develop, the 4-month-old infant can bilaterally reach to mid-line with either the upper or lower extremities in supine. Lifting the head and trunk from the supporting surface into flexion is not seen until about 5 months of age.

Balance between the flexors and extensors around any joint or body part such as the neck or trunk is crucial to the development of controlled movement. Flexion and extension of the trunk are combined unilaterally to produce lateral trunk flexion, whereas flexors and extensors on the opposite sides of the trunk combine to produce rotational movement.

MOBILITY-STABILITY

Controlled movement occurs within the framework of mobility and stability, or movement and posture. The relationship between stability (holding a posture) and mobility (moving) is called "postural control." Mobility is present before stability. Once a stable posture is established, movement control develops. Static postural control develops before dynamic postural control. Key postures for mobility and stability were originally described by Rood and clarified by Attermeier (Stengel et al, 1984). They are shown in Figure 4–2.

Infants are very mobile and initially demonstrate random movements such as kicking in supine. These random movements occur within the available range of motion, and some postures are assumed briefly, such as head lifting in the prone position. Next, infants learn to hold postures such as prone extension and the prone-on-elbows position. Prone extension is an example of stability in tonic holding, in which the infant holds the position by contracting extensor muscles against gravity. The prone-on-elbows position is an example of stability in co-contraction in which anterior and posterior trunk muscles of the shoulder girdle contract to maintain the position. Stability patterns establish a stable base from which movement can occur. Infants and children are able to maintain a posture such as sitting before they are able to attain the posture independently or demonstrate the ability to preserve the posture if disturbed.

Some postures are inherently stable and require little or no muscular effort. A prime example is W-sitting, in which the legs are internally rotated, the pelvis is anteriorly tilted, and the knees are flexed. It is as if a peg (the trunk) has been placed in a puzzle hole (the pelvis). Biomechanically, the child is locked in place with no need for active trunk control and is free to use the hands for play rather than support. The child is exhibiting positional stability, the stability that comes from the mechanics of the position, not from muscular control of the trunk. The use of muscular control to maintain a position is termed "dynamic stability" and is related to postural reactions elicited in response to disturbed balance or a planned weight shift.

Infants learn to control movement by weight shifting in stable postures. Controlled mobility is exhibited in a posture when the limbs are loaded (weight bearing), as in a closed kinetic chain, and weight is shifted. All but the first two postures in Figure 4–2 can provide practice in controlled mobility. During controlled mobility, muscles are worked from their origins rather than from their insertions. For example, when one is shifting forward in the prone-on-elbows position, the biceps bring the shoulders forward because the elbow joint is loaded, thus fixing the bicep's insertion. Controlled weight shifting

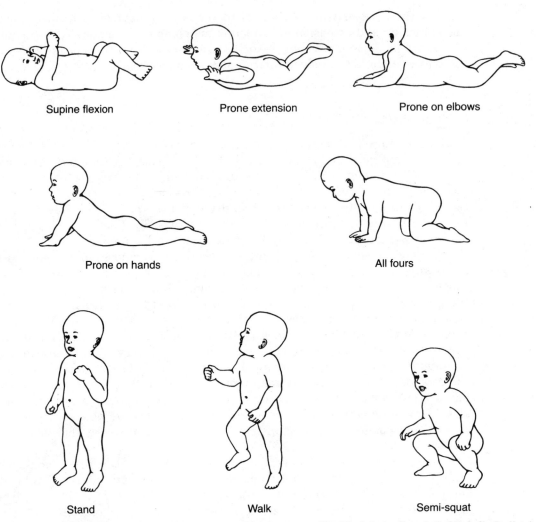

FIGURE 4–2. Rood's key developmental postures. (Modified from Campbell SK [ed]. *Pediatric Neurologic Physical Therapy*. Churchill Livingstone, New York, 1984, p 41.)

develops the dynamic stability needed to preserve the posture if balance is disturbed.

Skilled movement is defined as mobility superimposed on stability with the distal part free. In other words, the infant moves one part of the body while holding or stabilizing another part of the body, as in reaching for an object while prone on one elbow. In skilled movement, the limbs are unloaded and work in an open kinetic chain, and muscles move from insertion to origin, as in bringing something to the mouth while eating or in taking a step. Examples of skilled movements are creeping and walking. During gait, the stance phase leg performs controlled mobility, and the swing phase leg, upper extremities, and trunk perform skilled movement. In creeping, the weight-bearing limbs and the trunk perform controlled mobility and the moving limbs perform skilled movement. Dynamic postural control is necessary to move safely from one posture to another and can involve both controlled mobility and skill.

Reflex

Automatic movements include reflexes and postural reactions that are cued by sensation. Reflexes are stereotypical responses to sensory stimuli. Postural reactions are automatic responses to loss of balance. Reflexes occur early in developmental time, some appearing during gestation or shortly after birth, and are integrated by 4 to 6 months of age. A list of primitive, or early occurring, reflexes is found in Table 4–2. An infant's movements are intimately associated with reflexes for the first 3 months of life. Although a normally developing infant is not limited to only reflex motor behavior, reflexes do play a role in pairing sensory and motor action.

Many developmentalists have written about the possible functional implications of reflexes. The ATNR allows viewing of the infant's hand and may be the beginning of eye-hand coordination. Primitive withdrawal reflexes in the lower extremity and the Moro reflex may be seen as protective. Many reflexes (see Table 4–1) need to be suppressed in order to allow functional motor behavior to be expressed. The relationship of plantar grasp and walking has been studied (Effgen, 1982): those children who exhibited integration of the reflex achieved independent ambulation (walked), whereas those who did not integrate the reflex did not.

Hypothetically, as primitive reflexes fade, postural reactions and volitional movements appear, as shown in Figure 4–3. Some primitive reflexes disappear

Table 4–2. PRIMITIVE REFLEXES

Reflex	Age at Onset	Age at Integration
Suck-swallow	28 weeks' gestation	2–5 months
Rooting	28 weeks' gestation	3 months
Flexor withdrawal	28 weeks' gestation	1–2 months
Crossed extension	28 weeks' gestation	1–2 months
Moro	28 weeks' gestation	4–6 months
Plantar grasp	28 weeks' gestation	9 months
Positive support	35 weeks' gestation	1–2 months
Asymmetric tonic neck	Birth	4–6 months
Palmar grasp	Birth	9 months
Symmetric tonic neck	4–6 months	8–12 months

Data from Barnes MR, Crutchfield CA, Heriza CB. *The Neurophysiological Basis of Patient Treatment,* vol 2. Atlanta: Stokesville Publishing, 1982.

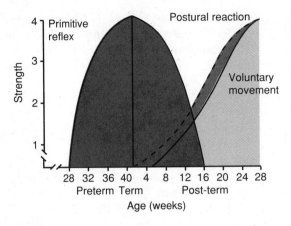
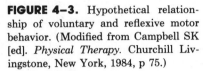

FIGURE 4–3. Hypothetical relationship of voluntary and reflexive motor behavior. (Modified from Campbell SK [ed]. *Physical Therapy*. Churchill Livingstone, New York, 1984, p 75.)

and others are integrated, allowing the postural reactions to organize functional movement. Postural reactions are the basis of voluntary movement. It is the postural reactions of protective extension, head- and trunk-righting, and equilibrium that provide the basis for posture, locomotion, and prehension. As listed in Table 4–1, righting reactions are needed as a foundation for certain motor behaviors such as achieving the prone-on-elbows position, rolling, and weight bearing on extended arms in prone position. Postural reactions occur in response to changes in the body's orientation to gravity and in the pattern of weight distribution and are affected by whether the center of gravity is within the base of support. Postural reactions provide a means of automatic postural adjustment to maintain or regain balance, making it safe to move voluntarily. There are three kinds of postural reactions: protective, righting, and equilibrium.

The earliest *protective reactions* are seen in response to quickly lowering the body toward a supporting surface. This downward response of the legs is seen at 4 months. Protective extension of the upper extremities becomes evident when the infant begins to sit with support. The infant can prop forward on extended arms if placed. A protective reaction is a response to a quick displacement of the center of gravity out of the base of support. Such displacement in sitting results in a brisk extension of the arm to "catch" and protect the person from falling. Protective reactions begin at 6 months in sitting and develop sequentially forward, sideways, and backward. They are generally completely developed by 10 months. These reactions become our backup system if we fail to regain our balance by use of an equilibrium reaction. Unfortunately, the use of these automatic responses can result in unintentional injury, as when an elderly individual sustains a Colles' fracture from falling on an outstretched arm.

Righting reactions begin at birth and exhibit peak occurrence at 10 to 12 months. These reactions can be elicited by any one of a number of sensory stimuli: vestibular, proprioceptive, visual, or tactile. Righting reactions become

Table 4-3. RIGHTING AND EQUILIBRIUM REACTIONS		
Reaction	**Age at Onset**	**Age at Integration**
HEAD-RIGHTING		
Neck (immature)	34 weeks' gestation	4–6 months
Labyrinthine	Birth–2 months	Persists
Optical	Birth–2 months	Persists
Neck (mature)	4–6 months	5 years
TRUNK-RIGHTING		
Body (immature)	34 weeks' gestation	4–6 months
Body (mature)	4–6 months	5 years
Landau	3–4 months	1–2 years
PROTECTIVE		
Downward lower extremity	4 months	Persists
Forward upper extremity	6–7 months	Persists
Sideways upper extremity	7–8 months	Persists
Backward upper extremity	9 months	Persists
Stepping lower extremity	15–17 months	Persists
EQUILIBRIUM		
Prone	6 months	Persists
Supine	7–8 months	Persists
Sitting	7–8 months	Persists
Quadruped	9–12 months	Persists
Standing	12–24 months	Persists

Data from Barnes MR, Crutchfield CA, Heriza CB. *The Neurophysiological Basis of Patient Treatment,* vol 2. Atlanta: Stokesville Publishing, 1982.

incorporated into equilibrium reactions and therefore persist as part of our automatic balance mechanism (Table 4–3).

Righting is defined as maintenance or restoration of the proper alignment of the head or trunk in space. One category of righting reactions produces movement in one plane; these movements are described as anterior, posterior, or lateral head-righting or trunk-righting. When held upright in vertical and tilted position in any direction, the head and trunk right or tilt in the opposite direction. Likewise, when one is in sidelying position, the tactile cue of the trunk on the supporting surface cues lateral head-lifting (righting). Head-righting develops during the first several months in response to gravity's effect on the vestibular system and through the body's contact (tactile cue) with the supporting surface.

A second category of righting reactions produces rotation around the body axis, as in rolling. These righting reactions of the head and trunk function to

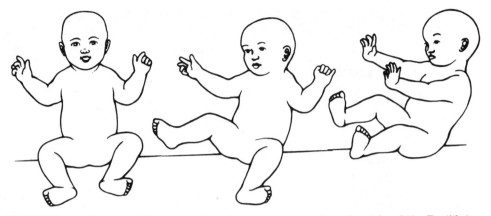

FIGURE 4–4. Sitting equilibrium reaction in response to a lateral weight shift. Equilibrium reactions in sitting mature when the infant begins creeping.

produce rotation around the long axis of the body and are an integral part of producing a smooth movement transition from one posture to another. Mature neck and body righting allow for the change from log rolling to segmental rolling seen in the 4- to 6-month-old infant.

Equilibrium reactions are more sophisticated than righting reactions and involve a total body response to a slow shift of the center of gravity outside the base of support. In a sitting equilibrium reaction, the head and trunk right, and the arm and leg abduct opposite the weight shift, followed by head and trunk rotation toward the abducted extremities (Fig. 4–4). Equilibrium reactions begin to appear at 6 months of age in the prone position, even as the infant is experiencing supported sitting. The remaining equilibrium reactions appear in an orderly sequence: prone, supine, sitting, quadruped, and standing. The maturation of the reactions in these postures lags behind the attainment of movement in the next developmental posture. For example, equilibrium reactions mature in sitting position when the child is creeping, and mature in quadruped position when the child walks.

LIFE SPAN CHANGES

Infancy

Motor skill development progresses sequentially over the first year of life, with the infant able to roll, sit, creep, pull to stand, and walk by 1 year. Reaching and prehension changes from swiping at objects at 5 months to discrete movement of the thumb and index finger by 10 months. Repetitive rocking, banging, and shaking movements of the trunk and extremities are also part of development during the first year of life, as seen in Figure 4–5 (Thelen, 1979). These "rhythmic stereotypies," a term used by Thelen, appear to be the

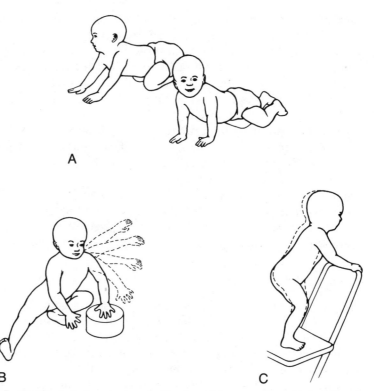

FIGURE 4–5. Rhythmical stereotypies. *A,* Hands-and-knees rocking. *B,* Arm-banging against a surface. *C,* Stand-bouncing. (Modified from Thelen E. Rhythmical stereotypies in infants. *Anim Behav* 27[3]:704, 706, 1979.)

precursors of significant changes in movement control. For example, the child rocks repetitively on hands and knees prior to creeping independently. These movements may represent transition behaviors because they seem to emerge as the infant is gaining control over a new posture.

Prior to achieving the ability to stand alone, the infant develops postural control in the prone position against gravity, in the supine position against gravity, and in the sidelying position against gravity. The infant learns in a fairly systematic way to keep the center of gravity within the base of support while moving around in the prone and supine positions. Major accomplishments in the development of balance include head and trunk control in prone, supine, sitting, quadruped, and standing positions, and the development of postural reactions in these positions.

As the infant learns the rules of moving, he or she learns postural control. Sensory information is used as feedback to refine movement accuracy. The infant needs to know how much force to generate, and when and in what direction to do so. Feedback allows refinement of movement parameters and assists the infant in organizing movement against gravity. The vestibular system processes sensory information related to gravitational orientation. Increased weight bearing through both upper and lower extremity joints provides proprioceptive information, as does movement itself. By 7 to 9 months of age, most infants are pulling to stand and beginning to cruise or walk sideways around low objects such as a coffee table. Independent upright ambulation is achieved anywhere from 9 to 15 months of age.

Vision is one of the primary sensory inputs used by children under 3 years of age to make balance or postural adjustments. Vision directs and motivates the infant's first reaching as well as crawling and creeping. The visual system matures after birth and requires input to complete its development. Visually impaired infants are normally delayed in their motor abilities because of the lack of visual information to guide and encourage movement. Auditory cues in addition to tactile information can be used to entice movement and provide directional information for the visually impaired infant.

Childhood and Adolescence

In early childhood (3 to 6 years), fundamental game-playing skills are learned. All children normally develop skill in running, jumping, throwing, and catching. These fundamental skills become the basis for more advanced movement skills such as playing soccer and learning ballet. The order in which the fundamental skills are acquired is sequential but varies with age. As the child's appreciation of proprioceptive input from joints and muscles increases during the 4th, 5th, and 6th years of life, the variability of the balance response in standing increases. By 7 years of age, the child depends primarily on input from proprioceptors for maintaining balance in standing. The vestibular and visual systems are used as secondary sources when there are conflicting data regarding the need for a postural response in standing.

Children improve their basic skill performance by increasing speed, accuracy, eye-hand coordination, strength, and balance. From 6 to 10 years of age, these skills become refined as the nervous system becomes more efficient in sending and processing neural impulses. Children become aware of the amount of force used and the reaction forces generated by their movements, such as in the relationship between the force of heel strike and the ground reaction to that heel strike. Better timing of movements and increased postural stability are combined with increases in strength and body size to improve the quality of the movements. A 10-year-old's speed in running a shuttle race or her form in performing a running broad jump is different than that of a younger child.

Generally, adult patterns of movement are attained between 6 and 10 years of age. By 10 years of age, the child is also able to demonstrate an adult balance strategy, the ankle strategy. This strategy is used in standing when the supporting surface is moved back and forth. The muscles around the ankle respond to maintain balance. This may be linked to the fact that the process of myelination of the nervous system is almost complete by 10 years of age.

The onset of puberty can have a short-term positive effect on motor performance of boys, which is related to an increase in adrenergic hormones. Boys that mature early demonstrate greater strength and endurance than boys that have not yet matured. The growth spurt seen in adolescent males is marked by a rapid gain in strength. Motor performance peaks during late adolescence, which for males occurs around 17 to 18 years of age.

The onset of puberty occurs 2 years earlier in girls than in boys. Static strength increases in females during adolescence, but gains do not show a spurt as they do in males. Although strength changes are related to skeletal maturity, such as peak height velocity (rate of fastest growth), motor performance is not (Malina & Bouchard, 1991). Although females demonstrate an increase in motor performance to around 14 years of age (Bailey et al, 1986), performance on tasks is highly variable during the remainder of adolescence, which is probably due to a complex interaction of strength, peak height velocity, and the onset of menses. Motivation, interest, and attitudes toward physical activity may also be factors.

The adolescent may continue to gain prowess in motor skills with practice. Parameters of performance such as speed, accuracy, form, and endurance can be changed, but the amount of change is highly variable and depends on practice and innate ability. The maximum degree of skill possible on most tasks is related to the individual's satisfaction with his or her own performance within the limits of cognitive, structural (physical), or sociocultural factors (Higgins, 1991). In other words, working with the resources at hand, the movement is as efficient as possible given the raw materials of the individual within the environment. Some improvement in motor performance is noted into the early twenties, but peak performance in most sports occurs relatively early.

Adulthood and Aging

Patterns of movement change with age, and movement patterns used by adults are highly variable. VanSant (1988) describes three common ways in which adults rise from the floor to a standing position. Although common forms of performance were detected in her study, only 25 per cent of the subjects used similar combinations of movements. The most consistent finding was the variability of the movements among the subjects. This has been confirmed in subsequent studies of adults in middle adulthood (VanSant et al, 1988) and in the task of rising from bed (VanSant, 1993).

It has been suggested that postural and balance skills decline with aging. Postural changes seen with aging can include forward head, kyphosis of the thoracic spine, and loss of lumbar lordosis. An increase in hip and knee flexion is also seen in many elderly persons. These changes appear to be related to alteration in the musculoskeletal system with age. Gait characteristics commonly seen in older adults such as an increase in base of support, a decrease of arm swing, an increase in double limb support, and slower cadence can be related to aging of the musculoskeletal and nervous systems.

Early studies that documented changes in the elderly used very simple tests for balance, which were generally not specific enough to discern the cause of the postural or balance problem. Also, the elderly subjects used for these studies were broadly defined as normal if they were over a certain age. Only recently have studies more rigorously defined normal as being free of musculoskeletal or neurologic pathology and without a history of falls (Gabell & Nayak, 1984). The normal elderly person in this study did as well as younger adults on measures of gait.

Postural sway in standing increases with age. The musculoskeletal system and the peripheral sensory systems show widespread decline with aging, which could account for the decrease in postural control. Processing of sensory information also slows with age. The fact that some elderly subjects were able to correct their postural responses over trials led Woollacott and colleagues (1988) to conclude that perhaps the delay in selection of an appropriate balance strategy was not simply a function of age. However, an adult over 60 is still more likely to exhibit decreased postural control and balance. Although the difficulties in this area are *not* all related to the normal aging process, the instability commonly found in the elderly may be due to associated changes in other body systems. In the elderly, an increase in instability cannot always be separated from some pathology (Horak et al, 1989), because with increasing age comes the increased probability that pathology may cause loss of balance and postural control.

SUMMARY

Motor behavior changes form to meet the needs of the individual. Needs are related to survival, safety, motivation, psychologic development, and societal and cultural expectations. The biologic foundation for motor skills is not stable over time. All of the body systems change at different times. Biologically, there are differences in (1) rate of growth, (2) magnitude of growth, (3) sensory processing, (4) flexibility, (5) strength, and (6) speed of response (VanSant, 1989). Environmentally, the variables are infinite and include (1) physical surroundings, (2) family structure, (3) access to motor learning, and (4) culture.

Motor development is both the change in motor behavior over the life span and the sequential, continuous, age-related process of change. Knowledge about the process of development is as important as knowledge about the product or motor skill. Roberton (1989) proposed that the dynamic system theory be applied to life span motor development research. If motor development is viewed as the study of change in motor behavior across a lifetime, age becomes a "marker variable" and may not be *the* cause of change. Altering the way in which we think about age may allow us (and researchers) to discover new information about why individuals move the way they do at different times in their lives. Motor development is as important to the clumsy child who wants to be included in activities on the playground as it is to the adult who wants to jog on a daily basis without injury, or to the elderly person who needs to adapt his or her movement to an aging body. Knowledge about motor development in the broadest sense is critical for us as health care professionals to be able to help people function at their optimal level regardless of age or occupation.

References

Bailey DA, Malina RM, Mirwald RL. Physical activity and growth of the child. In Falkner FT, Tanner JM (eds). *Human Growth: A Comprehensive Treatise,* vol 2, 2nd ed., New York: Plenum, 1986, pp 147–170.

Barnes MR, Crutchfield CA, Heriza CB. *The Neurophysiological Basis of Patient Treatment.* Atlanta: Stokesville Publishing, 1978.

Butterworth G, Hicks L. Visual proprioception and postural stability in infancy: A developmental study. *Perception* 6:255–262, 1977.

Cintas H. Cross-cultural variation in infant motor development. *Physical and Occupational Therapy in Pediatrics* 8:1–20, 1988.

Clark JE, Truly TL, Phillips SJ. Dynamical systems approach to understanding the development of lower limb coordination in locomotion. In Block H, Bertenhal BI (eds). *Sensorimotor Organization and Development in Infancy and Early Childhood.* Dordrecht: Kluever Publishing, 1990, pp 363–378.

Connor FP, Williamson GG, Siepp JM (eds). *Program Guide for Infants & Toddlers with Neuromotor and other Developmental Disabilities.* New York: Teacher's College Press, 1978.

Effgen SK. Integration of the plantar grasp reflex as an indicator of ambulation potential in developmentally disabled infants. *Phys Ther* 62:433–435, 1982.

Fitts PM. The information capacity of the human motor system in controlling the amplitude of movement. *J Exp Psychol* 47:381–391, 1954.

Gabell A, Nayak USL. The effect of age on variability in gait. *J Gerontol* 39:662–666, 1984.

Gesell A, Ilg FL, Ames LB, et al. *Infant and Child in the Culture of Today,* revised ed. New York: Harper & Row, 1974.

Gibson EJ. Introductory essay: What does infant perception tell us about theories of perception? *J Exp Psychol* 13(4):515–523, 1987.

Higgins S. Movement as an emergent form: Its structural limits. *Hum Movement Sci* 4:119–148, 1985.

Higgins S. Motor skill acquisition. *Phys Ther* 71:123–139, 1991.

Horak FB, Shupert CL, Mirka A. Components of postural dyscontrol in the elderly: A review. *Neurobiol Aging* 10:727–738, 1989.

Kellman PJ, Gleitman H, Spelke ES. Object and observer motion in the perception of objects by infants. *J Exp Psychol* 13(4):586–593, 1987.

Malina RM, Bouchard C. *Growth, Maturation and Physical Activity.* Champaign, IL: Human Kinetics, 1991.

McGraw M. *The Neuromuscular Maturation of the Human Infant.* New York: Hafner Publishing, 1945.

Milani-Comparetti A, Gidoni EA. Routine developmental examination in normal and retarded children. *Dev Med Child Neurol* 9:631–638, 1967.

Porter RE. Normal development of movement and function: Child and adolescent. In Scully RM, Barnes MR (eds). *Physical Therapy.* Philadelphia: JB Lippincott, 1989, pp 83–98.

Roberton MA. Motor development: Recognizing our roots, charting our future. *Quest* 41:213–223, 1989.

Schumway-Cook A, Woollacott MH. Growth of stability: Postural control from a developmental perspective. *J Motor Behav* 17(2):131–147, 1985.

Stengel TJ, Attermeirer SM, Bly L, et al. Sensorimotor dysfunction. In Campbell SK (ed). *Pediatric Neurological Physical Therapy,* 1st ed. New York: Churchill Livingstone, 1984, pp 13–87.

Thelen E. Rhythmical sterotypies in infants. *Anim Behav* 27(3):699–715, 1979.

Thelen E, Fisher DM. Newborn stepping: An explanation for a disappearing reflex. *Dev Psychol* 18:760–75, 1982.

VanSant AF. Rising from a supine position to erect stance: Description of adult movement and a developmental hypothesis. *Phys Ther* 68:185, 192, 1988.

VanSant AF, Cromwell S, Deo A, et al. Rising to standing from supine: A study of middle adulthood [Abstract]. *Phys Ther* 68:830, 1988.

VanSant AF. A life span concept of motor development. *Quest* 41:224–234, 1989.

Williams K, Haywood K, VanSant A. Movement characteristics of older adult throwers. In Clark JE, Humphrey JH (eds). *Advances in Motor Development Research,* vol 3. New York: AMS Press, 1990, pp 29–44.

Woollacott MH. Postural control mechanisms in young and old. In Duncan PW (ed). *Balance: Proceedings of the APTA Forum.* Alexandria, VA: APTA, 1990, pp 23–28.

Woollacott MH, Inglin B, Manchester D. Response preparation and posture control in the older adult. *Ann N Y Acad Sci* 525:42–53, 1988.

Chapter 5

Functional Assessment

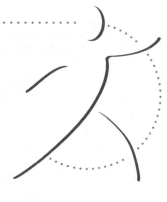

Objectives

AFTER STUDYING THIS CHAPTER, THE READER WILL BE ABLE TO:

1 Discuss the importance of functional assessment.
2 Identify well-developed, standardized assessment instruments.
3 Discuss reliability and validity issues of functional assessment measurement tools.
4 Compare and contrast commonly used functional assessment instruments.

As discussed in Chapter 1, an individual's success at meeting the challenges of everyday life reflects his or her functional independence. Is a small child capable of shopping for groceries, cooking, and managing finances? What about the older adult? Can an adult successfully balance the demands of work, home, family, and self? The answer to the first question is, of course, no. Within our society we care for children until they are capable of these activities. Children do, however, develop skills in mobility, dressing, and hygiene that allow them some degree of functional independence. We would hope that the answer to the latter two questions is yes. Adults and older adults want to live their lives as successfully and independently as possible. Occasionally, illness or injury may limit one's ability to physically function as independently as one would wish. At this point, an individual may turn to the health care community for support and assistance in regaining a self-sufficient lifestyle.

The primary task of health care professionals is to improve the health and functional independence of the client. In medical, surgical, psychosocial, and rehabilitation intervention, professionals strive to maintain or restore function. Health professionals in these areas of intervention hope to improve a person's functional capacity (Liang & Jette, 1981).

For the physical or occupational therapist, the focus of intervention is on physical functioning. The area of physical function includes the person's ability to move through the environment, perform self-care activities, successfully complete job tasks, and enjoy recreational pursuits (Guccione, 1993). How well can the patient move from place to place? Is the person able to successfully perform the tasks related to a profession or job? Can the person take care of basic daily tasks such as bathing, dressing, and eating? What about more difficult tasks such as shopping, taking a bus, or cleaning the house? By focusing intervention at these areas, the physical and occupational therapist can improve a client's ability to live as independently as possible.

For health care professionals to best serve their clients, they must be able to clearly, efficiently, and reliably identify at what level a client is able to perform important everyday tasks. Functional assessment provides this type of information and can be used to identify individuals needing intervention services, develop appropriate treatment plans, and evaluate the effectiveness of that treatment over time.

In looking at physical functioning, therapists often measure a patient's range of motion or muscle strength. These measures offer some degree of quantitative information that can be used to document a patient's need for services, or how well he or she has progressed in treatment. But do these measures in and of themselves reflect how that patient is functioning? If it is demonstrated that someone's range of motion in shoulder flexion has improved 5 degrees, progress has been made in range of motion, but it is unclear if that 5 degrees makes the difference in being able to put on a shirt or reach into the kitchen cabinets. To measure the success of intervention in these functional tasks, assessment must focus on function. Goniometry and muscle strength testing do not provide information on how function has changed. Instead, they may provide information on impairments, which ultimately affect function.

By using functional assessments, health care providers are more likely to develop meaningful treatment programs that will improve the quality of life for their clients (Haley et al, 1991). When appropriate assessment instruments are used as a basis for intervention, therapists can measure success in achieving the primary goal of therapy—improving the functional independence of their patients.

CHARACTERISTICS

A functional assessment can take many different forms and be implemented in many ways. Functional assessment is unique in that the activities and performance being assessed all relate to how well an individual can complete the necessary tasks of everyday life. Self-care activities such as dressing, washing, eating, and ambulating are referred to as *basic activities of daily living (BADL)*. More advanced activities that allow an individual to live independently in his or her community, such as shopping, using transportation, cooking, and cleaning, are referred to as *instrumental activities of daily living (IADL)*. Functional assessment needs to look at both of these categories of activities, as well as at abilities in job-related tasks and recreation. By addressing all areas of a person's life, the assessment reflects important aspects of how successfully a person can independently care for himself or herself.

In developing or choosing functional assessment strategies, the health care professional must be sure that the entire spectrum of activities performed during the client's day is represented. The assessment must address issues related to emotional, social, and environmental issues, not just physical functioning. How does a person interact with the environment? Can he or she easily commute to the workplace or get to the grocery store when necessary? Is it easy to move from place to place within the home regardless of whether the floor is carpeted or tiled? It must be clear that the goal of the assessment is to identify how the individual is functioning in everyday life, not to document the issues specific to the individual's medical problem such as weakness, depression, or confusion. It is important to understand how a person reacts to his or her medical problems and how medical issues interfere with successfully meeting the demands of daily life. All in all, a functional assessment must try to assess an individual's maximal functional potential, encompassing all domains of function (Jackson & Lang, 1989; Jette, 1985; Maguire, 1990).

Standardized Versus Nonstandardized Format

Functional assessments can be given in either a standardized or a nonstandardized format. Standardized assessment uses a formal functional assessment tool; the assessment is administered in the same way to everyone, every time it is used. The items included in a standardized assessment are carefully selected and very clearly defined. Nonstandardized assessment is more informal and includes a review of activities the evaluator considers important for an individual client.

Whenever a therapist works with a patient and evaluates how well that person can get out of bed, walk to the bathroom, or get dressed, the therapist is performing a functional assessment. When using this nonstandardized format, it is difficult to ensure that the assessment is complete. Have all important aspects of the patient's daily routine been included, or just the activities important to the therapist? When it is time to reassess the patient, can the initial evaluation be replicated? If not, how can the therapist accurately note patient progress? Use of nonstandardized assessments makes it difficult to effectively communicate patient status among health care professionals or to compare the functional status of patients with similar disabilities. Standardized assessment procedures can effectively minimize some of these problems. When standardized functional assessment instruments are being developed, care is taken to include information on all tasks that are important in defining a patient's functional status. Data obtained from the assessment are easy to communicate to other professionals familiar with the assessment instrument. Because standardized assessments are performed in the same way on repeated assessments, it is also easier to report on patient change.

Comprehensive functional assessment should contain both standardized and nonstandardized components. Using a formal standardized assessment provides the therapist with a body of reliable, valid information for all patients. Alone, this assessment strategy may not represent all activities that the client feels are important and meaningful in his or her everyday life. By also including a more individualized, nonstandardized component within the functional assessment, the therapist identifies important information unique to the client (Guccione, 1993).

Focus

Many of the formal functional assessment instruments in use today were developed to meet the needs of specific patient populations. For example, the Arthritis Impact Measurement Scale (AIMS) was developed to assess the status of adults with rheumatoid arthritis and includes not only items related to ability to complete functional tasks, but also information on pain (Meenan et al, 1980). As originally developed, it is not optimal for use with children, older adults, or individuals with other medical problems.

In reaction to this limitation, clinicians have developed other assessments better suited to their patient populations. A functional assessment tool for children with juvenile rheumatoid arthritis is the Juvenile Arthritis Functional Assessment Scale (Lovell et al, 1989). The GERI-AIMS (an adaptation of the Arthritis Impact Measure) was designed for use with older individuals with osteoarthritis or rheumatoid arthritis. It also assesses functional impairments related to other common medical problems of the elderly, independent of the arthritis-specific functional impairment (Hughes et al, 1991). Other types of instruments are available for individuals presenting with neurologic involvement. The Gross Motor Function Test was developed specifically for use with children with cerebral palsy (Russell et al, 1989). General functional assessments, such as the Functional Status Index (FSI), look at a wide variety of basic and instrumental activities of daily living (Table 5–1) and are useful for patients with chronic disabilities (Guccione et al, 1988).

Care must be taken when choosing an assessment instrument to ensure that the measurement tool is appropriate for the patient. Instruments that are developed for specific patient populations are good in that they can specifically focus on issues particular to a disease process that limits function, such as the pain of the arthritic patient. However, these instruments are not necessarily appropriate for use with other patient populations, because they may not be sensitive enough to other problem areas of the patient's performance. Also, instruments developed for use with a specific age group may not address issues important for individuals who are older or younger than that group. In general, functional assessment instruments may not be valid for use in patient populations other than those for which they were developed.

Perhaps the need of health care professionals to measure change in functional activities may best be met by developing additional assessment instruments. It would be helpful if the assessment could be used with patients of all ages, regardless of type of disease process or functional limitation. A more generic type of assessment would encourage more widespread clinical use of standardized functional assessments because clinicians would not have to learn a separate assessment for each patient population. Age-independent assessment would also make it possible to longitudinally follow the functional im-

Table 5-1. CATEGORIES OF THE FUNCTIONAL STATUS INDEX (FSI)	
Gross Mobility Walking inside Stair climbing Chair transfers	**Personal Care** Washing all parts of body Putting on pants Putting on a shirt Buttoning a shirt
Hand Activities Opening containers Writing Dialing a phone	**Home Chores** Doing laundry Reaching into low cupboard Doing yardwork Vacuuming a rug
Interpersonal Activities Driving a car Visiting family or friends Attending meetings Performing your job	

From Jette AM. Functional Status Index: Reliability of a chronic disease evaluation instrument. *Arch Phys Med Rehabil* 60:395–401, 1988.

pact of disability on development over time. One assessment developed to meet the challenge for a generic functional assessment is the Tufts Assessment of Motor Performance (Gans et al, 1988).

Design

Not only must the clinician decide on which assessment instrument best assesses a specific patient's functional skills and limitations, but the clinician must also decide which type of assessment can best be used with the patient. Three basic types of functional assessment designs are interview assessments, self-administered assessments, and performance-based assessments (Guccione et al, 1988).

The *interview assessment* is completed by a trained interviewer asking the client a set of standard questions and recording the answers in a standardized format. The information gleaned from this type of assessment is most useful when the interviewer has had training in how to administer and score the assessment. It is important that the interviewer not expand on questions or prompt answers to avoid influencing the client's answers.

Self-administered assessments are generally presented as questionnaires. The directions for completion of the questionnaire and questions themselves must be clearly written, so that the individual can understand what is being asked. It is also important to ensure that the way questions are asked or focused does not bias the person's answers. The accuracy of these types of assessments depends on the quality of the instrument itself and the person's ability to complete the questionnaire.

Both interview and self-administered assessments are based on a patient's self-report of their functional status. Studies comparing the validity of self-report to direct observation assessments have shown that agreement between the patient's report and the direct observation is good to excellent in BADL. A study showed that skill in IADL activities was slightly under-reported in patient self-reports (Harris et al, 1986). The validity of self-report measures makes them attractive for use in health care settings, especially because they are easy and relatively inexpensive to administer.

Performance-based assessments are those in which an evaluator observes the client's performance in functional tasks. This type of assessment does report someone's ability to complete BADL but is not as easily applied to the evaluation of IADL. Because the assessment is completed in a structured test environment, performance in the home environment may not be reflected. Direct observation assessment is also a time-consuming and therefore expensive process. The type of information gathered from this type of assessment may be most useful for developing and evaluating the success of therapeutic intervention programs.

Rating Performance

Functional assessments vary in how they rate an individual's performance. In the simplest rating format, a skill is noted as being present or absent, thereby documenting if something can be done. Checklist-type assessments favor this type of rating format but do not address the quality of that performance. It cannot be determined if the skill is accomplished efficiently, consistently, or to the degree necessary for functional independence within a wide variety of environments. For example, if the client can walk 20 to 30 feet with a cane in the therapy department and can ascend the stairs in the therapy department, he would certainly pass a checklist assessment including these tasks. However, what happens if the individual then goes home and encounters thick, plush carpeting or a steeper flight of stairs with higher steps than those in the therapy department? His ability to get into his apartment and walk from room to room may be very different from the performance seen in the therapy department. From another perspective, if while an individual walks with a cane the other arm becomes stiff and the hand clenches, the quality of ambulation may not be sufficient for her to perform daily tasks such as carrying a plate to the table or bringing in the newspaper.

Another common rating format for assessment instruments is to use a rank-ordered scale to categorize the individual's performance. Numeric or letter ratings are used to reflect where in the ranking a person's performance falls. Teachers use this type of system to rate classroom performance, achievement, degree of improvement, and so on. Another common example of this system is the rating of muscle strength. Depending on the muscle test format used, letter or numeric grades are assigned according to performance. In functional testing, it is difficult to use well-defined rank order systems to accurately reflect a person's performance. Everyone does things a little differently, adapting to his or her unique limitations and environmental demands. It is

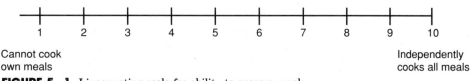

FIGURE 5–1. Linear rating scale for ability to prepare meals.

often difficult to fit a person's performance into the definitions of a specific category.

A similar rating system uses a visual analog scale. An individual is asked to rate his or her performance on a linear scale, on which one end of the line reflects one extreme and the other end the other extreme of performance. The person responding in such a system places a mark on the line at the point he or she feels best represents his or her performance. This system allows the individual to express his or her level of skill in a functional task at some point between being fully dependent and fully independent. An example is given in Figure 5–1.

Other scales use a summative rating system, in which different items are weighted such that independent completion of all tasks represented in the assessment results in a total score of 100. In developing this type of scale, weighting of items is generally based on professional judgment. Therefore, this scale reflects the developer's values about the importance of different functional skills, not necessarily how important certain skills are in a person's life. The client's performance of each task is evaluated and scored to reflect total or partial completion of the task independently. Scores for all tasks are added and compared to the perfect total score of 100. A score of 100 does not necessarily reflect normal performance, just as a score of 85 does not mean that someone is functioning within 15 per cent of normal. Another confusing aspect of summative scale formats is that scores can be compared mathematically. When an individual achieves a score of 10 on the initial assessment and a score of 50 on a subsequent assessment, it is not necessarily true that he or she is performing five times better than initially. One must remember that the score can be compared only within the context of the assessment instrument. This type of rating scale is good for measuring if change has occurred over time or with intervention (Guccione et al, 1988).

Another approach to rating performance is to rate the quality of performance of a skill. This approach is especially useful when using performance-based assessment strategies. For instance, it is possible to measure the efficiency with which a task is performed by measuring someone's heart rate before and after an activity. An evaluator can also use time tests to see how long it takes someone to walk 30 feet. This is important information when assessing someone's ability to efficiently cross a street, or to get from one high school class to another (Campbell, 1991; Guccione et al, 1988).

When choosing an assessment instrument, a therapist must consider all of the factors discussed above. For what patient population is the assessment appropriate? What type of assessment will best and most accurately measure a person's functional skills? How does the assessment rate the performance? What type of assessment and rating system gives the best information to identify clients needing services, develop treatment plans, or assess the effectiveness of intervention? Even after answering all of these questions, the therapist must consider additional aspects of assessment instruments that contribute to their effectiveness as measurement tools and affect the interpretation of the data they provide. These aspects include the reliability and validity of the instrument, as well as the measurement scale used to record data.

Measurement Issues

Several characteristics of assessment instruments affect their ability to accurately measure functional skills. Well-developed assessment strategies incorporate the principles of measurement science into their format. Measurement science involves the use of specific rules to evaluate a situation. By adhering to rules in the evaluation process, several important properties of measurement science are supported, including (1) standardization, (2) reliability, (3) validity, and (4) precision.

Standardization refers to the rules regarding the method of conducting the assessment and recording findings. By consistently using standardized testing procedures, one improves the reliability and validity of the assessment. *Reliability* refers to the ability of the test instrument to report findings in a consistent and repeatable fashion. *Validity* implies that the assessment is doing its intended job. Information regarding the reliability and validity of published functional assessments should be reported in assessment manuals or research reports. The health care professional should use the reported information to determine if the tool has been proven reliable and valid. Another measurement property is *precision,* which refers to the ability to detect appropriate levels of change (Liang & Jette, 1981).

Validity

In developing assessment tools that will be used widely by clinicians or that will be used in research projects, care must be taken to ensure that the instruments really measure what they say they will measure, a property referred to as "validity." Four issues have been identified that may diminish the validity of functional assessment instruments (Kaufert, 1983):

1. Effect of the use of aids, adaptations, or helpers to achieve a functional task.
2. Situational variation (i.e., between home and hospital settings) and individual motivation.
3. Professional perspective of the rater.
4. Role expectations of the patient.

For example, an individual may not be able to walk independently to the bathroom unless she uses a cane. If the assessment does not allow the person to use an assistive device, she will inaccurately be rated as unable to perform a basic functional task. On the other hand, a person who can independently use the bathroom in the hospital that is furnished with grab bars and/or an elevated toilet seat may not be as independent in his home environment without similar environmental modifications. Motivation also plays a role. If someone feels good about the prospect of going home or living independently, he or she may perform much differently than another individual who is depressed about the need to live in a long-term care facility. With regard to role expectation, if an assessment measures an individual's ability to cook or clean and this is not part of that person's social responsibility, he or she is not as likely to perform independently in these tasks. The professional perspective of the rater is another issue affecting validity. If the rater is a physical therapist, his or her impressions of functional independence in certain tasks may be very different from the impressions of a social worker.

Several types of validity exist. *Face validity* implies that the assessment tests what it is supposed to test. For instance, a test of BADL measures ability to perform self-care activities, not muscle strength. *Concurrent validity* is studied by comparing an instrument to another well-established instrument measuring the same parameters. If an individual is evaluated using two functional assessment instruments and performs consistently on the two assessments, those instruments are said to have good concurrent validity. *Content validity* is frequently determined by consensus of a panel of experts and reflects whether the instrument contains an adequate sample of activities and measures the intended content. *Predictive validity* reflects the degree to which the test can predict future outcomes. Finally, *construct validity* reflects how well the instrument measures its hypothetic framework.

Reliability

The assessment instrument must also have consistency and must reliably report information, a property referred to as "reliability." All items or parts of an assessment should measure similar things, improving the precision of the measurement instrument. This is a type of reliability called *internal consistency*. The assessment should also yield very similar results when given to the same client by two different therapists *(inter-rater reliability)* or when given by the same therapist on two separate administrations within a short time frame *(intra-rater reliability)*. Consistency between two administrations of the same test within a short period is also called *test-retest reliability*. In the latter instance, the tests must be given within a time frame that is short enough to eliminate the effects of treatment or development, but long enough to limit the influence of learning or familiarity with the test.

Measurement Scale

In using principles of measurement science to record findings, one quantifies observations by assigning a number score to them. For example, a score of 1 may indicate that someone is totally dependent in performing a task such as tooth-brushing. In contrast, a score of 5 may indicate complete independence in the task. Measurement scales used in assessments should be appropriate for quantifying the type of information collected. Data can be recorded on four types of measurement scales: nominal, ordinal, interval, and ratio.

Nominal scales record data that imply existence of a phenomenon or condition. Numbers are used purely as labels for the condition and therefore do not reflect magnitude. For example, males may be delineated by the number 1 and females by the number 2. Pass/fail tests also result in nominal data, with a score of 0 meaning a task cannot be completed and a score of 1 meaning it is completed.

Ordinal scales are rank-ordered rating scales. Numeric scores reflect order, but the interval between scores is not implied to be equal. This type of scale is used in manual muscle testing to differentiate between levels of muscle strength. A score of 4 in muscle testing does not reflect twice as much strength as a score of 2.

Interval scales reflect an order of magnitude or performance, similar to ordinal scales. An important characteristic of interval scales is that equal distances are being measured between scores. This means that scores can be added and subtracted from each other. For example, 3 inches plus 3 inches is 6 inches.

Ratio scales are characterized by one additional characteristic as compared to interval scales. They also include an absolute zero point, which allows scores to be added, subtracted, multiplied, or divided. If someone walks 30 feet in 10 seconds, his or her performance is twice as fast as someone who can perform the same task in 20 seconds.

It is important for clinicians to understand what type of data scale has been used in an assessment and what type of statistical analysis the data can therefore undergo. Nominal and ordinal data cannot undergo mathematical calculations and can be analyzed using only nonparametric statistical methods. Interval and ratio data, on the other hand, can be subjected to mathematical calculations and can withstand more rigorous parametric statistical analysis. Both types of statistical findings are valid and important methods of reporting results in research studies, but only if data undergo the appropriate form of analysis.

SURVEY OF MEASUREMENT INSTRUMENTS

In this section, a sample of standardized functional assessment instruments is reviewed. This selection represents only a small number of the assessments available to clinicians. These specific instruments were chosen because they are assessments appropriate for individuals of different ages or because they are commonly used in the clinic.

Pediatric Evaluation of Disability Index

The Pediatric Evaluation of Disability Index (PEDI) assesses the capability and performance of functional skills by children between the ages of 6 months and 7.5 years in the areas of self-care, mobility, and social function. It is meant to be used to detect functional deficits of individual children, monitor the child's progress in rehabilitation, and assist in program evaluation. The PEDI can be administered in a structured interview format with the child's parents (which is reported to take 45 to 60 minutes) or by recording the judgment of therapists and teachers as to the child's abilities (which is reported to take 20 to 30 minutes). Three different aspects of the child's functional performance are assessed: (1) the child's functional skill level, (2) the need for modification or adaptive equipment to achieve the task, and (3) the amount of physical assistance the child requires (Feldman et al, 1990; Haley et al, 1992).

The PEDI was used to assess 412 nondisabled children from New England. This normative sample represented all age groups for whom the test is appropriate and attempted to reflect demographics of the U.S. Census in 1980 (Haley et al, 1992). Results from this study have provided some information on the development of functional skills in children and permit comparisons between children with and without disabilities. The normative scores also allow the nominal data recorded in the PEDI to be converted to ratio scales reflecting item difficulty.

Good reliability and validity of the PEDI has been demonstrated. High internal consistency has been reported. Using a structured interview administration format, researchers have documented good inter-rater reliability. Concurrent validity of 0.70 to 0.73 between the PEDI and Batelle Developmental Inventory Screening Test (BDIST) has been demonstrated, implying that the two tests address similar but not the same issues. Good concurrent validity between the PEDI, BDIST, and Wee-FIM (pediatric version of the Functional Independence Measure) has also been demonstrated with a population of children with severe disabilities. The PEDI has demonstrated the ability to correctly discriminate between disabled and normal populations, and to detect change over time with intervention. Construct validity is achieved because the PEDI supports the assumptions that functional behaviors change with age and that attainment of a functional skill precedes independence in that skill. The latter assumption implies that the degree of caregiver assistance is an important changeable dimension to monitor in a functional assessment framework (Feldman et al, 1990; Haley et al, 1992).

Gross Motor Function Measure

The Gross Motor Function Measure is designed to be used with children with cerebral palsy. It evaluates motor functions such as rolling, crawling, sitting,

Table 5-2. TUFTS ASSESSMENT OF MOTOR PERFORMANCE ITEMS		
Mobility	**ADL**	**Communication**
Transfer to mat	Pouring	Talking
Sit to supine	Drinking	Writing
Sit to prone	Cutting putty	Typing
Prone to quadriped	Jacket on	Paper in envelope
Quadriped to supine	Zipper	
Supine to long sit	Snap	
Long sit to short sit	Button	
Mat to chair	Unsnap	
Propel wheelchair	Unbutton	
Sit to stand	Unzip	
Walk	Jacket off	
Walk on ramp	Shoes off	
Wheelchair ramp	Shoes on	
Upstairs		
Downstairs		

From Gans BM, et al. Description and interobserver reliability of the Tufts Assessment of Motor Performance. *Am J Phys Med Rehabil* 67:202–210, 1988.

standing, walking, running, stair use, and jumping. A four-point ordinal scale of measurement is used to assess each item. A score of 0 indicates the task cannot be done; 1 indicates the task can be initiated ($<10\%$ completion); 2 indicates partial completion of the task (10 to $<100\%$ completion); and 3 indicates the task can be completed. Summary scores can also be calculated, resulting in ratio data. Inter-rater and test-retest reliability are reported to be excellent (>0.80). Content and construct validity are also reported to be good. The measure is felt to be sensitive to changes in performance in functional tasks, making it an effective tool for documenting change in the motor performance of children with cerebral palsy (Russell et al, 1989).

Tufts Assessment of Motor Performance

The Tufts Assessment of Motor Performance (TAMP) is a standardized assessment of functional motor skills in mobility, activities of daily living, and physical aspects of communication (Table 5–2). It can be used with children or adults with any type of disability. Each functional activity is broken down into its component tasks. Performance on these tasks is then rated in comparison to predetermined criteria. The technique used to achieve a functional task is assessed, including movement patterns used, time taken to complete the task, and proficiency. The level of assistance necessary is also recorded. Items can be assessed individually, or summary scores can be calculated. The summary scores make it possible to document functional performance and quality of performance. Because the assessment looks at functional skills in a detailed manner, it is sensitive to small increments of change in performance.

This degree of precision makes it useful in treatment planning and in evaluating the effectiveness of intervention (Gans et al, 1988).

Early inter-rater reliability studies of the TAMP indicated fair to good reliability (Gans et al, 1988). Comparisons have also been made to assess use of the TAMP with pediatric and adult populations. Consistency of performance between the populations was reported to be good, but some tasks were more difficult for one age group than for the other. Because of this finding, it was recommended that parallel versions of the TAMP be developed (Haley & Ludlow, 1992).

Katz Index of Activities of Daily Living

This instrument was originally designed to measure how independently patients in institutional settings could perform BADL including bathing, dressing, toileting, continence, feeding, and transfer skills (Katz, 1963). Ambulation, or patient mobility, was not measured, limiting the usefulness of this tool. The original instrument has been adapted for use with community-based patients, adding two functional categories of ambulation and grooming, and deleting continence (Branch et al, 1984). Reliability studies have shown the instrument to have fair to good reliability. Agreement scores of 0.68 to 0.98 between raters have been demonstrated. Test-retest reliability coefficients range from 0.61 to 0.78 (Liang & Jette, 1981). Predictive validity of some of the Katz items has also been demonstrated with an elderly population living in senior housing or at home (Reuben et al, 1992).

Patients are rated as to whether they can complete tasks in the six functional areas independently, with some assistance, or totally dependently. Both patient self-report and direct observation are used to score the assessment. According to which of the six basic activities the patient performs independently, a letter score of A, B, C, D, E, F, or G is assigned. For example, the patient who is independent in all six tasks receives a score of A. The patient who is independent in all but bathing and one additional function receives a score of C. The items and scoring format of the Katz Index of Independence in Activities of Daily Living are illustrated in Figure 5–2.

Functional Independence Measure (FIM)

The FIM was developed by the Uniform Data System for Medical Rehabilitation at the State University of New York at Buffalo (1990) to assess functional skills of adults. A pediatric version, Guide for the Functional Independence Measure for Children (Wee-FIM), is also available (Uniform Data System for Medical Rehabilitation, 1991). A person's degree of independence or dependence in self-care activities, bowel and bladder management, mobility, locomotion, communication, social adjustment, and problem-solving is rated. Self-care activities include dressing, eating, grooming, and bathing. Transfers from the bed to chair, to the toilet, and to the tub/shower are included in the

Name _____ Day of evaluation _____
For each area of functioning listed below, check description that applies. (The word "assistance" means supervision, direction, or personal assistance.)

Bathing—either sponge bath, tub bath, or shower.

☐ Receives no assistance (gets in and out of tub by self if tub is usual means of bathing)

☐ Receives assistance in bathing only one part of the body (such as back or a leg)

☐ Receives assistance in bathing more than one part of the body (or not bathed)

Dressing—gets clothes from closets and drawers—including underclothes, outer garments and using fasteners (including braces if worn)

☐ Gets clothes and gets completely dressed without assistance

☐ Gets clothes and gets dressed without assistance except for assistance in tying shoes

☐ Receives assistance in getting clothes or in getting dressed, or stays partly or completely undressed

Toileting—going to the "toilet room" for bowel and urine elimination, cleaning self after elimination, and arranging clothes

☐ Goes to "toilet room," cleans self, and arranges clothes without assistance (may use object for support such as cane, walker, or wheelchair and may manage night bedpan or commode, emptying same in morning)

☐ Receives assistance in going to "toilet room" or in cleansing self or in arranging clothes after elimination or in use of night bedpan or commode

☐ Doesn't go to room termed "toilet" for the elimination process

Transfer

☐ Moves in and out of bed as well as in and out of chair without assistance (may be using object for support such as cane or walker)

☐ Moves in and out of bed or chair with assistance

☐ Doesn't get out of bed

Continence

☐ Controls urination and bowel movement completely by self

☐ Has occasional "accidents"

☐ Supervision helps keep urine or bowel control; catheter is used, or is incontinent

Feeding

☐ Feeds self without assistance

☐ Feeds self except for getting assistance in cutting meat or buttering bread

☐ Receives assistance in feeding or is fed partly or completely by using tubes or intravenous fluids

The Index of Independence in Activities of Daily Living is based on an evaluation of the functional independence or dependence of patients in bathing, dressing, going to toilet, transferring, continence, and feeding. Specific definitions of functional independence and dependence appear below the index.

A—Independent in feeding, continence, transferring, going to toilet, dressing, and bathing.
B—Independent in all but one of these functions.
C—Independent in all but bathing and one additional function.
D—Independent in all but bathing, dressing, and one additional function.
E—Independent in all but bathing, dressing, going to toilet, and one additional function.
F—Independent in all but bathing, dressing, going to toilet, transferring, and one additional function.
G—Dependent in all six functions.
Other—Dependent in at least two functions, but not classifiable as C, D, E, or F.

Independence means without supervision, direction, or active personal assistance, except as specifically noted below. This is based on actual status and not on ability. A patient who refuses to perform a function is considered as not performing the function, even though he is deemed able.

Bathing (sponge, shower, or tub)
Independent: assistance only in bathing a single part (as back or disabled extremity) or bathes self completely
Dependent: assistance in bathing more than one part of body; assistance in getting in or out of tub or does not bathe self

Dressing
Independent: gets clothes from closets and drawers; puts on clothes, outer garments, braces; manages fasteners; act of tying shoes is excluded
Dependent: does not dress self or remains partly undressed

Going to toilet
Independent: gets to toilet; gets on and off toilet; arranges clothes; cleans organs of excretion (may manage own bedpan used at night only and may or may not be using mechanical supports)
Dependent: uses bedpan or commode or receives assistance in getting to and using toilet

Transfer
Independent: moves in and out of bed independently and moves in and out of chair independently (may or may not be using mechanical supports)
Dependent: assistance in moving in or out of bed and/or chair; does not perform one or more transfers

Continence
Independent: urination and defecation entirely self-controlled
Dependent: partial or total incontinence in urination or defecation; partial or total control by enemas, catheters, or regulated use of urinals and/or bedpans

Feeding
Independent: gets food from plate or its equivalent, into mouth (precutting of meat and preparation of food, as buttering bread, are excluded from evaluation)
Dependent: assistance in act of feeding (see above); does not eat at all or parenteral feeding

FIGURE 5–2. Katz ADL Index. (From Guccione AA, Cullen KE, O'Sullivan SB. Functional assessment. In O'Sullivan SB, Schmitz TJ [eds]. *Physical Rehabilitation: Assessment and Treatment,* 2nd ed. Philadelphia: FA Davis, 1988. Adapted from Katz S, et al. Progress in the development of the Index of ADL. *Gerontologist/J Gerontol* 10:20, 1970.)

mobility section. Locomotion includes walking, managing stairs, and propelling a wheelchair.

Barthel Index

The Barthel Index was developed to measure improvement in patients with chronic disability who were participating in rehabilitation (Figure 5–3). BADL are assessed, including toileting, bathing, eating, dressing, continence, transfers, and ambulation. Patients receive numeric scores based on whether they require physical assistance to perform the task or can complete it independently. The total number of possible points on the assessment is 100. Items are weighted according to the professional judgment of the developers. A patient scoring 0 points would be dependent in all assessed activities of daily living, whereas a score of 100 would reflect independence in these activities (Mahoney & Barthel, 1965).

Specific reliability and validity studies have not been reported, but Barthel Index scores of adult patients who have had a stroke or have severe disabilities have been reported to correlate with clinical outcomes and functional status (Granger & Haley et al, 1979; Granger, Albrecht, & Hamilton, 1979). Specific, detailed instructions are provided, supporting standardized use of the measure (Jette, 1985).

Functional Status Index

The Functional Status Index (FSI) was derived from the Katz Index for use with individuals with arthritis. As seen in Figure 5–4, both basic and instrumental activities of daily living are assessed, making this an appropriate tool for use with community-dwelling, chronically disabled populations. Not only is the degree of dependence in achieving the task measured, but the amount of pain experienced with each activity and the patient's perceived difficulty in completing the task are rated.

Either the interviewer- or self-administered format can be used. Reliability studies have indicated fair inter-rater and test-retest reliability coefficients, ranging from 0.61 to 0.81. Construct validity has also been supported (Jette, 1980; Jette & Deniston, 1978; Liang & Jette, 1981).

SUMMARY
. . . .

This chapter presents a rationale supporting the importance of functional assessment in clinical practice. The primary goal of physical and occupational therapy intervention is to improve the functional skills of the clients served. This factor alone supports the need for therapists to incorporate functional assessment into their practices. Functional outcome measures can easily be developed into functional goals for the patient. By emphasizing functional

Date _____
Initial _____

FEEDING
10 = Independent. Able to apply any necessary
     device. Feeds in reasonable time.
 5 = Needs help (e.g., for cutting).   _____
BATHING
 5 = Independent   _____
PERSONAL TOILET
 5 = Independently washes face, combs hair,
     brushes teeth, shaves (manages plug if electric).   _____
DRESSING
10 = Independent. Ties shoes, fastens fasteners,
     applies braces.
 5 = Needs help, but does at least half of work in
     reasonable time.   _____
BOWELS
10 = No accidents. Able to use enema or
     suppository, if needed.
 5 = Occasional accidents or needs help with enema
     or suppository.   _____
BLADDER
10 = No accidents. Able to care for collecting device
     if used.
 5 = Occasional accidents or needs help with device.   _____
TOILET TRANSFERS
10 = Independent with toilet or bedpan. Handles
     clothes, wipes, flushes or cleans pan.
 5 = Needs help for balance, handling clothes or
     toilet paper.   _____
TRANSFERS—CHAIR AND BED
15 = Independent, including locks wheelchair, lifts
     footrests.
10 = Minimum assistance or supervision.
 5 = Able to sit, but needs maximum assistance to
     transfer.   _____
AMBULATION
15 = Independent for 50 yards. May use assistive
     devices, except for rolling walker.
10 = With help 50 yards.
 5 = Independent with wheelchair for 50 yards if
     unable to walk.   _____
STAIR CLIMBING
10 = Independent. May use assistive devices.
 5 = Needs help or supervision.   _____
                                          Totals _____

FIGURE 5–3. Barthel Index. (From Guccione AA, Cullen KE, O'Sullivan SB. Functional assessment. In O'Sullivan SB, Schmitz TJ [eds]. *Physical Rehabilitation: Assessment and Treatment,* 2nd ed. Philadelphia: FA Davis, 1988. Adapted from Mahoney FI, Barthel DS. Functional evaluation: The Barthel Index. *Md State Med J* 14[2]:61–65, 1965.)

outcomes, intervention focuses on the patient's independence, not the attainment of normality (Haley et al, 1991).

Several characteristics of assessment instruments should be considered when deciding which tools to use. A functional assessment should encompass activities that are important throughout a client's day and should consider social, emotional, environmental, and cognitive issues relevant to that client.

KEY: ASSISTANCE: 1 = independent; 2 = uses devices; 3 = uses human assistance; 4 = uses devices and human assistance; 5 = unable or unsafe to do the activity

PAIN: 1 = no pain; 2 = mild pain; 3 = moderate pain; 4 = severe pain

DIFFICULTY: 1 = no difficulty; 2 = mild difficulty; 3 = moderate difficulty; 4 = severe difficulty

Time frame: On the average during the past 7 days

ACTIVITY	ASSISTANCE (1–5)	PAIN (1–4)	DIFFICULTY (1–4)	COMMENTS
Mobility				
Walking inside	_____	_____	_____	
Climbing up stairs	_____	_____	_____	
Rising from a chair	_____	_____	_____	
Personal care				
Putting on pants	_____	_____	_____	
Buttoning a shirt/blouse	_____	_____	_____	
Washing all parts of the body	_____	_____	_____	
Putting on a shirt/blouse	_____	_____	_____	
Home chores				
Vacuuming a rug	_____	_____	_____	
Reaching into low cupboards	_____	_____	_____	
Doing laundry	_____	_____	_____	
Doing yardwork	_____	_____	_____	
Hand activities				
Writing	_____	_____	_____	
Opening container	_____	_____	_____	
Dialing a phone	_____	_____	_____	
Social activities				
Performing your job	_____	_____	_____	
Driving a car	_____	_____	_____	
Attending meetings/ appointments	_____	_____	_____	
Visiting with friends and relatives	_____	_____	_____	

FIGURE 5–4. Functional Status Index (FSI). (Courtesy of Alan M. Jette.)

The mode of administration, scoring format, and measurement characteristics of reliability and validity of the instrument should also be considered. To assist clinicians in their exploration of functional assessment instruments, a sample of instruments has been reviewed.

Once it has been established that a client is not functioning at optimal capacity, intervention can be designed to address that person's individual needs. From the framework of the standardized assessment, the clinician must decide what domains of function are involved and which components of function are limiting performance. Strength, endurance, balance, mobility, or coordination may be the factor limiting physical performance. Specific therapeutic programs can be designed to address any of the factors involved.

For the therapist to thoroughly understand physical function and the factors that influence it, he or she must have a working knowledge of the human body. The next unit of this book explores the role of each of the body systems involved in movement and discusses the effect of life span development on these systems.

References

Branch LG, Katz S, Kneipmann K, Papsidero JA. A prospective study of functional status among community elders. *Am J Public Health* 74:266–268, 1984.

Feldman AB, Haley SM, Coryell J. Concurrent and construct validity of the pediatric evaluation of disability inventory. *Phys Ther* 70:602–610, 1990.

Gans BM, Haley SM, Hallenborg SC, Mann N, Inacio CA, Faas RM. Description and interobserver reliability of the Tufts Assessment of Motor Performance. *Am J Phys Med Rehabil* 67:202–210, 1988.

Granger CV, Albrecht GL, Hamilton BB. Outcome of comprehensive medical rehabilitation: Measurement by PULSES Profile and Barthel Index. *Arch Phys Med Rehabil* 60:145–154, April, 1979.

Granger CV, Dewis LS, Peters NC, Sherwood CC, Barrett JE. Stroke rehabilitation: Analyses of repeated Barthel Index measures. *Arch Phys Med Rehabil* 60:14–17, 1979.

Guccione AA. Functional assessment of the elderly. In Guccione AA (ed). *Geriatric Physical Therapy.* St. Louis: Mosby, 1993, pp 113–123.

Guccione AA, Cullen KE, O'Sullivan SB. Functional assessment. In O'Sullivan SB, Schmitz TJ (eds). *Physical Rehabilitation: Assessment and Treatment,* 2nd ed. Philadelphia: FA Davis, 1988, pp 219–235.

Haley SM, Coster WJ, Ludlow LH. Pediatric functional outcome measures. *Phys Med Rehabil/Clin North Am* 2(4):689–723, 1991.

Haley SM, Coster WJ, Ludlow LH, Haltiwanger JT, Andrellos PJ. *Pediatric Evaluation of Disability Inventory (PEDI).* Boston: New England Medical Center Hospital and PEDI Research Group, 1992.

Haley SM, Ludlow LH. Applicability of the hierarchical scales of the Tufts Assessment of Motor Performance for school-aged children and adults with disabilities. *Phys Ther* 72:191–209, 1992.

Harris BA, Jette AM, Campion EW, Cleary PD. Validity of self-report measures of functional disability. *Top Geriatr Rehabil* 1(3):31–41, 1986.

Hughes SL, Edelman P, Chang RW, Singer RH, Shuette P. The GERI-AIMS: Reliability and validity of the arthritis impact measurement scales adapted for elderly respondents. *Arthritis Rheum* 34:856–865, 1991.

Jette AM. State of the art in functional status assessment. In Rothestein J (ed). *Measurement in Physical Therapy.* New York: Churchill Livingstone, 1985, pp 137–168.

Jette AM. Functional Status Index: Reliability of a chronic disease evaluation instrument. *Arch Phys Med Rehabil* 61:395–401, 1980.

Jette AM, Deniston OL. Inter-observer reliability of a functional status assessment instrument. *J Chron Dis* 31:573–580, 1978.

Katz S, Ford AB, Moskowitz RW, Jackson BA, Jaffe MW. Studies of illness in the aged—The Index of ADL: A standardized measure of biological and psychosocial function. *JAMA* 185(12):914–919, 1963.

Kaufert JM. Functional ability indices: Measurement problems in assessing their validity. *Arch Phys Med Rehabil* 64:260–267, 1983.

Liang MH, Jette AM. Measuring functional ability in chronic arthritis: A critical review. *Arthritis Rheum* 24:80–86, 1981.

Lovell DJ, Howe S, Shear E, Hartner S, McGirr G, Schulte M, Levinson J. Development of a disability measurement tool for juvenile rheumatoid arthritis: The Juvenile Arthritis Functional Assessment Scale. *Arthritis Rheum* 32:1390–1395, 1989.

Mahoney FI, Barthel DW. Functional evaluation: Barthel Index. *Md State Med J* 14:61–65, 1965.

Meenan RF, Gertman PM, Mason JH. Measuring health in arthritis: The Arthritis Impact Measurement Scale. *Arthritis Rheum* 23:146–152, 1980.

Reuben DB, Sui AL, Sokkun K. The predictive validity of self-report and performance-based measures of function and health. *J Gerontol* 47:(4)M106–M110, 1992.

Russell DJ, Rosenbaum PL, Cadman DT, Gowland C, Hardy S, Jarvis S. The gross motor function measure: A means to evaluate the effects of physical therapy. *Dev Med Child Neurol* 31:341–352, 1989.

Uniform Data System for Medical Rehabilitation. *Guide to the Uniform Data Set.* New York: State University of New York at Buffalo, 1990.

Uniform Data System for Medical Rehabilitation. *Guide for the Functional Independence Measure for Children (Wee-FIM).* New York: State University of New York at Buffalo, 1991.

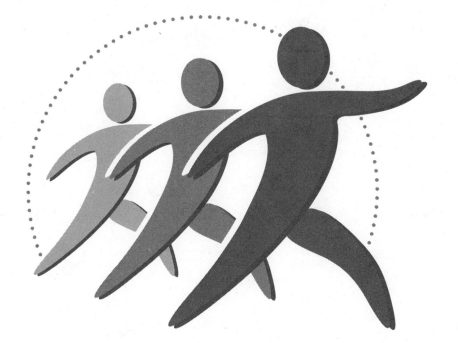

Unit Two

Body Systems Contributing to Functional Movement

Chapter 6

Skeletal System Changes

Objectives

AFTER STUDYING THIS CHAPTER, THE READER WILL BE ABLE TO:

1   Describe the structure of the components of the skeletal system.

2   Identify the function of bone and cartilage in supporting posture and movement.

3   Discuss unique structural and functional characteristics of the skeletal system in the developing fetus, infant, child, adolescent, adult, and older adult.

4   Relate the age-related characteristics of the skeletal system to functional movement abilities and risk factors.

5   Incorporate issues of life span development of the skeletal system into patient assessment and treatment planning.

The ability to walk, run, lift, and manipulate objects is influenced by the strength and resilience of the skeletal system. A young infant cannot walk, climb stairs, push a stroller, or tie shoes. Not only do infants lack the experience and practice necessary for these tasks, their immature skeleton does not provide a structural framework on which these movements can take place. Older adults may not have the spring in their step, power in their tennis serve, or manual dexterity they enjoyed when they were younger. The changes in the skeletal system that occur with aging may contribute to decreased efficiency of movement.

The skeletal system, as discussed in this chapter, consists of the bony skeleton and cartilage. The skeleton provides a structure on which muscles can work. The size and shape of the bones and location of muscular attachments form an efficient system of levers and struts. Cartilage acts as a shock absorber and protects joint surfaces from wear and tear. An understanding of the role of the skeletal system components and their changing properties throughout development is necessary to appreciate the contribution of the skeletal system to functional movement.

COMPONENTS OF THE SKELETAL SYSTEM

Cartilage

Cartilage, a type of connective tissue, can tolerate mechanical stress and acts as a supporting structure in the body. It provides a mechanism for shock absorption, acts as a sliding surface for the joints, and plays a role in the development and growth of bone. During fetal development, a cartilage model is laid down from which the long bones of the body will develop. The ends of immature long bones also contain cartilage plates, which are the site of bone growth.

Three types of cartilage exist, each meeting different functional needs. *Hyaline cartilage* is the most abundant and rigid. It is found at the articular surfaces of joints and the walls of respiratory passages such as the trachea and bronchi. Hyaline cartilage also makes up the fetal model of the future long bones and can be found at the epiphyseal growth plates of immature bone. *Fibrocartilage* is found at the acetabulum, intervertebral disks, menisci, and tendinous insertions. It is more pliable than hyaline cartilage but still provides strength and support to the skeletal system. Fibrocartilage fibers are arranged parallel to the stress forces that the tissue experiences. *Elastic cartilage* is the most pliable cartilage and can be found at the larynx, ear, and epiglottis, where it provides support with flexibility (Bacon & Niles, 1983). This chapter focuses primarily on hyaline cartilage.

Hyaline cartilage covers the ends of the bones that make up synovial joints, and in this capacity it is called *articular cartilage*. It is responsible for facilitating motion at the joints and can tolerate a variety of loading forces. Synovial fluid and the compression of fluids from within the surface of the articular cartilage contribute to the lubrication of the joint. Articular cartilage provides a low friction surface and allows joints to move freely and easily for 80 or even 100 years (Chrisman, 1984; Gradisar & Porterfield, 1989). Years of microtrauma, isolated instances of more severe joint trauma, and aging of the cartilaginous tissue eventually result in a breakdown of articular cartilage, which contributes to the development of osteoarthritis.

PROPERTIES

Cartilage consists of water, collagen fibers, cartilage cells (chondrocytes), and a ground substance in which the collagen fibers are embedded. Elastic cartilage also contains elastin fibers. The fibers and ground substance make up the extracellular matrix surrounding the chondrocytes. Differences in the extracellular matrix and amount of water in the tissue help to differentiate the three types of cartilage. For example, the water content of articular cartilage is 80 per cent but of fibrocartilage is only 50 per cent (Gradisar & Porterfield, 1989).

Cartilage has no nerve supply and no vascular supply of its own. Oxygen and nutrients must be obtained from surrounding tissues. Most cartilage is covered by a layer of dense connective tissue called the *perichondrium*. The perichondrium is vascularized and supplies nutrients to the cartilage via diffusion. Articular cartilage is not covered with perichondrium and depends on diffusion of nutrients from synovial fluid. In articular cartilage, periods of compression and decompression facilitate the exchange of fluids. During decompression, diffusion can occur; during compression, fluids can be squeezed out (Gradisar & Porterfield, 1989; Pickles, 1989). Both processes are necessary to maintain adequate nutrition of the cartilage.

FORMATION

Cartilage is derived from embryonic mesoderm, as is other connective tissue. Cartilage growth occurs by two different processes, interstitial growth and appositional growth. Interstitial growth occurs within the cartilage by mitotic division of the existing chondrocytes. It occurs in the early phases of cartilage development to increase tissue mass, at the epiphyseal plates of long bones, and at articular surfaces. In appositional growth, new cartilage is laid down at the surface of the perichondrium. In this process, chondroblasts of the perichondrium, which are precursers to chondrocytes, form an extracellular matrix and develop into mature chondrocytes (Junqueira et al, 1989). Nonarticular cartilage loses the capacity for interstitial growth early and then undergoes only appositional growth.

In the formation of articular cartilage, collagen fibers of the extracellular matrix weave together and form a loop parallel to the joint surface (Fig. 6–1). These collagen fibers are embedded in the subchondral bone or deep cartilage tissue. This structural arrangement helps the cartilage to retain water and to maintain its shape (Gradisar & Porterfield, 1989; Pickles, 1989).

Mechanical loading, including compression, is necessary to maintain healthy articular cartilage. In the absence of mechanical loading, atrophy of

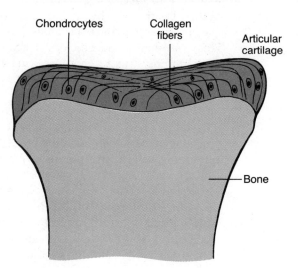

FIGURE 6–1. Arrangement of articular cartilage collagen fiber loops parallel to the joint surface.

the articular tissue may be seen. Constant compression, however, leads to a thinning of cartilage, and excessive compression contributes to degeneration of the cartilage (LeVeau & Bernhardt, 1984). With use, cells of the articular surface are worn away, the cartilage thins, and eventually the surface changes. Cartilage repair depends on interstitial growth and the ability of chondrocytes to synthesize and maintain the extracellular matrix. Chrisman (1984) reports that articular cartilage has the ability to repair itself, undergo limited mitosis, metabolize nutrients, and maintain its matrix even during aging. He concludes that aging articular cartilage has less capacity for repair than younger cartilage because of decreased ability to synthesize new extracellular matrix. For example, a young individual with chondromalacia is able to recover from articular cartilage damage with rest. In the older individual, similar cartilage degeneration cannot be repaired, and osteoarthritis results. Others report that articular cartilage has poor ability for repair, except in infancy (Gradiser & Porterfield, 1989). They suggest that damaged articular cartilage is replaced by scar tissue or fibrocartilage, whose mechanical properties are not optimal for providing low friction joint motion under high mechanical loads. Most authors do agree that wear and tear over time result in a worn, less efficient articular surface.

AGING

The composition of cartilage changes with age. Water content of cartilage decreases from 80 to 90 per cent in the fetus to 70 per cent in the adult (VanderWeil, 1983). The extracellular matrix becomes more rigid and eventually calcifies, making diffusion of nutrients more difficult. If cartilage nutrition cannot be maintained, chondrocytes die (Leeson et al, 1988).

Whitbourne (1985), Chrisman (1984), and Pickles (1989) suggest that thinning of articular cartilage occurs with age. Decreased numbers of cells are seen throughout the cartilage, especially at weight-bearing surfaces. Repeated exposure to mechanical loading wears away the cartilage and compromises its ability to protect the articulating bony surfaces. The extracellular matrix of the articular cartilage becomes hard and brittle, resulting in decreased resiliency, strength, and efficiency. Friction increases during joint movement with the thinning, fraying, and cracking of articular cartilage.

Bone

The bony skeleton accounts for 14 per cent of adult weight and for 97 to 98 per cent of total height (Sinclair, 1985). Intervertebral disks contribute to the remaining height. In humans, bone has several functions, including (1) protection of vital organs, (2) support of body weight, (3) storage for minerals, (4) structural leverage for movement, and (5) bone marrow storage.

Bony protection of the central nervous system is provided by the skull, which forms a vault around the brain, and by the vertebral column, which encases the spinal cord. The rib cage protects the lungs and heart. The bones of the vertebral column, shoulder girdle, pelvic girdle, upper extremities, and lower extremities are arranged to effectively support the body weight in upright postures. Muscles are strategically attached to this bony framework, allowing efficient movement to occur with muscular contraction.

In addition to providing protection and support, bone is a storage site for materials used by the body. Bone marrow, which is important in the formation of blood cells, is stored in bone. Calcium, phosphate, and other ions are stored in bone as crystalline salts. These salts contribute to the strength of the bone and its ability to withstand the compressive forces of weight bearing. The stored minerals are also used to maintain blood mineral levels when changes in diet or metabolic demand occur. If the blood levels of calcium and phosphate drop, these minerals are accessed from the bone. Likewise, after a meal, calcium is deposited in bone or excreted rather than increased in blood levels (Guyton, 1987; Lanyon, 1989; Junqueira et al, 1989).

The structure of bone, as well as its stiffness and strength, allow it to meet the functional demands of everyday activities. Throughout development, bone must be produced and maintained in sufficient quantity to withstand a lifetime of weight bearing, movement, and functional activity.

GENERAL STRUCTURE AND FORM

Bone is a connective tissue composed of bone cells and bone matrix. These elements are held together by a ground substance. The bone matrix is a hard, calcified substance made up of collagen fibers and mineral salts. It surrounds the primary bone cell, the osteocyte, which functions to maintain the nutrition and mineral content of the bone matrix. Two other types of bone cells are the osteoblast, active in the formation of new bone, and the osteoclast, associated with resorption of bone. Osteoblasts are found on the surface of bone and synthesize new bone matrix. As they are encased in sufficient bone matrix, they become osteocytes. Osteoclasts are found in areas of bone resorption, where they break down the bone matrix and release minerals into the circulation (Junqueira et al, 1989; Malina & Bouchard, 1991).

The external surface of bone, except at articular surfaces, is covered with periosteum. The periosteum is made up of collagen fibers and bone-forming cells, which provide a source of osteoblasts. The internal surface of bone, the endosteum, is thinner than the periosteum, but also supplies osteoblasts for bone growth and repair. Both surfaces are vascularized and play a role in nutrition of bone.

All bones are made up of two types of bone tissue, *compact bone* and *spongy bone,* also called *cancellous bone.* Compact bone, which is hard and dense, makes up the shaft of long bones and provides a thin outer covering to areas of spongy bone. It is formed when thin plates of bone (lamellae) are arranged concentrically around a channel containing blood vessels and nerves (haversian canals). This vascular channel is formed when new bone matrix surrounds existing blood vessels. Four to twenty lamellae surround a haversian canal, making up an osteon (haversian system). Osteons provide a mechanism to maintain nutrition of the bone. They are continuously being destroyed and

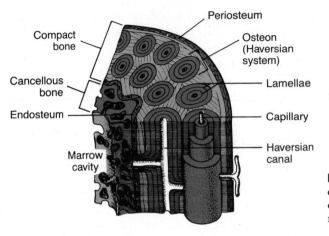

FIGURE 6–2. Cross section depicting compact bone with osteons, cancellous bone, and marrow cavity.

rebuilt throughout the life span. Spongy bone, made up of loosely woven strands of bone tissue (trabeculae), is found at the ends of the long bones and surrounds the inner bone marrow cavity of the shaft. The open spaces of the spongy bone house the bone marrow and vessels that nourish the bone (Leeson et al, 1988). Figure 6–2 shows compact bone surrounding a portion of spongy bone.

The general form of each bone, its muscular attachments, and its anatomic relationships are all genetically determined. Heredity and the mechanical stresses placed on developing bone dictate the shape, size, and structure of the mature bone. Bone mass, girth, cortical thickness, curvature, density, and arrangement of trabeculae are influenced by the mechanical stresses produced during functional activities. Weight bearing and the pull of muscular attachments on bone during activities direct the arrangement of collagen fibers within bone trabeculae in the same direction as the stress forces (Smith DW, 1981). In the absence of functional loading of the bone, deficiencies in bone architecture and structure will result (Lanyon, 1989). The relationship between bone structure and the mechanical loads it experiences was identified by J. Wolff in 1892. According to Wolff's law of bone transformation, the structure of bone will change in response to the mechanical loads placed on it, according to certain mathematical laws (LeVeau & Bernhardt, 1984; Martin & Brown, 1989).

Nutrition and hormones are important factors in the growth and development process of bone. People who do not get enough protein, calcium, vitamin D, and vitamin C in their diet experience abnormal bone growth. Without adequate dietary protein, insufficient collagen is produced by the osteoblasts, leading to poor calcification of the bone matrix. In vitamin C deficiency, the cartilage formed for bone growth also lacks collagen. In severe vitamin C deficiency (scurvy), decreased rate of growth at the cartilage growth plates of the long bones results in deficient bone formation. Vitamin D deficiency in children causes rickets. In this disorder, growth in the region of the cartilage growth plate is distorted because calcification of the cartilage is deficient (Junqueira et al, 1989; Smith DW, 1981). The role of hormones in bone development is evidenced by the influence of growth hormone on growing bone. A rapid growth period accompanies the hormonal changes of adolescence. In contrast, accelerated loss of bone mineral content occurs immediately following menopause, again related to hormonal changes in the body.

DEVELOPMENT

In embryologic development, bone forms from the mesoderm. Fetal bone is made of primary or woven bone tissue. Woven bone consists of an irregular array of collagen fibers and is less mineralized than mature bone. As osteons form, mineralization of the bony matrix increases and mature bone tissue replaces woven bone. A similar process can be seen throughout development as new, woven bone is laid down and other bone tissue is resorbed. Therefore, woven bone, mature bone, and areas of bone resorption are all found in adult bone tissue.

Bone develops by one of two different processes, intramembranous ossification or endochondral ossification. *Intramembranous ossification* takes place directly within mesenchyme tissue, beginning near the end of the embryonic period and proceeding rapidly. Mesenchymal cells produce an organic matrix called *osteoid,* which is composed of collagen fibers. Calcium phosphate crystals accumulate on the collagen fibers, resulting in ossification (Gould & Davies, 1985). In this process, numerous ossification centers are formed, which fuse into spongy bone tissue. With time, some of this spongy bone will become compact bone (Leeson et al, 1988; Junqueira et al, 1989). The skull, carpals, tarsals, and part of the clavicle are formed by intramembranous ossification.

In *endochondral ossification,* a hyaline cartilage model of the bone is laid down first and then replaced by bone in an orderly fashion. Endochondral bone growth is seen in the long bones of the body and is the method by which bones increase in length. The parts of the long bone are listed below and depicted in Figure 6–3.

Diaphysis: shaft of the long bone. The portion of bone formed by the primary center of ossification.

Epiphysis: ends of the long bones. The portion of bone formed by secondary centers of ossification.

Epiphyseal plate: growth zone of the bone, which is composed of hyaline cartilage.

Metaphysis: wider part of the shaft of the long bone, adjacent to the epiphyseal plate. Metaphysis consists of spongy bone during development. In adults, it is continuous with the epiphysis.

Endochondral bone development is illustrated in Figure 6–4. Primary centers of ossification form at the center of the diaphysis. First a bony collar

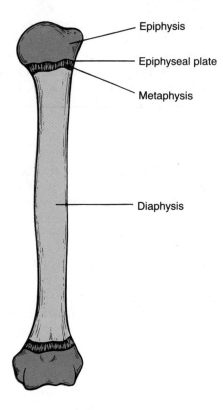

Epiphysis

Epiphyseal plate

Metaphysis

Diaphysis

FIGURE 6–3. The structural components of a long bone.

is laid down around the center of the diaphysis via intramembranous ossification of the perichondrium (Junqueira et al, 1989). Cartilage cells in the central diaphysis then become hypertrophied and are destroyed. As the remaining cartilage matrix becomes calcified, the area is infiltrated by osteoblasts and capillaries. The osteoblasts lay down ossified bone matrix. Ossification proceeds toward the ends of the diaphysis. Secondary ossification centers form in the epiphysis. Ossification radiates in all directions from the secondary ossification center. Endochondral ossification is also seen in the vertebrae, as depicted in Figure 6–5.

A growth (epiphyseal) plate, composed of hyaline cartilage, is formed between the diaphyses and epiphyses. This is the site of longitudinal bone growth. Interstitial growth of the hyaline cartilage continues at the surface of the epiphysis. The new cartilage undergoes endochondral ossification in the metaphysis. As the bone approaches its adult length, chondrocyte formation slows while endochondral ossification at the metaphysis continues. The epiphyseal plate narrows and eventually closes (Brashear & Vanderweil, 1983; Malina & Bouchard, 1991).

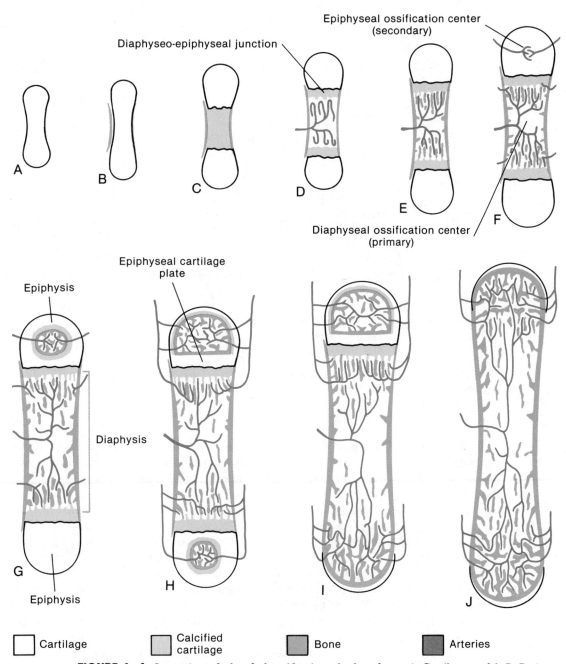

FIGURE 6–4. Stages in endochondral ossification of a long bone. *A*, Cartilage model. *B*, Periosteal bone collar appears. *C*, Cartilage begins to calcify. *D*, Vascular mesenchyme enters the calcified cartilage matrix. *E*, Vascular mesenchyme divides the cartilage matrix into two zones of ossification. *F*, Blood vessels and mesenchyme enter the upper epiphyseal cartilage. *G*, The epiphyseal ossification center develops in the cartilage. A similar ossification center develops in the lower epiphyseal cartilage. *I*, The lower epiphyseal plate disappears. *J*, Then the upper epiphyseal plate disappears, forming a continuous bone marrow cavity. (Modified from Bloom W, Fawcett DW. *A Textbook of Histology,* 11th ed. London, Chapman & Hall, 1986.)

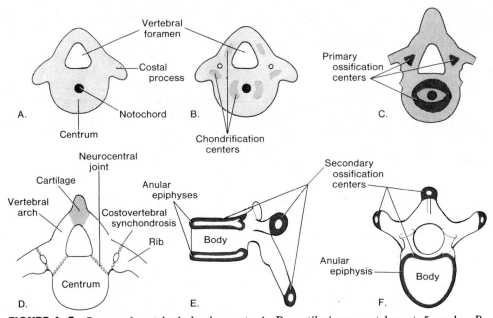

FIGURE 6–5. Stages of vertebral development. *A*, Precartilaginous vertebra at 5 weeks. *B*, Chondrification centers in a mesenchymal vertebra at 6 weeks. *C*, Primary ossification centers in a cartilaginous vertebra at 7 weeks. *D*, A thoracic vertebra at birth, consisting of three bony parts. Note the cartilage between the halves of the vertebral neural arch and between the arch and the centrum. *E* and *F*, Two views of a typical thoracic vertebra at puberty showing the location of the secondary centers of ossification. (From Moore, KL. *The Developing Human,* 5th ed. Philadelphia: WB Saunders, 1993, p 359.)

Mechanical loading of the epiphyseal plate effects longitudinal bone growth. The growth plate is usually aligned perpendicular to the load that crosses it (LeVeau & Bernhardt, 1984), and formation of new bone is stimulated as tension or compression forces are applied. If the compression or tension forces are too great, they may inhibit bone growth. Unequal forces along the epiphyseal plate may stimulate a change of direction of bone growth, whereas torsional forces at the growth plate may result in rotational changes. The changes in angle of inclination between the femoral neck and shaft from approximately 150 degrees in infancy to 125 degrees in the adult and 120 degrees in the older adult provide an example of directional change in normal bone development (Fig. 6–6). Figure 6–7 illustrates torsional changes in the femur, from retroversion prenatally to 25 to 30 degrees of anteversion at birth and 8 to 16 degrees of anteversion in the adult (Norkin & Levangie, 1983). Table 6–1 summarizes some of these changes in lower extremity structure. It should also be noted that shearing forces applied across the epiphyseal plate may contribute to displacement of the growth plate. Therapeutically this is an important consideration when working with individuals whose skeleton has not reached maturity, because displacement of the epiphyseal plate interferes with normal growth.

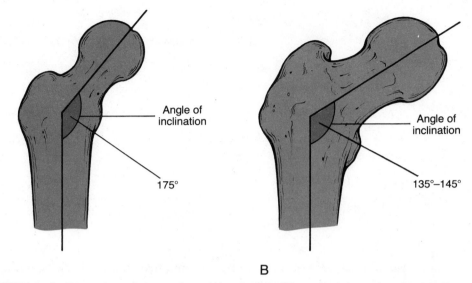

A

B

FIGURE 6-6. Comparison of the newborn *(A)* and adult *(B)* proximal femoral angle of inclination.

Cartilaginous growth plates are found not only at the ends of long bones, but also at points of muscular attachment, where they are called *traction epiphyses* or *apophyses.* Muscle contraction places a traction force on the bone and stimulates bone growth. This is demonstrated at the proximal femur. Figure 6-8 reflects the effects of muscle pull on the greater trochanter and lesser trochanter of the femur. The greater trochanter has broad muscular attachments, whereas the lesser trochanter has only the attachment of the iliopsoas tendon. The traction force exerted by the muscular activity stimulates varying degrees of bone growth at these locations, helping shape the developing bone into its mature form. Muscle weakness can affect bone growth, as demonstrated in Figure 6-8. Muscle weakness also affects apposi-

FIGURE 6-7. Comparison of the newborn *(A)* and adult *(B)* femoral angle of torsion. In both views a superior perspective *(left),* looking down from the head/neck of femur to the femoral condyles, and an anterior perspective *(right)* are provided.

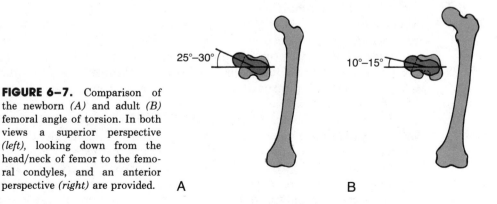

A

B

Table 6-1. DEVELOPMENTAL CHANGES IN LOWER EXTREMITY ALIGNMENT			
	Birth	**3 Years**	**Adult**
Acetabular roof	7° from vertical	17° from vertical	
Femur			
Angle of inclination	135°–145°		125%
Angle of torsion	25°–30° anteversion		8°–16° anteversion
Tibial torsion	5°–10° internal tibial torsion		20°–25° external tibial torsion
Calcaneus	22° varus		0°–3° varus

Data from Bernhardt DB. Prenatal and postnatal growth and development of the foot and ankle. *Phys Ther* 68:1831–1839, 1988.

tional bone growth. It can result in diminished diameter of bone, as well as a 5 to 10 per cent decrease in bone length, as exemplified by the shortened affected limbs of a person with hemiplegia (Smith, 1981).

Bones grow not only in length, but also in diameter. New bone is laid down on the outer surface of the bone and is absorbed from the inner surface, determining the thickness of bone and size of the marrow cavity within the bone. This process is called *appositional growth* and continues throughout life, but the proportion of bone formation to resorption varies. In childhood and adolescence, formation is greater then resorption, increasing bone diameter and thickness. Throughout early and middle adulthood, equilibrium between the two processes maintains bone size. In later adult life, resorption exceeds formation, resulting in loss of bone mass (Thibodeau, 1987). Because resorption occurs at the inner surface of the bone, the marrow cavity becomes larger and the bony shell surrounding it thinner (Fig. 6–9).

The ongoing reconstruction of bone tissue by resorption in some areas and subsequent formation of new bone in other areas is called *bone remodeling*. Through this process, bone achieves adult form, adapts its architecture to accommodate changes in mechanical loading, and renews its structure. Remodeling of bone improves its mechanical resilience and structural alignment. Mechanical strain, especially compression, is an important force in the bone remodeling process because it provides the stimulus for bone growth. Fibers within the bone tissue are aligned in response to mechanical stress, allowing the bone to withstand functional load bearing (Lanyon, 1989). Sufficient bone mass with optimal internal architecture is necessary to meet the demands of everyday life.

Because bone serves as the storage site for calcium, serum calcium levels will also affect bone remodeling. As the concentration of calcium in the blood changes, calcium in the bone is accessed by one of two processes. In the first process, calcium is quickly transferred into or out of younger, less calcified lamellae, adjusting to food intake or functional demands of the body. The second process is slower and depends on stimulation of calcium-regulating

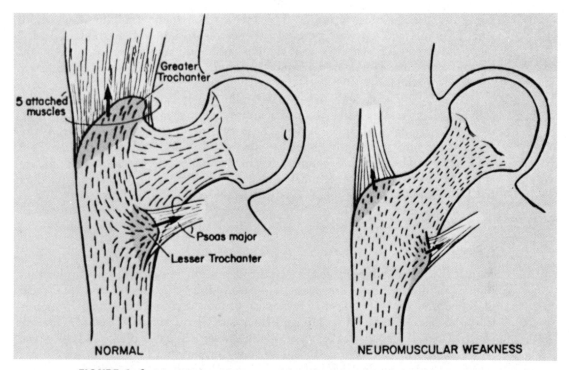

FIGURE 6–8. Muscular attachments to immature bone shape bone growth: normal compared to muscle weakness. (From Graham JM: Smith's *Recognizable Patterns of Human Deformation*. Philadelphia: WB Saunders, 1988, p 147.)

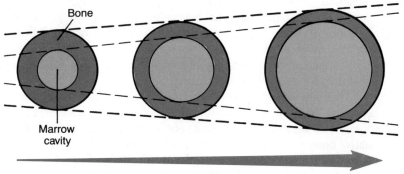

FIGURE 6–9. Effect of appositional bone growth over time—an increase in diameter of bone. Because resorption is greater than production, bone thickness is decreased and the width of the marrow cavity is increased.

hormones. Parathyroid hormone is released when blood calcium levels drop. This hormone activates osteoclasts to begin resorption of bone matrix, which releases the calcium stores in well-established bone matrix. Calcitonin, another thyroid hormone, is released as blood calcium levels increase, inhibiting resorption (Junqueira et al, 1989).

Bone is an adaptable tissue, responding to hormonal demands and the mechanical stresses placed on it. To maintain bone mass and architecture, a balance must be achieved between these two processes. Good nutrition and exercise are important throughout the life span to build and maintain maximal bone mass and structural competence of the skeleton. Many studies of the effect of exercise on bone mass suggest that increased functional loading results in increased bone mass, whereas decreased functional loading results in bone loss (Lanyon, 1989).

AGING

As just discussed, adaptation of bone through remodeling continues throughout life. Skeletal maturity, however, as measured by closure of the epiphyseal plate, occurs within the first two decades of life. Maximal bone mass, which is the total bone growth in length and thickness, is obtained between 20 and 30 years of age (Duncan & Parfitt, 1984). Between the ages of 35 and 40 years, bone resorption can begin exceeding bone formation (Thibodeau, 1987). Increasing the mechanical load placed on bone through physical activity appears to help maintain a balance between bone formation and resorption even at older ages. Bone loss appears to vary between racial groups and the sexes. Bone loss is less severe in African-American adults than it is in Caucasian adults. Women also appear to begin losing bone mass earlier than men (Duncan & Parfitt, 1984). A decrease in mass eventually results in a more fragile bone, which is less able to withstand mechanical forces such as compression and bending.

Other changes involved in the aging of bone include cross-linkage and the architectural rearrangement of collagen fibers, and excessive mineralization of trabecular bone. Fibrils are arranged more longitudinally. Osteons become shorter and narrower as the haversian canals become wider. Excessive mineralization of bone occurs as bone matrix deteriorates because, as the bone becomes more porous, more sites for mineral deposition are provided (Klein & Rajon, 1984). These changes increase the brittleness of bone and compromise its ability to withstand mechanical loads.

Throughout life, the body must maintain the necessary serum calcium level. Intestinal absorption of calcium declines with age, increasing the amount of calcium that must be retrieved from bone to meet the body's needs. As a result, bone mass is gradually lost because bone resorption frequently occurs faster than new bone can be formed. The loss of bone tissue during remodeling leaves the bone thinner and more susceptible to injury. The increased brittleness due to internal changes in bone structure also increases the risk of fracture.

SKELETAL SYSTEM DEVELOPMENT THROUGH THE LIFE SPAN

This section reviews pertinent issues of skeletal system development as they relate to the age of the developing individual.

Prenatal Period

As discussed earlier, bone and cartilage are differentiated from the mesoderm layer early in the gestational period. Development of bone, by either intra-membranous or endochondral ossification, begins in the embryonic period (3rd to 8th gestational weeks). By 5 weeks gestational age, mesenchymal models of bones appear in the extremities, with upper extremity development preceding lower extremity development. In the 6th week, mesenchymal cells have differentiated into chondroblasts, which form the cartilage model of the long bones. As seen in Figure 6–10, primary centers of ossification appear as early as the 7th to 8th week; by the 12th week of gestation, they have appeared in almost all bones of the extremities (Moore, 1988). The diaphyses are fairly well ossified by birth, but the epiphyses remain cartilaginous. A few secondary ossification centers begin to appear late in fetal development, as shown in Figure 6–10.

Vertebral development also begins in the embryonic period. Cartilage models of the vertebrae are formed from mesenchymal cells located around the notochord. By the 7th to 8th gestational week, three ossification centers have formed in the vertebrae model. As Figure 6–5 shows, these bony parts remain connected by cartilage at birth (Moore, 1988).

The confined intrauterine environment in the later weeks of gestation limits the fetus's positioning options and applies forces to the fetal skeletal system. Intrauterine molding of the developing skeletal system can occur and results in deformities such as congenital hip dislocation, tibial bowing, meta-tarsus adductus, calcaneus varus, and extreme ankle dorsiflexion. Some of these deformities will spontaneously improve in the first few years of life. Others, such as congenital hip dislocation, require early orthopedic management—applying corrective mechanical forces to the skeleton during infancy (Hensinger & Jones, 1982).

Functionally, early intramembranous ossification of the skull serves to protect the developing brain. The bones of the skull are not fused, as evidenced by the "soft spots," called *fontanelles.* Expansion and molding of the cranium accommodate brain growth. The lack of fusion of the bones of the skull also allows adaptation of the cranium to the intrauterine environment and passage through the birth canal.

Infant and Child

As mentioned above, the diaphyses of the long bones are fairly well ossified at birth. Secondary ossification centers in the epiphyses continue to appear through adolescence (see Fig. 6–10). Throughout infancy and early childhood, bone growth occurs rapidly. Factors such as genetic makeup, nutrition, general

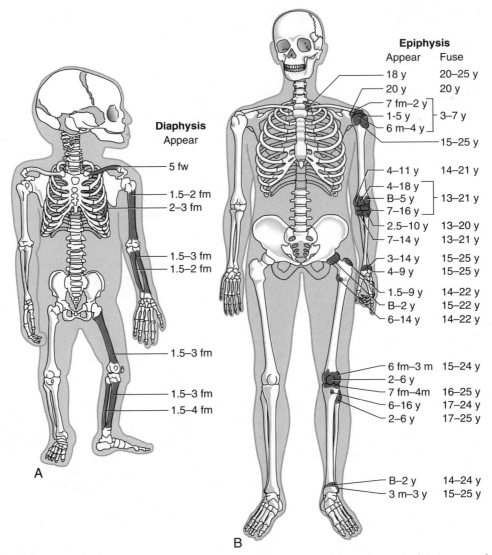

FIGURE 6–10. Appearance of primary and secondary ossification centers. *A*, Appearance of diaphyses. *B*, Appearance and fusion of epiphyses. fw = fetal weeks, fm = fetal months, m = postnatal months, y = years, B = birth. (Modified from Anson B. *Morris' Human Anatomy*, 12th ed. New York: McGraw-Hill, 1966.)

health, and hormonal levels affect the rate of bone growth and time of appearance of the secondary ossification centers (Hensinger & Jones, 1981). The appearance of centers of ossification and fusion of the epiphyses occur earlier in girls than in boys (Porter, 1989). The dynamic quality of bone growth contributes to the spontaneous correction of skeletal abnormalities and the responsiveness to orthopedic treatment seen in children. The infant born with congenital bony deformities, such as metatarsus adductus or club foot, may benefit greatly from early orthopedic intervention. Corrective forces can be applied with casting or taping procedures to correct bony alignment. Bleck (1982) reports that all but 5 to 15 per cent of childhood lower extremity deformities resolve spontaneously. Abnormal skeletal development also occurs if unbalanced muscle action around a joint is present, as in cerebral palsy or spina bifida. For example, bone growth will proceed in response to the strong adduction and internal rotation forces exerted by muscles at the hip of the child with cerebral palsy. This abnormal force interferes with normal development of the acetabulum, femoral torsion, and the femoral neck/shaft angle. The hip can become unstable, and the risk for dislocation is increased.

The epiphysis is an active site for new bone formation and plays an important role in early skeletal development. During periods of rapid growth, forces acting on the epiphysis can have dramatic effects. Injury or infection to the epiphysis can result in abnormal bone growth and limb length deficiencies (Hensinger & Jones, 1982). The newborn infant is especially susceptible to infection of the epiphysis because the epiphyseal plate is very thin at this age and does not provide a significant barrier between the metaphysis and the epiphysis. Blood vessels easily cross the growth plate, allowing infection to be spread from the metaphysis to the epiphysis. As the epiphyseal plate becomes thicker, the blood vessels can no longer cross it, eliminating the possibility for transmission of infection. Fractures of the epiphyseal plate will interfere with bone growth patterns, resulting in asymmetric bone growth or the cessation of growth.

Structural differences between growing and adult bone make children more susceptible to injuries such as plastic deformation of the bone, greenstick fractures, and apophyseal avulsion (avulsion of muscle tendon from its insertion) (Wojtys, 1987). In general, growing bone is less dense and more porous than adult bone. As a result, it is more sensitive to both compressive and tensile stress. The cortex of the metaphysis is also thinner than that of the diaphysis, making it less resistant to compressive forces. The periosteum, however, is thicker than in adult bone and less readily torn, resulting in less displaced fractures.

Areas of Bone Growth. The head and trunk of the newborn infant make up a proportionately larger part of the total skeleton than in the adult. During childhood, the growth of the axial skeleton does not contribute as much to a child's increasing height as does the growth of the lower extremities.

The lower extremities and pelvis undergo angular, rotational, and length changes as the infant learns to move. At birth, the ilia and sacrum are more upright than they are in the adult. Once the infant starts walking, the curvature of the sacrum increases, the ilia thicken, and acetabular depth increases (Sinclair, 1985). The acetabular roof rotates from a relatively vertical position to one of more forward inclination (Bernhardt, 1988). Bernhardt describes changes throughout the developing lower extremity (see Table 6–1). The femoral angle of inclination decreases (see Fig. 6–6), creating a better lever arm for force production of the hip abductors. The femoral angle of torsion also changes (see Fig. 6–7), decreasing the amount of anteversion from birth to adulthood. Different rates of growth in the three epiphyseal zones of the proximal femur contribute to the angular and rotational changes of the bone (Bernhardt, 1988). By 8 years of age, the proximal femur has attained its adult form (Ogden, 1983).

Angular and torsional changes also take place in the tibia and ankle/foot complex. External tibial torsion increases from the newborn period to adulthood. The relationship between the femur and tibia changes from a position of bow legs (genu varum) in infancy to one of knock knees (genu valgus) by 3 years of age. The degree of valgus then decreases to normal adult values. The newborn's foot also is in a position of varus at the calcaneus and forefoot, which slowly decreases until adult values are reached. Slight forefoot varus may persist until 2 years of age. Weight bearing and the torsional forces of muscles actively contracting during creeping (four-point), standing, and walking contribute to these changes.

Not only does the lower extremity skeleton undergo transformation as the infant develops functional movement skills, but changes also are seen in the spine. In the newborn, the anteroposterior spinal curve is relatively concave. The cervical lordosis is present at birth, possibly because of early ossification of the occipital bone, but it becomes more evident by 3 months of age, when the infant has developed head control. The lumbar lordosis develops as the infant learns to sit. Iliopsoas tightness from fetal positioning combined with antigravity work in prone, four-point, and kneeling positions may contribute to development of the lumbar lordosis (LeVeau & Bernhardt, 1984; Walker, 1991). Orthopedic management of spinal deformities, such as scoliosis and kyphosis, can be achieved by bracing the immature skeleton.

Adolescence

During adolescence, bone continues to grow and remodel in response to mechanical loading stresses. The adolescent experiences sudden increases in height and weight, with growth of the trunk exceeding the lower extremities. The adolescent growth spurt of girls begins at an average of 12 to 13 years of age, preceding that of boys by approximately 2 years. A growth spurt in bone width is seen through adolescence in boys and up to age 14 in girls. The width of the bone cortex increases in both boys and girls, but boys also demonstrate an increase in width of the central marrow cavity (Malina & Bouchard, 1991). Rapid bone growth frequently outpaces increases in muscle length, resulting in decreased flexibility. Injuries can result if adolescents do not modify their activities to accommodate these changes in flexibility.

Skeletal system problems such as scoliosis often become obvious and may progress rapidly during adolescence. Mild scoliosis of 5 degrees or less is seen in 10 per cent of children during puberty; boys and girls are equally represented. Only a small percentage of scoliotic curves progress to greater than 15 degrees (Staheli, 1983).

The rapid growth spurt seen during adolescence increases the vulnerability of the open epiphysis and may be related to the occurrence of slipped capital femoral epiphysis in this population (Ogden, 1983). Although the etiology is unknown, it is suspected that growth imbalances, hormone level changes, and stress on the epiphysis contribute to the slipping (Staheli, 1983). The epiphysis is also less stable than the joints, making epiphyseal injury likely when the joint area is involved. Apparent joint sprains in this age group should be critically evaluated to rule out involvement of the epiphysis.

Stress fractures and apophyseal avulsion fractures are also seen, especially in the adolescent athlete when activity or training level changes. These injuries are related to overuse and stress on the system beyond the ability for self-repair. Common sites for stress fracture in the adolescent are the lumbar spine, tibia, and fibula. Gymnasts or individuals performing repetitive activities that place an axial load on an extended spine are at risk for lumbar spondylolysis, a stress fracture of the pars interarticularis (Smith AD, 1988). Long distance runners frequently present with fractures at the tibia or fibula (Wojtys, 1987).

Apophyseal avulsion fractures occur when traction forces are applied at the apophysis and it is pulled away from the bone. Common sites for avulsion fractures are the anterior superior iliac spine, anterior inferior iliac spine, lesser trochanter, and ischium (Smith AD, 1988). Osgood-Schlatter disease may also be associated with avulsion of the apophysis at the tibial tuberosity following a traction injury. The definite etiology of this disease is unknown, but it affects adolescent boys (10 to 15 years of age) and girls (8 to 13 years of age) (Wojtys, 1987). Physical conditioning programs, thorough preseason screening examinations, and appropriate supervision during athletic activities are important to prevent these stress-related injuries.

Cartilage injury can also be seen in adolescence. Chondromalacia of the patella, with softening and fibrillation of the cartilage, results from stress on the kneecap. Rotational or angular malalignment of the patella is usually seen. Restriction of overactivity allows the cartilage to repair itself.

Attainment of Skeletal Maturity. Skeletal maturity is attained when the epiphyseal plates close. Epiphyseal closure begins in childhood and is usually complete by 25 years of age (see Fig. 6–10). Fusion of the vertebral arches is seen in the cervical spine in the first year of life and in the lumbar spine by 6 years of life. Fusion of the vertebral arch and centrum occurs between 5 and 8 years of age. Secondary centers of ossification in the vertebrae do not unite until the 25th year (Moore, 1988).

Adulthood

After the epiphyses have closed, the bones no longer lengthen. Throughout adulthood, only bone remodeling occurs. Weight bearing and muscle contraction continue to stimulate bone remodeling and increase bone density (Whitbourne, 1985). Both men and women attain their maximal bone mass by 20 to 30 years of age. Bone formation and resorption remain balanced until 35 to 40 years of age (LeVeau & Bernhardt, 1984; Whitbourne, 1985; Martin & Brown, 1989). After that time, bone loss is greater than bone replacement. In the adult skeleton, cortical bone loss has been reported to begin in the fourth decade and cancellous bone loss to begin in the third decade of life (Borner et al, 1988).

Several different estimates of the amount of bone loss with aging are reported in the literature. Raab and Smith (1985) estimate that women lose 1 per cent of bone mass per year prior to menopause. For the 4 to 5 years after menopause, 2 to 4 per cent of bone mass per year is lost. After this time, the rate of loss returns to 1 per cent per year. Men are reported to lose 0.5 per cent of bone mass per year. This loss translates into a decline in bone strength, which increases the risk for spontaneous fractures and functional motor deficits.

Fibrous cartilage changes also become apparent in adulthood as the intervertebral disk loses water. The nucleus pulposus is primarily affected; most water content is lost in the second to fourth decades of life. Water loss continues slowly in older adulthood, during which time the annulus fibrosus also undergoes fibrotic changes. The intervertebral disk becomes flattened and less resilient. Considering the early changes in the disk, it is not surprising that the highest incidence of back pain is reported between the ages of 30 and 50 years (Koeller et al, 1986; Lewis & Bottomly, 1990).

Older Adulthood

With aging, the skeletal system becomes progressively more compromised. Loss of bone mass continues in older adulthood and can be related to osteopenia, osteomalacia, or osteoporosis. Osteopenia occurs when either organic or inorganic components of bone fail to develop. Osteomalacia refers to abnormal mineralization of the bone matrix because of calcium and phosphate deficiencies. It affects both recently formed and well established bone, decreasing the amount of mineral per unit of bone matrix. Osteoporosis refers to reduction of bone mass because of decreased formation of new bone and/or increased resorption while bone chemistry is normal (Junqueira et al, 1989; Pickles, 1989).

Age-related bone loss may also be related to the decreased activity level of elderly individuals, which limits both the mechanical loading of bone and circulation. Pickles (1989), MacKinnon (1988), and Borner and colleagues (1988) discuss several studies reporting effects of continued weight-bearing activities on bone density and conclude that physical activity can help to maintain bone density. Continued functional loading of the skeletal system appears to help balance bone formation and resorption.

	Table 6-2. AGE-RELATED SKELETAL SYSTEM CONCERNS RELATED TO PHYSICAL ACTIVITY	
Age Period	**Skeletal System Concern**
Prenatal	Intrauterine molding late in gestation
Newborn	Epiphyseal infection
Childhood	Epiphyseal injury
	Apophyseal avulsion
	Greenstick fracture
Adolescence	Scoliosis
	Epiphyseal injury
	Apophyseal avulsion
	Stress fracture
Adulthood	Back pain secondary to disk changes
Older adulthood	Osteoporosis
	Osteoarthritis

FUNCTIONAL IMPLICATIONS OF SKELETAL SYSTEM CHANGES

This section highlights the functional effects of skeletal system changes. Special areas of concern regarding functional activities of each age group have been discussed and are summarized in Table 6–2. The main topics covered in this section, osteoporosis and osteoarthritis, are common problems for older adults. Understanding the processes underlying these two disorders is important for developing prevention programs and possibly will limit the functional losses experienced by older adults.

Osteoporosis

Osteoporosis due to the progressive loss of bone mass with aging is referred to as *senile* or *involutional osteoporosis.* Pathologic conditions such as poor nutrition, metabolic disorders, neoplasm, and hormonal influences can also be related to the development of osteoporosis. Physical inactivity related to aging, long periods of bedrest, and exposure to weightless environments have been identified as factors contributing to osteoporosis. The individual most at risk for the development of osteoporosis is the slightly built, sedentary, Caucasian female.

The clinical features of osteoporosis are pain, loss of height, kyphosis, and decreased function, because bone is unable to withstand the compression forces of weight bearing. MacKinnon (1988) reports that 40 per cent of normal bone strength should be adequate to withstand normal mechanical loading. When the amount of bone mass is no longer sufficient to support the body during activity, spontaneous fracture may result. The most frequent sites for spontaneous fracture secondary to osteoporosis are the spine, proximal femur, and wrist. Anterior compression fractures of the vertebrae result in wedge-shaped vertebrae and lead to kyphotic posturing. Central collapse of adjacent vertrabrae lead to fish-shaped vertebrae, decreasing the disk space and skeletal height. In general, the microfractures related to osteoporosis cause pain and lead to a flexed posture. No specific criteria exist for the diagnosis of osteoporosis. It is generally felt that when bone mass content falls below 2 standard deviations of the mean bone mass content for young normal persons, osteoporosis is present (Borner et al, 1988).

Two categories of involutional osteoporosis exist. One category, related to decreased intestinal absorption of calcium, is seen in both men and women and affects both cortical and cancellous bone. For these individuals, clinical management with dietary calcium is reportedly beneficial (Kauffman, 1987). However, Borner and colleagues (1988) review other studies that question the effectiveness of calcium supplementation. The second category of involutional osteoporosis is associated with menopause and affects primarily cancellous bone. When estrogen secretion decreases with menopause, the bone is thought to become more sensitive to parathyroid hormone, increasing the rate of bone resorption (MacKinnon, 1988). Calcium and fluoride supplements combined with estrogen therapy are of some value for women with this type of osteoporosis (Borner et al, 1988).

Good nutrition and a lifelong commitment to exercise may influence the maximal bone mass attained in early adulthood and maintenance of that bone mass. Exercise programs may effectively slow or prevent the bone loss associated with aging or even increase the bone mass (Martin & Brown, 1989; Borner et al, 1988; MacKinnon, 1988). In planning exercise programs, one should include weight-bearing and strengthening activities. Weight-bearing activities such as walking and running provide mechanical loading to the bones of the lower extremities and spine. Twisting, explosive, and stacatto movements should be avoided because of the forces they place on bone tissue. Spinal extension exercises should be emphasized because flexion exercises may be problematic, contributing to anterior wedging and compression fractures of the vertebrae (MacKinnon, 1988). Although previous studies emphasized the need for weight-bearing activities, one study reported increased vertebral and radial bone density in male swimmers as compared to their peers who did not exercise. No differences were noted between women swimmers and nonexercisers (Orwoll et al, 1989).

Osteoarthritis

Osteoarthritis refers to the degeneration of articular cartilage with age. It affects 70 per cent of people at some point in their life and most adults over 70 years of age (Gradisar & Porterfield, 1989). The cartilage thins, and clefts and cracks form, leaving the surface uneven and unable to efficiently provide frictionless joint motion. Underlying bone, which is innervated, becomes exposed to mechanical stress, resulting in pain. Bony spurs or outgrowths covered with hyaline cartilage may also develop in the joint. The individual suffering from osteoarthritis experiences pain with movement and limited range of motion.

Treatment for osteoarthritis is limited to protecting affected joints from undue stress, minimizing joint range of motion limitations, and relieving pain. Anti-inflammatory medications offer some relief. Individuals with osteoarthritis also benefit from participating in exercise programs that emphasize balanced loading of the joint surface. The exercises should address improvement of muscle strength, preservation of joint range of motion, and improved efficiency when performing everyday tasks so that loading forces on the cartilage are equalized (Friedman et al, 1983). Prolonged jogging or impact exercises should be avoided, because they put high loads on the cartilage and may increase tissue destruction. When conservative treatment approaches do not relieve symptoms, surgical debridement of the joint surface or joint replacement is considered.

SUMMARY
· ·

This chapter has focused on the lifetime development of two components of the skeletal system, cartilage and bone. Together these elements provide a structural base on which movement can take place. Optimal, healthy development of the skeletal system depends not only on genetics and nutrition, but also on an active lifestyle. The mechanical stresses of everyday, functional activities and exercise help the system achieve its most efficient form and maintain its stability. Lifelong commitment to good nutrition and exercise helps the young adult attain his or her maximal bone mass and maintain a strong skeletal system well into older adulthood.

References

Bacon RL, Niles NR. *Medical Histology—A Text-Atlas with Introductory Pathology.* New York: Springer Verlag, 1983.

Bernhardt DB. Prenatal and postnatal growth and development of the foot and ankle. *Phys Ther* 68:1831–1839, 1988.

Bleck EE. Developmental orthopedics III: Toddlers. *Dev Med Child Neurol* 24:533–555, 1982.

Borner JA, Dillworth BB, Sullivan KM. Exercise and osteoporosis: A critique of the literature. *Physiother Can* 40(3):146–155, 1988.

Brashear RH, VanderWeil CJ. Histology and growth of bone. In Wilson FC (ed). *The Musculoskeletal System: Basic Processes and Disorders,* 2nd ed. Philadelphia: JB Lippincott, 1983, pp 89–96.

Chrisman OD. The aging of cartilage. In Nelson CL, Dwyer AP (eds). *The Aging Musculoskeletal System—Physiologic and Pathological Problems.* Lexington, MA: DC Heath, 1984.

Duncan H, Parfitt AM. The biology of aging bone. In Nelson CL, Dwyer AP (eds). *The Aging Musculoskeletal System—Physiologic and Pathological Problems.* Lexington, MA: DC Heath, 1984.

Freidman MA, Eisenberg RA, Wright PH. Osteoarthritis. In Wilson, FC (ed). *The Musculoskeletal System—Basic Processes and Disorders,* 2nd ed. Philadelphia: JB Lippincott, 1983.

Gould J, Davies G. *Orthopedic and Sport Physical Therapy.* St. Louis: CV Mosby, 1985.

Gradisar IA, Porterfield JA. Articular cartilage: Structure and function. *Top Geriatr Rehabil* 4(3):1–9, 1989.

Guyton AC. *Human Physiology and Mechanisms of Disease.* Philadelphia: WB Saunders, 1987.

Hensinger RN, Jones EJ. Developmental orthopedics I: The lower limb. *Dev Med Child Neurol* 24:95–116, 1982.

Hensinger RN, Jones ET. *Neonatal Orthopedics.* New York: Grune & Stratton, 1981.

Junqueira LC, Carneiro J, Kelley RO. *Basic Histology,* 6th ed. Norwalk, CT: Appleton & Lange, 1989.

Kauffman T. Posture and age. *Top Geriatr Rehabil* 2(4):13–28, 1987.

Klein L, Rajan JC. The biology of aging human collagen. In Nelson CL, Dwyer AP (eds). *The Aging Musculoskeletal System—Physiologic and Pathological Problems.* Lexington, MA: DC Heath, 1984.

Koeller W, Muehlhaus S, Meier W, Hartmann F. Biomechanical properties of human intervertebral discs subjected to axial dynamic compression—Influence of age and degeneration. *J Biomech* 19(10):807–816, 1986.

Lanyon LE. Strain related bone modeling and remodeling. *Top Geriatr Rehabil* 4(2)13–24, 1989.

Leeson TS, Leeson CR, Papara AA. *Text/Atlas of Histology.* Philadelphia: WB Saunders, 1988.

LeVeau BF, Bernhardt DB. Developmental biomechanics. *Phys Ther* 64(12):1874–1882, 1984.

Lewis CB, Bottomley, JM. Musculoskeletal changes with age: Clinical implications. In Lewis CB (ed). *Aging: The Health Care Challenge,* 2nd ed. Philadelphia: FA Davis, 1990.

MacKinnon JL. Osteoporosis— A review. *Phys Ther* 68(10):1533–1540, 1988.

Malina RM, Bouchard C. *Growth, Maturation and Physical Activity.* Champaign, IL: Human Kinetics, 1991.

Martin AD, Brown E. The effects of physical activity on the human skeleton. *Top Geriatr Rehabil* 4(2):25–35, 1989.

Moore KL. *The Developing Human—Clinically Oriented Embryology,* 4th ed. Philadelphia: WB Saunders, 1988.

Norkin C, Levangie P. Joint structure and function: A comprehensive analysis. Philadelphia: FA Davis, 1983.

Ogden JA. Development and growth of the hip. In Katz JF, Siffert RS (eds). *Management of Hip Disorders in Children.* Philadelphia: JB Lippincott, 1983.

Orwoll ES, Ferar J, Oviatt SK, McClung MR, Huntington K. The relationship of swimming exercise to bone mass in men and women. *Arch Intern Med* 149:2197–2200, 1989.

Pickles B. Biological aspects of aging. In Jackson O (ed). *Physical Therapy of the Geriatric Patient,* 2nd ed. New York: Churchill Livingston, 1989, pp 27–76.

Porter RE. Normal development of movement and function: Child and adolescent. In Scully RM, Barnes MR (eds). *Physical Therapy.* Philadelphia: JB Lippincott, 1989.

Raab DM, Smith EL. Exercise and aging: Effects on bone. *Top Geriatr Rehabil* 1(1):31–39, 1985.

Sinclair D. *Human Growth After Birth,* 4th ed. London: Oxford University Press, 1985.

Smith AD. Children and sports. In Scoles P (ed). *Pediatric Orthopedics in Clinical Practice,* 2nd ed. Chicago: Year Book, 1988.

Smith DW. Recognizable patterns of human deformation. Identification and management of mechanical effects on morphogenesis. *Major Probl Clin Pediatr* 21:1–151, 1981.

Staheli LT. Orthopedics in adolescence. *Dev Med Child Neurol* 25:806–818, 1983.

Thibodeau GA. *Anatomy and Physiology.* St. Louis: Mosby, 1987.

Vanderweil CJ. Chemistry and biochemistry of cartilage and synovial fluid. In Wilson FC (ed). *The Musculoskeletal System—Basic Processes and Disorders,* 2nd ed. Philadelphia: JB Lippincott, 1983.

Walker J. Musculoskeletal development: A review. *Phys Ther* 71:878–889, 1991.

Whitbourne SK. *The Aging Body—Physiological Changes and Psychological Consequences.* New York: Springer Verlag, 1985.

Wojtys EM. Sports injuries in the immature athlete. *Orthop Clin North Am* 18(4):689–708, 1987.

Chapter 7

Muscle Development and Function

by PATRICIA A. WILDER

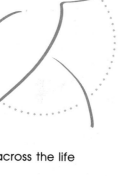

Objectives

AFTER STUDYING THIS CHAPTER, THE READER WILL BE ABLE TO:

1   Define the basic characteristics of skeletal muscle morphology and organization.
2   Describe the basic physiology of skeletal muscle contraction.
3   Understand the development changes in skeletal muscle across the life span.
4   Provide the functional implications of age-related changes in skeletal muscles.

This chapter discusses the basic components of skeletal muscle, how skeletal muscle changes over time, and the functional implications of these changes.

GENERAL CHARACTERISTICS OF MUSCLE

Muscle is the largest tissue mass in the body. There are three types of muscles: voluntary (skeletal) muscle, involuntary (smooth) muscle, and cardiac muscle. These three types of muscle are further divided into two subtypes: striated muscle and nonstriated muscle. Smooth muscle is the single example of the nonstriated type and is found in the walls of the digestive system, urinary bladder, and blood vessels. The main purpose of smooth muscle contraction in these structures is to decrease their diameter. The cells are 10 to 600 μm in length and 2 to 12 μm in diameter. They are spindle shaped and have a single, centrally placed nucleus.

Striated muscle consists of cardiac and skeletal muscle. Cardiac muscle is a special form of striated muscle found only in the heart. Its arrangement of contractile proteins is identical to that of skeletal muscle, but the arrangement of fibers is different. Cardiac cells are joined together by specialized intercellular junctions that are visible in the light microscope as dark heavy lines between the cells. The cells are irregularly shaped and usually contain a single, centrally placed nucleus.

Skeletal muscle, the focus of this chapter, is generally considered the main energy-consuming tissue of the body and provides the propulsive force to move about and perform physical activities. Skeletal muscle is also known as voluntary, striated, striped, or segmental muscle. Of the energy produced during contraction, only about 20 per cent is used to produce movement; the rest is lost as heat.

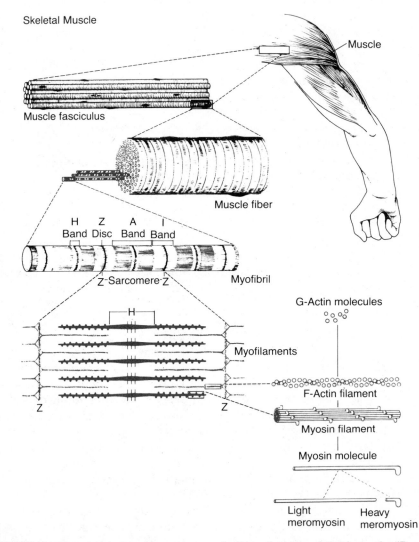

FIGURE 7–1. Macroscopic to microscopic organization of mature skeletal muscle. (Drawing by Sylvia Colard Keene. Modified from Fawcett DW. *Bloom and Fawcett: A Textbook of Histology.* London: Chapman & Hall, 1986.)

There are more than 500 skeletal muscles in the body. On a microscopic level, muscle cells are considered to be cylindric. They range from 1 to 40 μm in length and from 10 to 100 μm in diameter. The cells are multinucleated, with the nuclei located at the periphery of the cell or just beneath the *sarcolemma,* or plasma membrane. External to the sarcolemma is a highly glycosylated layer (i.e., it also contains proteins that function as enzymes) of collagen fibers called the *external lamina;* it is the external lamina that completely ensheathes each cell.

Organization of Mature Skeletal Muscle

The organization of skeletal muscle from macroscopic to microscopic levels is illustrated in Figure 7–1. A more detailed view of micro-organization is provided in Figure 7–2. The entire muscle is encased in a thick connective sheath of collagen fibers and fibroblasts called the *epimysium.* Extensions of this sheath extend into the interior of the muscle, subdividing it into small bundles or groups of myofibers called *fasciculi.* Each bundle or fasciculus is surrounded by a layer of connective tissue called the *perimysium.* Within the fasciculus, each individual muscle myofibril is surrounded by a layer of connective tissue called the *endomysium.* The endomysium is rich in capillaries and, to a lesser extent, nerve fibers. All connective tissue coverings ultimately come together at the tendinous junction; the tendon transmits all contractile forces generated by the muscle fibers to the bone.

As seen in Figure 7–1, each individual myofiber is filled with cylindric bundles of myofibrils that are made up of myofilaments. Each myofilament is divided into segments called *Z lines* or *Z bands;* these Z lines are actually actin and myosin filaments that slide over each other during muscle contraction. These organized, repeating units of actin and myosin are called *sarcomeres.* The sarcomere is the basic contractile unit of the muscle fiber and extends from Z line to Z line. The alternating light and dark pattern in the sarcomere reflects the amount of overlap of the actin and myosin filaments.

Figure 7–3, a sagittal section of a muscle bundle, shows the arrangement

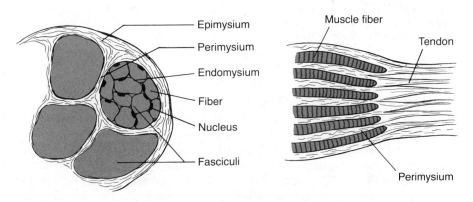

FIGURE 7–2. Micro-organization of skeletal muscle.

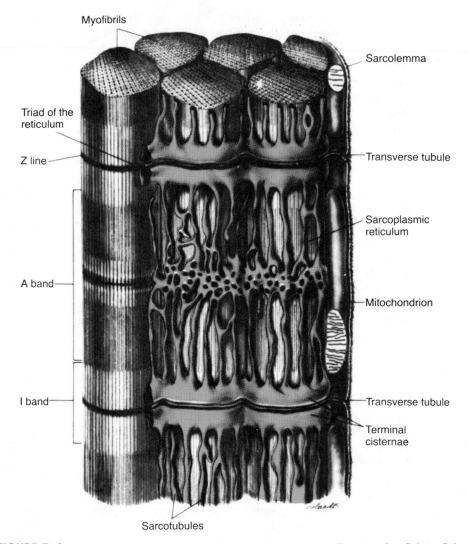

Myofibrils

Sarcolemma

Triad of the
reticulum

Z line

Transverse tubule

Sarcoplasmic
reticulum

A band

Mitochondrion

I band

Transverse tubule

Terminal
cisternae

Sarcotubules

FIGURE 7–3. Transverse tubule sarcoplasmic reticulum system. (Drawing by Sylvia Colard Keene. From Fawcett DW. *Bloom and Fawcett: A Textbook of Histology.* London: Chapman & Hall, 1986. Modified from Peachey. *J Cell Biol* 25:209, 1965.)

of the *sarcoplasmic reticulum (SR),* a system of membranous anastomosing channels intimately associated with the surface of each myofibril. Calcium ions (Ca^{++}) necessary for muscle contraction are released from the SR and then resorbed by the SR. Figure 7–3 also illustrates the arrangement of the *transverse tubular system (T tubules).* T tubules are extensions of the sarcolemma deep into the interior of the muscle fiber. At certain junctions, the invaginations of the T tubules become intimately associated with expansions of the SR; these junctures are called *terminal cisternae.* The function of the T tubules

FIGURE 7–4. The contraction apparatus: Combination of many myosin molecules to form a myosin filament. Also shown are the cross-bridges and the interaction between the heads of the cross-bridges and adjacent actin filaments. (From Guyton AC. *Human Physiology and Mechanisms of Disease,* 5th ed. Philadelphia: WB Saunders, 1992, p 58.)

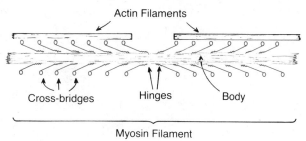

is to extend the wave of depolarization that initiates muscle contraction throughout all the myofibrils of the muscle.

Contractile Apparatus

As depolarization occurs for muscle contraction, Ca^{++} activates the attractive forces between the filaments of actin and myosin. However, the process of contraction will continue only if there is energy; this energy is derived from the high-energy bonds of adenosine triphosphate (ATP), which is degraded to adenosine diphosphate (ADP). As illustrated in Figure 7–4, in the relaxed state the bulbous heads of the myosin filaments are in close association with the actin filaments but do not touch them. However, in the presence of Ca^{++} and ATP, the heads of the myosin molecules form cross-bridges with active sites on the thin filaments of actin. The head of the myosin contains adenosinetriphosphatase (ATPase), which breaks down the ATP. The resulting energy produces a conformational change in the myosin head region that exerts a directional force on the actin filament. As a result, the actin filaments are drawn toward the center of the sarcomere, overlapping the myosin filament. The net result is shortening of the sarcomere, or contraction of the muscle.

Excitation of the Contractile Apparatus

The *neuromuscular junction,* the point of contact between the nerve and surface of the muscle fiber, has a number of morphologic and biochemical specializations. These specializations directly mediate the transfer of the electric impulse of the nerve to the myofiber. Figure 7–5 illustrates the expansion of the axon into a foot plate that comes to rest in a depression of the surface of the myofiber called a *junctional fold.* The membranes of the nerve and muscle fiber do not come into contact but are separated by a narrow space called the *synaptic cleft.*

The foot plate contains large numbers of small membrane-bound vesicles called *synaptic vessels;* these vessels contain the chemical transmitter *acetylcholine (ACh).* When an action potential passes down the motor axon and reaches the nerve ending, the synaptic vesicles fuse with the presynaptic

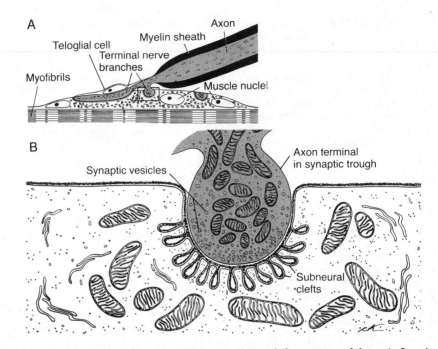

FIGURE 7-5. Neuromuscular junction: Different views of the motor endplate. *A*, Longitudinal section through the endplate. *B*, Electron micrographic appearance of the contact point between one of the axon terminals and the muscle fiber membrane, representing the rectangular area shown in *A*. Modified from R. Couteaux. From Fawcett DW. *Bloom and Fawcett: A Textbook of Histology.* London: Chapman & Hall, 1986. In Guyton AC. *Human Physiology and Mechanisms of Disease,* 5th ed. Philadelphia, WB Saunders, 1992, p 68.)

membrane, thereby emptying their contents, ACh, into the synaptic cleft. Most of the ACh is immediately hydrolyzed by *acetylcholinesterase (AChE)*. The remaining ACh molecules diffuse across the synaptic cleft, where they bind to *ACh receptors* in the muscle membrane. This bonding induces the formation of an action potential that sweeps down the surface of the myofiber.

In summary, the major physiologic events leading to muscle contraction are as follows:

1. A wave of depolarization spreads down the motor axon to the nerve terminal.
2. ACh is released from the synaptic vesicles.
3. ACh diffuses across the synaptic cleft.
4. ACh combines with receptors in the sarcolemma of the muscle fibril.
5. Depolarization of the sarcolemma occurs because of the change in membrane permeability.
6. Depolarization of the T tubules occurs.
7. Depolarization of the SR occurs.
8. Ca^{++} is released from the SR.

9. Cross-bridges are formed between the myosin and actin heads, and ATP breaks down.

10. There is a conformational change of the myosin molecule leading to sliding of the actin filaments across the myosin, a shortening of the sarcomere. Result: contraction of the muscle.

11. AChE hydrolyses ACh to stop the wave of depolarization.

12. SR resorbs all Ca^{++}, cross-bridge formation ceases, and the muscle relaxes.

Isotonic Twitch Curve and Fiber Types

The sequence of events summarized above can be visualized through a recording of the rise to peak tension of a muscle after nerve stimulation. The isotonic twitch curve is a record of the contractile event from the time of stimulation to final total relaxation time (Fig. 7–6).

All muscle fibers respond with the characteristic isotonic twitch curve when stimulated. However, the course of the cycle is not the same for all muscle fiber types. If the isotonic twitch curve were measured in a large population of muscle fibers, each fiber would fall into one of three major groups based on contraction time. These groups have a variety of names in the literature; I shall refer to them as fast-twitch (IIb and IIa), slow-twitch (I), and slow. Fast-twitch and slow-twitch fibers make up virtually all muscles in humans. Slow fibers are found only in extraocular and middle ear muscles.

All human muscles are a mixture of all three fiber types, type IIb, type IIa, and type I (Rose & Rothstein, 1982). Type IIb fibers have large diameters and are glycolytic. They tend to build up an oxygen debt and have a high capacity for anaerobic metabolism. Type IIb fibers have few mitochondria and narrow Z lines. Type IIa fibers are very similar; these fibers use both anaerobic and aerobic metabolism. Both of these fast-twitch fibers are suited for short bursts of powerful activity, although the type IIa fibers are more fatigue resistant. The gastrocnemius muscle has a preponderance of fast-twitch fibers. This gives the muscle its capacity for very forceful and rapid contractions, which are used for jumping. The slow-twitch, type I fibers have a small diameter, with large amounts of oxidative enzymes and an extensive capillary

FIGURE 7–6. Isotonic twitch curve. S = point of stimulation of the motor nerve, a = start of contraction, b = point of maximal contraction, c = point of maximum relaxation, I = latency period of time from stimulation to start of contraction, II = contraction period, or time from start of contraction to peak tension, III = relaxation period, or time from peak contraction to total relaxation.

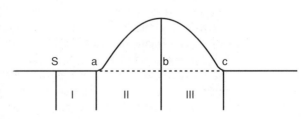

density. Type I fibers are best suited for activities required in repetitive, lower-force contractions and are considered fatigue resistant. Most "postural" muscles, such as those associated with the spinal column or the lower extremities, are composed predominantly of slow-twitch, or type I, fibers. The soleus muscle has a preponderance of slow-twitch muscle fibers and therefore is considered a postural muscle used for prolonged lower extremity activity.

Motor Unit

The functional unit of a muscle is the motor unit, which is defined as a single nerve cell body and its axon plus all muscle fibers innervated by the axon's branches. All the muscle fibers of a motor unit are of the same fiber type. Each muscle fiber receives innervation from one neuron. The intensity of a muscle contraction is graded by the number of motor units recruited. The number of muscle fibers in a motor unit varies according to the muscle. For example, in the large muscles of the lower limb, motor units range in size from approximately 500 to 1000 fibers. In contrast, the small muscles in the hand or the extraocular muscles have motor units that range in size from approximately 10 to 100 fibers. These muscles are capable of producing very fine movements (e.g., typing, tying a bow, making small adjustments of the eye).

SKELETAL MUSCLE DEVELOPMENT

Prenatal

To understand some of the age-related changes in skeletal muscle, it is important to study the events of skeletal muscle development. The muscular system develops from mesoderm, except for the muscles of the iris, which develop from the ectoderm. The events of mesenchymal tissue differentiation into muscle fiber are depicted in Figure 7–7. The important cell types to be considered are myoblasts, myotubes, myofibers, fibroblasts, and satellite cells (Colling-Saltin, 1978).

The *myoblast* is the major cell type found in areas of muscle formation. Myoblasts are spindle-shaped cells with centrally placed elongated nuclei. These cells do not contain organized contractile proteins. During development, myoblasts align into chain-like configurations parallel to the long axis of the limb. Subsequent to alignment, the plasmalemmas of the myoblasts fuse to form large, multinucleated cells called myotubes. Each syncytium (the multinucleate mass of protoplasm produced by cell merging) contains a variable number of nuclei ranging up to several hundred. Cellular fusion as described is the only mechanism by which muscle cells become multinucleated.

The *myotubes* are the immature multinucleated muscle cells. Nuclei are centrally located in these elongated cylindric cells. Contractile proteins are rapidly synthesized and become evident as striated fibrils in the peripheral cytoplasm. *Myofibers* are the mature multinucleated muscle cells. Myofibers

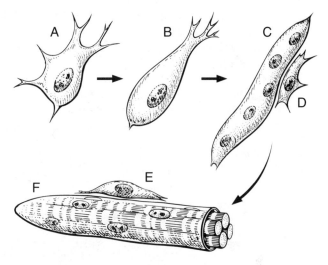

FIGURE 7–7. The differentiation of mesenchymal tissue into muscle fiber: A, mesenchymal cell, B, myoblast, C, myotube, D, fibroblast, E, satellite cell, F, muscle fiber.

contain the characteristic striations of skeletal muscle, or sarcomeres. All nuclei are peripherally located and are closely apposed to the sarcolemma (or "plasma membrane") of the cell.

The *fibroblasts* are the flattened, irregularly shaped cells found in association with the developing myofibers. During the early stages of development, these cells provide an extracellular matrix on which the connective tissue framework of a muscle is developed.

The last fiber type to be discussed is the *satellite cell*. These mononucleated, spindle-shaped cells are closely associated with the surface of the myofibers. They are found between the plasmalemma and external lamina of the myofibers and can be positively identified only with the electron microscope. The position of the satellite cell is shown in Figure 7–7. Satellite cells play an important and integral role, both in normal muscle growth during the postnatal period and in the repair of muscle following injury. At birth, satellite cell nuclei account for over 30 per cent of the total myofiber nuclei (Schultz & Lipton, 1982).

The role of the satellite cells during normal postnatal growth is to supply nuclei to the enlarging fibers. Although myoblasts constitute a rapidly proliferating cell population during embryonic development, once incorporated into the syncytium of a myofiber, they no longer replicate their DNA or divide. The nuclei are permanently postmitotic once they become part of the syncytium. Nevertheless, when myofibers increase in size during growth, their number of nuclei increases, in some cases over 100 times. This increase in myonuclei depends on the satellite cells associated with the fiber. These cells are continually dividing; after a mitotic division, one or both of the daughter cells fuse with the fiber, thereby injecting an additional nucleus into the syncytium. Likewise, in the event of massive injury to the muscle, the myofibers usually die. Surviving satellite cells are activated—they start proliferating and recapitulate the embryonic events leading to muscle formation. In this manner the damaged muscle is repaired or replaced. The satellite cells play an integral role in muscle growth and in regeneration following injury (Gibson & Schultz, 1976).

As stated previously, muscle tissue develops from primitive cells called myoblasts, which are derived from mesenchymal cells. The skeletal muscles of the trunk—those that surround the vertebral column—are formed from mesoderm called *paraxial mesoderm* (Fig. 7–8). Paraxial mesoderm further differen-

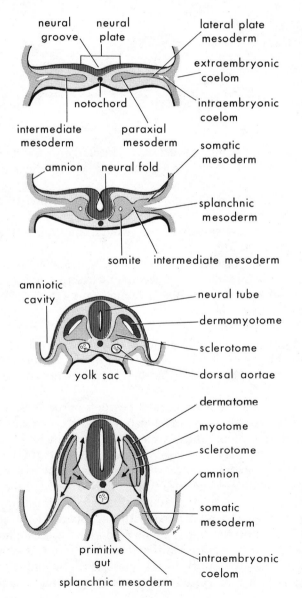

FIGURE 7–8. Transverse sections through an embryo (18 days to 4 weeks) depicting the development of somites from paraxial mesoderm, which includes the development of dermomyotome and scleratome. (From Moore KL. *Before We Are Born*. Philadelphia: WB Saunders, 1993.)

tiates into *somites;* somites are paired structures of mesoderm tissue that ultimately give rise to the muscles and bony segments that make up the vertebral column and to the skin that covers the vertebral column. The muscles of the extremities develop from myoblasts located within the limb region, in situ. It is generally believed that there is no migration of myoblasts from the region of the vertebral column to the region of the limbs.

CHANGES IN FIBER TYPES

Most muscle fibers are undifferentiated prior to 30 weeks of gestation. However, some type I fibers can be distinguished as early as 21 weeks. Type II fibers generally cannot be identified until 30 or 31 weeks of gestation. Studies have concluded that between 31 weeks and 37 weeks of gestation, type II fibers constitute about 25% of the muscle fibers present in the fetus (Malina & Bouchard, 1991).

DEVELOPMENT AND MIGRATION OF FIBERS

Nearly all the skeletal muscles are present, and in essence have their mature form, in a fetus of 8 weeks. Approximately six fundamental processes occur up to the 8th week that involve the gross development of muscle. The formation of a muscle is the result of one or more of these processes. These six fundamental processes are described by Crelin (1981):

1. The direction of the muscle fibers may change from the original craniocaudal orientation in the myotome. Only a few muscles retain their initial fiber orientation (parallel to the long axis of the body); examples of these are the rectus abdominis and the erector spinae. Examples of muscles that undergo a change in direction are the flat muscles of the abdominal wall (the rectus abdominis) and the external and internal oblique muscles.
2. Portions of successive myotomes commonly fuse to form a composite single muscle. An example of this process is the rectus abdominis. This muscle is formed by the fusion of the ventral portions of the last six or seven thoracic myotomes. The intercostal muscles are the derivatives of single myotomes.
3. A myotome may split longitudinally into two or more parts that become separate muscles; examples of this process are the trapezius and the sternocleidomastoid muscles.
4. The original myotome masses may split into two or more layers. The external and internal intercostal muscles and the abdominal oblique muscle are examples of this process.
5. A portion of the muscle or all of the muscle may degenerate. The degenerated muscle leaves a sheet of connective tissue known as an *aponeurosis.* The epicranial aponeurosis connecting the frontal and occipital portions of the occipitofrontalis muscle is an example of this particular process.
6. The last process concerning muscle migration is the migration of a myotome to regions more or less remote from its site of formation. The forma-

tion of the muscles of the upper chest is an example of this process. The serratus anterior muscle migrates to the thoracic region and attaches ultimately to the scapula and the upper eight or nine ribs. This muscle migration takes with it the spinal nerve innervation of the 5th, 6th, and 7th cervical spinal nerves. The migration of the latissimus dorsi muscle is even more extensive. This migration carries with it its 7th and 8th cervical spinal nerve innervations to attach ultimately to the humerus, the lower thoracic and lumbar vertebrae, the last three or four ribs, and the crest of the ilium of the pelvis.

In muscle development, a wide range of variation of these six processes can occur without interfering with an individual's normal functional ability.

Controls of Muscle Development and Differentiation. Differentiation and growth of muscles are the concern of many hypotheses. Most researchers would agree that genetic coding is a component of muscle development. Evidence suggests that it might be important to consider an intact sensible afferent inflow as well as the impact of mechanical loading (Colling-Saltin, 1978a). There is disagreement, however, over the question of whether the nerve has any influence during the fetal period. Some researchers identify contact between nerve and muscle starting as early as the 13th fetal week (Colling-Saltin, 1978b). However, at this early age, it is difficult to determine whether the contact is functional. Perhaps the muscle fiber itself has the most influence over what type of nerve is establishing functional contact. Control of development and differentiation of the muscle cell, during both the fetal period and the neonatal period, is strongly determined by what is inherited and genetically coded in the nucleus of the muscle cell (Colling-Saltin, 1978b); however, the importance of nervous system influence on the development of muscle cannot be dismissed. Gibson and Schultz (1982) discuss "neurotrophic" substances, which are thought to have some influence on differentiation of muscle. It is unclear whether the influence of a neurotrophic substance is present during development. The studies that have been done were conducted on adults and revealed that, by switching a nerve from a glycolytic muscle to an oxidative muscle, the oxidative muscle became glycolytic.

Infancy to Adulthood

The growth of skeletal muscles is the result of an increase in both the number of muscle fibers and the size of the individual fibers. The greatest increase in the number of muscle fibers occurs before birth. After birth, the growth of the muscle comes mainly from the increase in size of individual fibers. In the male, there is a 14-fold increase in fiber number from 2 months to 16 years of age. During this time, there is a rapid spurt at 2 years and a maximum rate of increase from 10 to 16 years of age; from 10 to 16 years, the fiber number doubles (Crelin, 1981). The fiber size increases linearly from infancy to adolescence and even beyond for the male. In the female, the increase in fiber number is more linear than in the male, with a tenfold postnatal increase. In the female the increase in fiber size is more rapid than in the male after 3 1/2 years, reaching a plateau at 10 1/2 years. This increase in fiber size with age is associated with an increase in the number of nuclei in the muscle cell. The estimated number of nuclei in developing muscles has been estimated from measurements of DNA content in samples of muscle tissue in children. Both sexes continue to increase their fiber number until the age of 50 years, after which there is believed to be a steady decline (Crelin, 1981).

At or around birth, skeletal muscles tend to be predominantly fast-twitch, and have a high speed of contraction and a short relaxation time. At about 1 to 2 years of age, the characteristics of slow-twitch fibers—slow speed of contraction and longer relaxation times—are acquired. Type I and type II fibers gradually increase in number during the first postnatal year (Colling-Saltin, 1978b). The undifferentiated fibers (fibers not identified as either type I or type II) decrease. By 1 year, there is little difference in the relative fiber distribution in the muscle tissue of children and adults. Proportions of different types of fibers also vary considerably among individuals for a given skeletal muscle. For example, a standard deviation of about 15 per cent is observed in the percentage of type I fibers in the vastus lateralis muscle of young adult males (the mean is about 50 per cent) (Malina & Bouchard, 1991). Overall, the contractile properties of skeletal muscle mature early in infancy.

Older Adulthood: The Development of Muscular Atrophy

The muscle wasting associated with the aging process is generally referred to as *senile muscular atrophy* (Schultz & Lipton, 1982). No distinct patterns of muscular atrophy for this age group are apparent. Some reports state that muscle loss is greater in the lower extremities, with the thigh muscles exhibiting greatest loss. However, functional patterns of the subjects involved in these reports were not well controlled. Actually, because the various muscles of the body are composed of different proportions of the three basic fiber types and are subjected to different degrees of functional demands, it should not be surprising that different muscles show different rates and magnitudes of muscle atrophy. The degree of atrophy associated with aging may be completely related to the activity level of the individual.

MECHANISMS OF MUSCLE ATROPHY

Atrophy of a muscle can result from a decrease in the number of fibers, a decrease in the diameter of myofibers, or a combination of both. The exact nature of the change in human muscle is unknown, but there are two schools of thought concerning changes that take place with age (Schultz & Lipton, 1982).

One theory states that in glycolytic (white) muscles, the diameter of IIb fibers decreases, but their number remains constant. There is a concurrent decrease in the number of IIa fibers, but their diameter remains the same. In oxidative muscles, there is a loss in the number of type IIa fibers. The other theory states that for all muscles there is a loss in the number of type II fibers such that the ratio of IIb/IIa remains constant and the ratio of II/I decreases. There is a small decrease in the diameter of all fibers. Although the two versions are on the surface quite different, it is important to point out that the net result of each one is an increased percentage of type I, or slow-twitch-oxidative, fibers in all muscles.

These morphologic changes are generally consistent with biochemical changes in the muscles with age. There is a reduction in virtually all enzymes per milligram of muscle with advanced age. Anaerobic enzymes exhibit the greatest reduction, which is consistent with the relative increase in type I fibers. However, with advanced age, the oxidative (slow-twitch) fibers rely more heavily on glycolysis. Functionally, the net result of these changes is first a reduction in strength based on the morphologic changes, and later a reduction in endurance because of biochemical changes within the fibers (Cress et al, 1984).

POSSIBLE CAUSES OF MUSCULAR ATROPHY OF OLDER ADULTS

The possible causes of senile muscular atrophy are many. Several of these will be presented.

Neural Factors. Many of the changes observed in the muscles of older adults resemble those changes found in denervated muscle; consequently, many investigators have speculated that some of the age-related changes may be the result of perturbations in the peripheral nervous system.

The hypothesis that aged muscle undergoes a "functional denervation"—that is, if there is inactivity and a muscle is not used, neural degeneration occurs, which promotes functional degeneration—continues to be the most popular among investigators attempting to explain the mechanism behind age-related atrophic changes (Schultz & Lipton, 1982).

Vascular Changes. Some investigators have suggested that age-related deterioration in skeletal muscle is related to a decrease in blood flow to the muscles. This suggestion is substantiated by morphologic studies that indicate a decrease in the ratio of capillaries to muscle fiber. An additional factor is the increase in the amount of connective tissue. Interestingly, the greatest increase in the laying down of additional connective tissue with age is in the area of the endomysium, the location of the capillary bed. In addition, the basement membrane increases in thickness around both the capillary and the myofiber. The net result of these changes (all mainly at the level of the endomysium) is an increase in diffusion distances, possibly producing an "age-related hypoxia." It is unknown whether chemical changes in the basement membrane, for example, may produce a selective barrier to certain essential molecules required by the muscle fibers. Little work has been carried out to actually measure muscular blood flow and verify any significant change with age.

Other Changes With Age

Collagen. The amount of connective tissue increases, mostly at the level of the endomysium. Collagen obtained from old muscle is less soluble and exhibits increased resistance to degradative enzymes such as collagenase. These changes in the collagen are all consistent with increased cross-linking or additional bonds between the collagen molecules and would explain the increase in "stiffness" of old muscle.

Motor Endplate. A number of morphologic changes are described for the aging neuromuscular junction (NMJ). The number of synaptic vesicles is increased with age, but they are found in tight clusters, suggesting that they have undergone agglutination. The synaptic cleft becomes enlarged, and the enlarged area is filled with thickened basal lamina. In addition, the junctional folds appear unfolded, and the plasma membrane of the muscle fiber appears thickened.

EFFECTS OF ANATOMIC AND PHYSIOLOGIC CHANGES ON THE ISOTONIC TWITCH CURVE

In general, in the older adult the three phases of the isotonic twitch curve are prolonged (see Fig. 7–6). The amplitude of the curve is also reduced. Table 7–1 summarizes factors contributing to the phase changes.

In phase I, the latency period of the twitch curve is prolonged. A major factor contributing to the increased latency period is a 10 to 15 per cent reduction in nerve conduction velocity. Once the impulse reaches the nerve terminal, portions of the following scenario may also play a role in further increasing the latency period. The nerve impulse should cause the release of

Table 7–1. FACTORS CONTRIBUTING TO PROLONGATION OF THE PHASES IN THE ISOTONIC TWITCH CURVE IN OLDER ADULTS

Phase I: Latency Period	Phase II: Contraction Phase	Phase III: Relaxation Period
Decreased conduction velocity	Disorganization of myofilaments	Decreased AChE at NMJ to inhibit muscle contraction
Agglutination of synaptic vesicles: Slowed release of ACH Decreased amount of ACH	Decreased ATPase activity	
	Decreased creatine phosphate levels	
Enlarged synaptic cleft	Decreased uptake of calcium by sarcoplasmic reticulum	
Decreased number of postsynaptic receptor sites		
Increased basement membrane thickness		

ACh from the synaptic vesicles. However, because many of the vesicles are clumped, the process of release is slowed, and the amount of ACh ultimately released is reduced. Because the synaptic cleft is enlarged, it takes longer for the substance to diffuse across the cleft to the postsynaptic membrane. The increased basement membrane material adds a further diffusion barrier. Once the ACh molecules have reached the postsynaptic membrane, there are fewer receptors for binding because of the unfolding of the synaptic folds. Membrane characteristics of the thickened sarcolemma may have changed sufficiently to decrease conduction velocity of muscle depolarization.

Phase II, the contraction phase, is also prolonged. Maximum contraction potentials are prolonged up to six times in aged individuals. Several factors may contribute to this increase. A disorganization of the myofilament lattice has been observed with the electron microscope and may indicate disruption of the contractile process at the molecular level. Calcium-activated ATPase activity is decreased with age. In addition, the levels of creatine phosphate are reduced with age. Creatine phosphate is a high-energy compound that transfers organic phosphate to ADP to produce ATP (creatine phosphate + ADP = ATP + keratin). Creatine phosphate is responsible for maintaining sufficiently high levels of ATP for muscle contraction to take place. Interestingly, although creatine phosphate decreases with age, the levels of creatine remain constant. Thus, the rate at which creatine is rephosphorylated is compromised with age. Finally, there is a reduced uptake of calcium by the sarcoplasmic reticulum.

Phase III, the relaxation period, is also prolonged. The amount of AChE at the NMJ is reduced. The net result is an increase in the time required to hydrolyze the ACh, allowing depolarization of the sarcolemma to continue.

FUNCTIONAL IMPLICATIONS

This section discusses the functional implications of the changes occurring in the development of skeletal muscle tissue across the life span. Muscle strength and endurance are emphasized.

Muscle strength is an expression of muscular force, or the individual's capacity to develop tension against an external resistance. The literature defines several types of strength: static, explosive (power), and dynamic (Rose & Rothstein, 1982). *Static strength* is referred to as isometric strength and is the force exerted against an external resistance without any change in muscle length. It is generally measured for specific muscle groups (e.g., grip strength of the hand, flexion or extension of the knee). *Explosive strength* or *power* is the ability of muscles to produce a certain amount of force in the shortest amount of time. It is measured as a function of strength and is thought to be more of an indicator of functional ability than static strength testing is. *Dynamic strength* is the force generated by repetitive contractions of muscles.

Muscle endurance is the ability to repeat or maintain muscular contractions over time. It is believed that the capacity of a muscle to increase in muscular endurance is related to the ability of the muscle to transport oxygen, or the *oxidative metabolism* of the muscle. This ability is related to the individual's maximal oxygen uptake, or *VO$_2$ max,* levels, This is defined as the transport of oxygen (O$_2$) from the atmosphere for utilization by the mitochondria of the muscle and is related to individual cardiovascular function (Frontera & Evans, 1986). Further discussion is found in Chapter 15.

Infancy to Adolescence: Static and Dynamic Strength

Information on strength measures is not very extensive for the early childhood and preschool ages. More information is available for the middle childhood and adolescent years. It is clear that muscular strength increases gradually during early infancy and early childhood. Sex differences in the early years are not significant. Thelen and colleagues (1984) hypothesize that certain reflexes (e.g., the stepping reflex) do not "disappear" or become "integrated" solely because of the maturation of the central nervous system, but are simply not seen during certain months of development because the infant is not strong enough to overcome gravity and produce the movement pattern. Thelen's research provides evidence that the "stepping reflex" observed in the upright posture is the same pattern of movement as the "kicking" pattern observed when the infant is placed in supine position. When an infant is no longer observed stepping in the upright posture, this same infant is observed kicking in the supine position. When the movement pattern of stepping is seen again, the infant has developed the muscular strength to overcome gravity. The central nervous system has matured, but so has the muscle bulk and strength of the infant. When the movement pattern reappears, it is more organized and appears to be under more voluntary control.

Strength is seen to increase linearly between the ages of 6 and 18 years (Figure 7–9). Boys appear to have a strength spurt during the adolescent years, which is due to hormone development. With increasing age, the percentage of girls whose performance on strength tests equals or exceeds that of boys declines considerably. After age 16, the average strength of boys is greater than the average strength of girls. Although growth studies generally stop at age 18, strength continues to increase into the third decade of life, especially for males.

Infancy to Adolescence: Muscular Endurance

Muscular endurance improves linearly with age from 5 to 13 or 14 years of age in boys, followed by a spurt similar to that for static muscular strength. Muscular endurance also increases with age in girls, but there is no clear evidence of a spurt as seen in the boys (Malina & Bouchard, 1991).

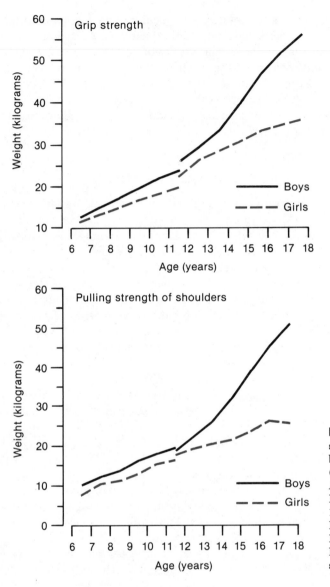

FIGURE 7–9. Mean grip strength and pulling strength between 6 and 18 years of age. (From *Growth, Maturation and Physical Activity.* [p. 191] by R.M. Malina and C. Bouchard, 1991. Champaign, IL: Human Kinetics. Copyright 1991 by Robert M. Malina and Claude Bouchard. Reprinted by permission.)

Adulthood and Aging: Strength

Strength in men is maximal between the ages of 30 and 35 years. Certain authors state that strength remains relatively constant until around 50 years of age, at which time it declines (Larsson et al, 1982; Asmussen, 1981). Others describe a loss in strength of approximately 1 per cent per year, starting at about age 30 years (Larsson, 1978; Sperling, 1980).

Researchers agree that the rate of decline in muscular strength with age appears to be slightly less in the upper extremities (i.e., small muscle groups) than in the back and legs (i.e., large muscle groups) (Asmussen, 1981; Grimby et al, 1982). Larsson et al (1982) evaluated 114 males, ages 11 to 70 years, for both static and dynamic lower extremity strength. Both strength and speed of contraction were found to decline with age. Studies of women indicate similar findings—that muscle strength, both static and dynamic, decreases with age. In women, this decrease in muscle strength may be observed earlier than in men (Grimby et al, 1982). It is generally considered that about 50 per cent of an individual's muscle strength is lost by the age of 70 years. Strength values of individuals (males or females) over the age of 75 years are very limited. Much of the strength loss in individuals apparently depends on individual activity level or fitness level. If the individual remains active, the amount of muscle strength loss may be less.

The majority of strength studies have measured isometric strength, which does not relate highly to functional skills (Aniansson & Gustafsson, 1981). Muscle power *does* relate to the ability to perform functional skills. As stated above, power diminishes with age. The loss of power with age may be the result of a loss of the fast-twitch muscle fibers. It remains unclear how significant this loss is to overall functional ability in the older adult. The degree of functional loss depends on many factors; the activity level of the individual is thought to be one of the more important factors (Aniansson et al, 1981; Aniansson & Gustafsson, 1981). It is generally thought that the decrease in strength is the result of a decrease in muscle quantity (reduction in muscle fiber numbers), whereas a decrease in muscle power is the result of altered muscle quality; however, this speculation remains to be documented.

Chapman and colleagues (1972) have demonstrated that elderly subjects who exercise can achieve increases in strength that are similar in magnitude to those one would expect in much younger subjects. Moritani and DeVries (1979) have suggested that much of the demonstrable strength gain in older individuals is the result of learning to recruit a larger number of motor units. Regardless of the mechanisms involved, it appears that the elderly can improve muscular strength and endurance and substantially improve their functional capacity.

Adulthood and Aging: Muscle Endurance

Numerous authors have reported that adaptation to endurance training is minimal for persons over 60 years of age (Berested, 1968; Wilmore et al, 1970). Other studies (DeVries, 1970; Sidney & Shephard, 1978) have documented significant strength and endurance improvements for older adults with resistive training. The improvement is especially seen when the older adult has had a sedentary lifestyle and when the improvement is expressed as a percentage of initial strength levels.

Endurance training of muscle is usually associated with training to increase oxidative capacity of aged skeletal muscle. Several studies have shown a significant increase in Vo_2 max in older men and women (Verg et al, 1985;

Heath et al, 1981). Verge and associates (1985) observed a 25 per cent increase in Vo_2 max after 1 year of training in a group of older individuals with a mean age of 63 years. Thomas and co-workers (1985) found that the best predictor of an elderly subject's Vo_2 max after 1 year of training is the initial Vo_2 max.

Heath and colleagues (1981) calculated that trained master athletes (males) have a decline in Vo_2 max of 5 per cent per year, whereas untrained older adults have a decline of 9 per cent per year. These findings support the hypothesis that the age-related decline in aerobic capacity is in part due to modifiable factors such as inactivity. Maximum aerobic power determines, to a large extent, an individual's capacity to perform the activities of daily living (ADL) without undue fatigue. The question is, can endurance training alter or slow the aging process? Current research suggests a positive answer to this question. However, more research is needed to further determine which factors are age-related and which factors are related to activity level or other non-age factors.

SUMMARY

Many factors can influence muscle development both before and after birth (i.e., genetics, nutrition, and activity levels). What is interesting is that muscle morphology changes only minimally with age. Functional changes over the life span with respect to muscle are also minimal if activity is maintained. As we age, maintaining functional independence has a great deal to do with remaining physically active.

Age-related changes in muscle cannot be stopped, but they can be slowed. The only known way to slow them is to maintain a healthy nutritional status and exercise on a regular basis. Human muscle status will remain responsive to these factors through most of the life span. Even aged muscle is trainable with the appropriate endurance and resistance goals.

References

Aniansson A, Grimby G, Rundgren A. Isometric and isokinetic quadriceps muscle strength in 70 year old men and women. *Scand J Rehabil Med* 12:161–168, 1980.

Aniansson A, Grimby G, Nygaard E, et al. Muscle fiber composition and fiber area in various age groups. *Muscle Nerve* 2:271–272, 1981.

Aniansson A, Gustafsson E. Physical training in elderly men with special reference to quadriceps muscle strength and morphology. *Clin Physiol* 1:87–98, 1981.

Asmussen E. Aging and exercise. In Horvath SM, Yousef MK (eds). *Environmental Physiology: Aging, Heat and Altitude*. New York: Elsevier/North-Holland, 1981.

Berested AM. Trainability of old men. *Acta Med Scand* 178:321–327, 1968.

Chapman EA, DeVries HA, Swezey R. Joint stiffness: Effects of exercise on young and old men. *J Gerontol* 21:182–191, 1972.

Colling-Saltin AS. Enzyme histochemistry on skeletal muscle of the human foetus. *J Neurol Sci* 39:169–185, 1978a.

Colling-Saltin AS. Some quantitative biochemical evaluations of developing skeletal muscles in the human foetus. *J Neurol Sci* 39:187–198, 1978b.

Crelin ES. Development of the musculoskeletal system. In Estler IA (ed). *Clinical Symposia* 33(1):2–36, 1981.

Cress ME, Byrnes WC, Dickinson AL, et al. Modification of type II fiber atrophy and LCH isozyme consequent of an 8 week endurance training program in elderly women. *Med Sci Sports Exerc* 16:2:243–245, 1984.

DeVries HA. Physiological effects of an exercise training regimen upon men aged 52 to 88. *J Gerontol* 25:235–336, 1970.

Frontera WR, Evans WJ. Exercise performance and endurance training in the elderly. *Top Geriatr Rehabil* 2:17–32, 1986.

Gibson MC, Schultz E. Fine structure of satellite cells in growing skeletal muscle. *Am J Anat* 147:49–70, 1976.

Gibson MC, Schultz E. The distribution of satellite cells and their relationship to specific fiber types in soleus and extensor digitorum longus muscles. *Anat Rec* 202:329–337, 1982.

Grimby G, Danneskiold-Samsoe B, Hvid K, et al. Morphology and enzymatic capacity in arm and leg muscles in 78–81 year old men and women. *Acta Physiol Scand* 115:125–134, 1982.

Heath GW, Hagberg JM, Ehsani AA, et al. A physiological comparison of young and older endurance athletes. *J Appl Physiol* 51:634–640, 1981.

Larsson L. Morphological and functional characteristics of the aging skeletal muscle in man. A cross-sectional study. *Acta Physiol Scand* 457(Suppl):1–36, 1978.

Larsson L, Grimby G, Karlsson J. Muscle strength and speed of movement in relation to age and muscle morphology. *J Appl Physiol* 46:451–456, 1982.

Malina RM, Bouchard C. *Growth, Maturation and Physical Activity.* Champaign, IL: Human Kinetics, 1991.

Mauro A. Satellite cell of skeletal muscle fibers. *J Biophys Biochem Cytol* 9:493–498, 1961.

Moore, KL. *The Developing Human, Clinical Oriented Embryology.* Philadelphia: WB Saunders, 1977.

Moritani T, DeVries HA. Neural factors versus hypertrophy in the time course of muscle strength gain in young and old men. *Am J Phys Med* 58:115–130, 1979.

Rose SJ, Rothstein JM. Muscle mutability, Part I: General concepts and adaptations to altered patterns of use. *Phys Ther* 62:1773–1785, 1982.

Schultz E, Lipton BH. Skeletal muscle satellite cells: Changes in proliferation potential as a function of age. *Mech Aging Dev* 20:377–383, 1982.

Sidney KH, Shephard RJ. Frequency and intensity of exercise training for elderly subjects. *Med Sci Sports Exerc* 10:125–131, 1978.

Sperling L. Evaluation of upper extremity function in 70 year old males and females. *Scand J Rehabil Med* 12:139–144, 1980.

Thelen E, Fisher DM, Ridley-Johnson R. The relationship between physical growth and a new-born reflex. *Infant Behav Dev* 7:479–493, 1984.

Thomas SG, Cunningham DA, Rechnitzer PA, et al. Determinants of the training response in elderly men. *Med Sci Sports Exerc* 17:667–672, 1985.

Verg JE, Seals DR, Hagberg JM, et al. Effects of endurance exercise training on ventilatory function in older individuals. *J Appl Physiol* 58:791–794, 1985.

Williams PL, Warwick R. *Gray's Anatomy,* 36th ed. Philadelphia: WB Saunders, 1980.

Wilmore JH, Royce J, Girandola RN, et al. Physiological alterations resulting from a 10 week program of jogging. *Med Sci Sports Exerc* 2:7–14, 1970.

Chapter 8

Cardiopulmonary System Changes

Objectives

AFTER STUDYING THIS CHAPTER, THE READER WILL BE ABLE TO:

1 Describe structural and functional characteristics of the cardiopulmonary system as they relate to physical functioning.
2 Discuss age-related structural and functional characteristics of the cardiopulmonary system.
3 Relate age-related changes in the cardiopulmonary system to physical functioning.

Together, the cardiovascular and pulmonary systems deliver necessary nutrients and oxygen to body tissues, as well as remove waste products. Blood, moving through the vascular system, provides the transport system for these substances. Oxygen is delivered to the blood via the pulmonary system. This chapter presents the structure, function, and development of these two systems as they relate to physical functioning.

COMPONENTS OF THE CARDIOPULMONARY SYSTEM

Cardiovascular System

COMPONENTS

The cardiovascular system is made up of the heart and the vascular network. Its purpose is to pump blood and deliver it throughout the body. The blood is pumped from the heart through a high-pressure arterial system to the target organs. There, nutrients and waste products are exchanged between capillaries and tissue. The low-pressure venous system then returns blood to the heart. *Heart rate* refers to the number of times the heart beats per minute; *stroke volume* refers to the amount of blood that is pumped from the ventricle with each heart beat. By multiplying heart rate by stroke volume, one can determine the amount of blood pumped from the ventricles in 1 minute, which is referred to as *cardiac output.*

Heart. The heart is made up of four chambers and acts as the pump of the cardiovascular system. Each of the chambers, the right and left atria and ventricles, acts as an individual pump, but they are coordinated. Figure 8–1 depicts postnatal circulation through the heart, lungs, and periphery. The *atria* move blood into the *ventricles,* which then pump with sufficient force to deliver blood to the lungs and the periphery. The chambers of the right side of the heart receive blood from the periphery and pump it to the lungs to be oxygenated. The chambers on the left side of the heart then receive the oxygenated blood and pump it through the aorta to the systemic circulation. Valves in the heart ensure unidirectional blood flow. The *tricuspid* and *mitral valves,* found between the atria and ventricles, prevent blood from flowing back into the atria during ventricular contraction. The *aortic* and *pulmonary valves,* also called the semilunar valves, prevent blood from flowing back into the ventricles from the aorta and pulmonary artery (McArdle et al, 1991).

Structurally, the heart is made up of three layers, which are also called *tunics* (Fig. 8–2). The inner layer, *endocardium,* is made up of a single layer of squamous endothelial cells and a layer of connective tissue. The connective tissue contains blood vessels, nerves, and branches of the heart's conducting system. The middle layer, *myocardium,* is the thick muscular layer of the heart and is richly supplied with capillaries. Cardiac muscle cells in the myocardium are able to conduct electricity, but they also have a long refractory period, allowing them to maintain rhythmic heart contraction. The outer layer, *epicardium,* is made up of loose connective tissue and fat that is covered by simple squamous epithelium. Large blood vessels, such as the coronary arteries, and nerves supplying the heart are found in the epicardium (Bacon & Niles, 1983; Junqueira et al, 1989; Leeson et al, 1988).

Contraction of the heart muscle is controlled by the cardiac conducting system, which consists of the sinoatrial (SA) node, atrioventricular (AV) node, and atrioventricular bundle of His (Fig. 8–3). The conduction system contains specialized cardiac muscle cells that carry impulses faster than other myocardial cells. The stimulus for cardiac contraction originates in the *SA node,* the pacemaker of the heart. The SA node is supplied by the nodal artery, a branch of the right carotid artery. Autonomic nerve and ganglion cells are also found near and in the node. These circulatory and nervous system influences help regulate heart rate and contractility. The *AV node* receives the impulse from the SA node and delays it slightly, allowing the atria time to empty before the ventricles contract. The *AV bundle of His* and its branches then carry the stimulus to the ventricles. From there, the contractile stimulus is transmitted from one cardiac muscle fiber to another, resulting in a wave of cardiac contraction (Bacon & Niles, 1983; Junqueira et al, 1989; Leeson et al, 1988). The conduction system of the heart is a coordinating system. Each part of it can conduct or initiate an impulse on its own, but because the SA node fires

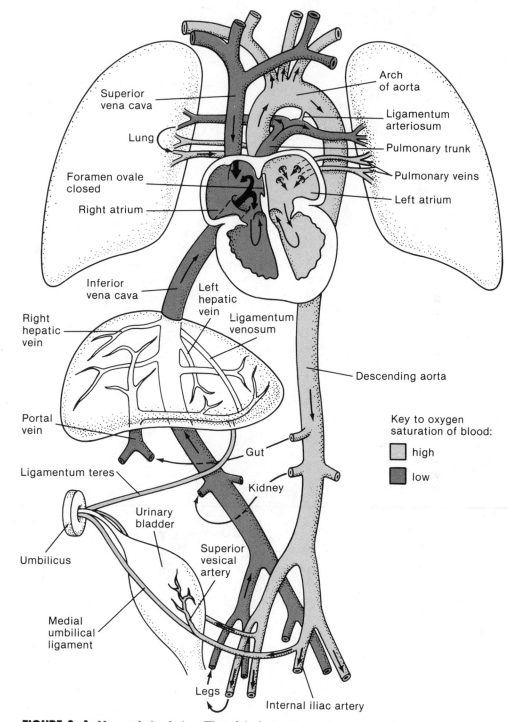

FIGURE 8–1. Neonatal circulation. The adult derivatives of the fetal vessels and structures that become nonfunctional at birth also are shown. The arrows indicate the course of the neonatal circulation. The organs are not drawn to scale. After birth, the three shunts that permitted blood to bypass the lungs during fetal life cease to function, and the pulmonary and systemic circulations separate. (From Moore KL. *The Developing Human,* 5th ed. Philadelphia: WB Saunders, 1993.)

Adventitia or pericardium

Media or myocardium

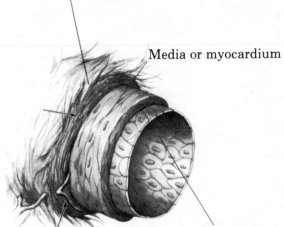

Intima or endocardium

FIGURE 8–2. Layers of the heart. (From Bacon RL, Niles NR. *Medical Histology: A Text-Atlas with Introductory Pathology.* New York: Springer-Verlag, 1983.)

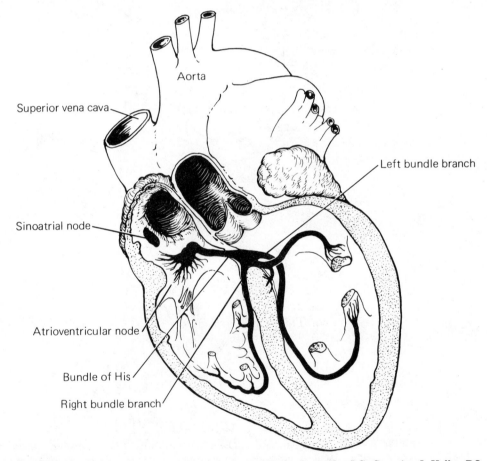

Aorta

Superior vena cava

Left bundle branch

Sinoatrial node

Atrioventricular node

Bundle of His

Right bundle branch

FIGURE 8–3. The conducting system of the heart. (From Junqueira LC, Carneiro J, Kelley RO. *Basic Histology,* 7th ed. Norwalk, CT: Appleton & Lange, 1992.)

first, the rhythm is controlled. When the SA node is not functioning properly, cardiac arrhythmias occur.

Vascular System. Three main types of vessels make up the vascular system: arteries, capillaries, and veins. Arteries and veins are structurally similar to the heart in that they are made up of three concentric layers (Fig. 8–4). The inner layer, *tunic intima,* is made up of a layer of endothelial cells and a subendothelial layer of elastic connective tissue. Some smooth muscle cells are also found in the subendothelial layer. The middle layer, *tunic media,* consists of concentric layers of smooth muscle cells, elastic fibers, collagen fibers, and proteoglycons. The outer layer, *tunic adventitia,* is made up of fibroelastic connective tissue. The fibers are arranged parallel to the vessel and become continuous with the connective tissue of the organ through which the vessel is running. Small blood vessels, *vasa vasorum,* are found in the media and adventitia layers of large vessels. They nourish the thicker layers of the vessel, where sufficient nutrition cannot be supplied by diffusion from the circulating blood.

Arteries carry blood from the heart to the rest of the body and minimize fluctuations in pressure caused by the heart beat. For instance, when the ventricles contract, the arteries are stretched, decreasing pressure. When the ventricles relax, the arteries return to their original size and maintain the level of pressure.

Arteries can be divided into three groups. The large elastic arteries, called *conducting arteries,* include the aorta and its main branches. The tunic media of these vessels is made up of layers of elastic membrane, which makes them efficient at absorbing the pressure changes that accompany each heart beat. The number of layers increases from 40 layers in the newborn to 70 layers in the adult. The second category, the *muscular* or *distributing arteries,* are branches of the large elastic arteries that supply blood to the organs and extremities. The tunic media of the distributing arteries is made of up to 40 layers of smooth muscle cells that regulate blood flow in response to nervous system or hormonal input. Connective tissue, including elastic and collagen fibers, can be found between the muscular layers. The third category of arteries, the *arterioles,* are small vessels that deliver blood to the capillaries. The tunic intima of the arteriole consists of a layer of endothelium and an internal elastic membrane. The tunic media is made of one to five layers of smooth muscle cells and a few elastic fibers. Vasoconstriction and vasodilation of the arterioles control the systemic blood pressure so that only a slow steady stream of blood enters the capillaries. The arterioles are innervated by the autonomic nervous system and can quickly react to functional needs of the tissue (Bacon & Niles, 1983; Junqueira et al, 1989; Leeson et al, 1988).

Capillaries provide a site for the exchange of nutrients and waste products between the blood and the tissue, connect the arterial and venous systems, and contain a large volume of the blood in the body. The capillary itself is a small vessel, made up of a single layer of endothelial cells surrounded by a thin layer of collagen fibers. A very large network of capillaries branches off the arteriole

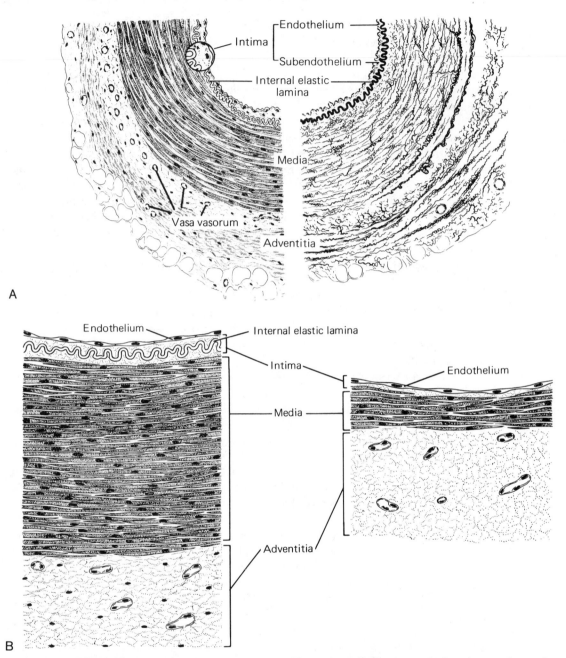

FIGURE 8–4. *A,* Three layers of an artery. The tunic media is composed of a mixture of smooth muscle and elastic fibers. The adventitia and the outpart of the media have small blood vessels (vasa vasorum) and collagenous fibers. *B,* Comparison of muscular artery (left) and accompanying vein (right). (From Junqueira LC, Carneiro J, Kelley RO. *Basic Histology,* 7th ed. Norwalk, CT: Appleton & Lange, 1992.)

system; the surface area of the capillary network is 6000 m² (Junqueira et al, 1989). Areas of the body with high metabolic needs, such as the lungs, liver, kidneys, and skeletal muscle, have large capillary networks.

Veins are responsible for carrying blood back to the heart and for transport of waste products from the tissue. Seventy per cent of the total blood volume can be found in the venous system of the body (Junqueira et al, 1989). Veins have larger diameters and thinner walls than arteries. Because of their size and the large number of veins that make up the venous system, blood flows back to the heart slowly and at low pressure.

Veins can be divided into three major categories by size. *Venules,* the smallest veins, receive blood from the capillaries. The diameter of the venule is greater than that of the capillary and serves to slow the rate of blood flow. As the venule size increases, layers of connective tissue and then smooth muscle cells are added. When the size of the venule is approximately 50 μm, elastic fibers and smooth muscle fibers can be found between the tunic intima and the tunic adventitia. At greater than 200 μm, muscle fibers make up the tunic media of the venule (Leeson et al, 1988). The next category of *small to medium-sized* veins includes most named veins in the body and their branches. These veins contain valves that maintain unidirectional flow of blood. The tunic intima and tunic media are thin, whereas the tunic adventitia is thick. The *large veins* make up the third category of veins and include the superior vena cava, inferior vena cava, portal vein, pulmonary veins, abdominal veins, and main tributaries. The tunic adventitia is the thickest and most developed component of these veins, containing longitudinal bundles of smooth muscle fibers. These muscle cells strengthen the venous wall and help to prevent distension (Junqueira et al, 1989; Leeson et al, 1988).

CONTROL

Regulation of heart rate and dilation/constriction of the vessels of the vascular system are influenced by the autonomic nervous system and by the presence of chemicals in the circulation. Nervous system control originates in the medulla and is carried via the sympathetic and parasympathetic branches of the autonomic nervous system.

Autonomic fibers are found within the cardiac conducting system. Sympathetic input to the heart increases the rate and strength of cardiac contraction via release of catecholamines (epinephrine and norepinephrine). Sympathetic innervation of smooth muscle cells in the tunic media of the arteries and the tunic media and tunic adventitia of the veins stimulates vasoconstriction. Parasympathetic input to the heart is received via the vagus nerve and slows the heart rate by releasing acetylcholine. Skeletal muscle arteries also dilate in response to parasympathetic input.

The vascular system relates sensory information to the nervous system through the stretch-sensitive baroreceptors, found in the aorta and carotid sinus, and the chemoreceptors, found in the carotid and aortic bodies. These receptors react to changes in blood pressure, levels of oxygen and carbon dioxide in the circulating blood, and acidity (pH) of the blood (Bacon & Niles, 1986; Junqueira et al, 1989).

MECHANICS OF CIRCULATION

Blood flow is regulated by pressures exerted by the various structures in the system. Within the heart, *preload* is the amount of pressure necessary to stretch the ventricles during cardiac filling. *Afterload* is the amount of pressure that must be exerted by the ventricles to overcome aortic pressure, open the aortic valve, and push the blood out toward the periphery. The vessels then continue to control blood flow, not only because of the neural and chemical influences described above, but also because of their physical properties. Length and diameter of the vessels help determine peripheral vascular resistance and influence the speed of blood flow. Blood pressure is actually the pressure exerted by the blood on the vessels as it flows through them.

For efficient mechanical control of blood flow, the blood pressure must be sufficient for blood to flow through the system and must stretch the ventricles during preload. It must likewise not be so high that afterload is increased, making the ventricles work harder to overcome aortic pressure and empty. In individuals with hypertension (high blood pressure), the chronic increased aortic pressure eventually leads to left ventricular hypertrophy because the ventricle has been working so hard to maintain adequate stroke volume. This can eventually contribute to congestive heart failure.

Pulmonary System

COMPONENTS

The pulmonary system consists of the lungs and the structures that connect the lungs to the external environment. It is a closed system, open to the external environment only at the nose and mouth. The system can be divided into two major functional parts, the conducting portion and the respiratory portion (Fig. 8–5).

The *conducting portion* of the pulmonary system provides a pathway for air to travel between the environment and the lungs. In this portion no gas exchange takes place, but the air is cleaned, moistened, and warmed. The conducting portion of the pulmonary system includes the nose, pharynx, larynx, and trachea and portions of the bronchial tree in the lungs. The conducting portion of the bronchial tree includes the two main bronchi, bronchi to the main lobes and to the segments of the lungs, and bronchioles. The diameter of these conducting tubes decreases with each successive branching, helping to regulate the flow of air during inspiration and expiration. The *bronchi* are made up of hyaline cartilage and smooth muscle cells. The muscle cells are arranged in spirals and increase in number closer to the respiratory portion of the pulmonary system. The *bronchioles* are made of smooth muscle cells and elastic fibers. Sympathetic nervous system input via the vagus nerve influences

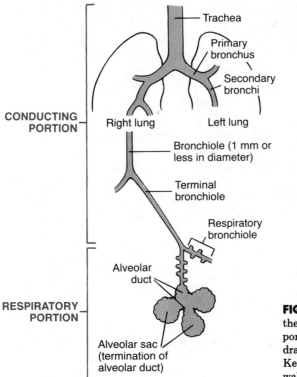

CONDUCTING PORTION

Trachea

Primary bronchus

Secondary bronchi

Right lung

Left lung

Bronchiole (1 mm or less in diameter)

Terminal bronchiole

Respiratory bronchiole

Alveolar duct

RESPIRATORY PORTION

Alveolar sac (termination of alveolar duct)

FIGURE 8-5. The main divisions of the pulmonary system: the conducting portion and the respiratory portion. (Redrawn from Junqueira LC, Carneiro J, Kelley RO. *Basic Histology,* 7th ed. Norwalk, CT: Appleton & Lange, 1992.)

contraction of the smooth muscle cells, and conducting vessels in the bronchial tree change in length and diameter.

The *respiratory portion* of the pulmonary system includes the remaining branches of the bronchial tree, alveolar ducts, alveolar sacs, and alveoli. As air is moved through these structures, gas exchange takes place. Respiratory bronchioles differ from conducting bronchioles because they have alveoli along their walls. *Alveoli* are small air sacs where gas exchange can take place because only a very thin barrier is found between the air and the circulating blood. Alveoli are not found only in the respiratory bronchioles; large numbers of alveoli branch off of the alveolar ducts and alveolar sacs. If the total alveolar surface could be flattened out, 150 m² of surface area would be available for gas exchange (Leeson et al, 1988). *Alveolar sacs* (clusters of alveoli) and alveoli branch off of *alveolar ducts,* which contain smooth muscle cells, elastic fibers, and collagen fibers. Elastic and reticular fibers are found where the alveoli arise from the respiratory bronchioles, alveolar ducts, or alveolar sacs. The elastic fibers help to open the alveoli during inspiration and allow recoil during exhalation. Reticular fibers help maintain the shape of the alveoli.

Alveolar epithelium is made up of two types of cells. *Type I* alveolar cells are flat and thin respiratory epithelial cells, providing a large surface area for gas exchange. *Type II* cells are responsible for the production of *surfactant,* the detergent-like substance that mixes with water to decrease the alveolar surface tension. The decreased surface tension allows the alveoli to open more easily during respiration. This is especially important for the newborn—lack of surfactant in the premature infant results in respiratory distress. Surfactant is constantly produced and turned over throughout life.

Air can also move from one part of the respiratory system to another via collateral ventilation mechanisms. Two mechanisms of collateral ventilation are pores of Kohn and Lambert's canals. Little is known about these structures, so the functional significance of their absence can only be hypothesized. *Pores of Kohn* are gaps in the alveolar walls that provide an opening from one alveolus and its neighbor. *Lambert's canals* or *channels* are small pathways from the respiratory bronchi to nearby alveoli.

CONTROL/REGULATION

Ventilation is controlled by input from the respiratory center of the central nervous system, located in the brain stem. Chemoreceptors detect changes in blood levels of oxygen and carbon dioxide as well as the pH of the blood, stimulating appropriate respiratory changes. Proprioceptive input from stretch receptors in the lungs also stimulates respiration.

The pulmonary system is innervated by the parasympathetic and sympathetic branches of the autonomic nervous system. Parasympathetic input results in bronchial constriction, whereas sympathetic input results in bronchodilation. Sensory and motor nerve fibers are found in the lung to the level of the terminal bronchioles. Some studies have reported sensory endings to the level of the alveoli and suggest that these receptors are responsible for increased levels of surfactant secretion with nervous stimulation (Leeson et al, 1988).

MECHANICS OF VENTILATION

The lungs, thorax, intercostal muscles, and diaphragm provide a pumping action that transports gas between the alveoli and the environment. During inspiration, the intercostal muscles contract to elevate the rib cage. The diaphragm also contracts, increasing the diameter of the thoracic cavity. This muscle activity expands the pleural cavity and results in increased negative pressure in the thoracic cavity. Atmospheric air rushes in and the lungs expand. Bronchi and bronchioles increase in diameter. The expansion of the lungs activates stretch receptors, inhibiting inspiration. Exhalation occurs passively, with muscle relaxation and elastic recoil of the chest wall. Inhibitory input to inspiration is decreased, once again activating inspiration.

The ability of the musculoskeletal pump to transport inspiratory and expiratory gases is influenced by the compliance and resistance of the chest wall and lungs. Flexibility of the joints of the thoracic cavity contributes to

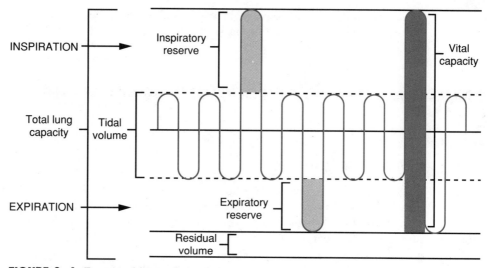

FIGURE 8–6. Functional lung volumes.

achieving optimal expansion of the space. Resistance and elasticity of the pulmonary tissues must be overcome by the contraction of the respiratory muscles, diaphragm, intercostals, and accessory muscles of respiration. Resistance of the conducting airways also affects the amount of work necessary to deliver oxygen to the tissues.

The amount of air contained in the lungs is defined by various functional volumes (Fig. 8–6). The amount of air moved during resting inspiration and exhalation is referred to as the *tidal volume (V_T)*. The additional inspired air that can be taken into the lungs with a deep breath is called the *inspiratory reserve volume (IRV)*; the additional air that can be pushed out of the lungs with forced exhalation is called the *expiratory reserve volume (ERV)*. The sum of these three volumes is called the *vital capacity (VC)*. The *residual volume (RV)* is the amount of air that is left in the lungs after exhalation. *Minute ventilation (MV)* is the total amount of air exchanged by the pulmonary system in 1 minute.

Resistance and compliance factors, the breathing rate, and the amount of air being moved with each breath determine the energy cost of breathing. The pulmonary system itself requires oxygen to fuel the work of breathing. The source of that oxygen is the bronchial arteries, which deliver blood from the aorta to the lung tissue. Blood is then returned to the heart via the pulmonary and bronchial veins.

A second source of pulmonary circulation originates in the pulmonary artery, which carries deoxygenated blood from the right ventricle to the lungs. This artery branches in conjunction with the bronchial tree to the level of the respiratory bronchioles. From here a capillary network is formed, accompanying the alveoli. Other branches from the pulmonary artery are sent to the periphery of the lungs. Pulmonary venules arise from the capillary network and branch into successively larger veins through the bronchial tree. The pulmonary veins carry the blood back to the heart.

CARDIOPULMONARY SYSTEM DEVELOPMENT ACROSS THE LIFE SPAN

Prenatal Period

CARDIOVASCULAR SYSTEM

The cardiovascular system is the earliest system of the body to function in the developing embryo, with blood circulation starting in the 3rd week of gestation. Functionally this circulation is necessary because the embryo has grown, and simple diffusion of nutrients and waste products across cell membranes can no longer meet nutritional demands.

The *heart* is developed as a recognizable structure between 20 and 50 gestational days. By the end of the 3rd week of gestation, a primitive heart tube has been formed from clusters of mesoderm cells. As this tube elongates, a series of dilatations and constrictions differentiate the vessel into an atrium, a ventricle, the truncus arteriosus, and the sinus venosus (Fig. 8–7). The *sinus venosus* functions early as the pacemaker of the conducting system of the heart and is the precursor to the sinoatrial node, atrioventricular node, and bundle of His. At approximately 4 weeks of gestation, areas of swelling form on the walls of the atrioventricular canal. These swellings, called *endocardial cushions,* grow together during the 5th week of gestation and begin to divide the heart into left and right chambers. The primitive atrium is also divided into two chambers by the formation of the septum primum and the septum secundum. An oval opening left between the interatrial septae, called the *foramen ovale,* is important for fetal circulation. Near the end of the 4th week of gestation, contractions of the heart coordinate unidirectional flow of blood. By the 7th week, the heart tube has become a four-chambered vessel (Fig. 8–8).

The embryo's primitive heart tube establishes links with its blood vessels and with the placenta as early as the 13th to 15th day of gestation. Circulation is then established between the mother and the embryo, ensuring exchange of nutrients and waste products. Maternal nutrients and oxygen are transported to the fetus via the *umbilical vein;* waste products and carbon dioxide are removed via the *umbilical artery.* By the 5th week of development, embryonic vessel formation is underway.

Fetal circulation is depicted in Figure 8–9. The fetus receives all necessary oxygen from the mother; little blood flow is necessary through the lungs. The foramen ovale and ductus arteriosus in the fetal heart allow blood to circumvent the pulmonary system. The *foramen ovale* shunts blood from the right to the left atrium. The *ductus arteriosus* shunts blood from the right ventricle to the pulmonary artery and the aorta. These two shunts will close at birth,

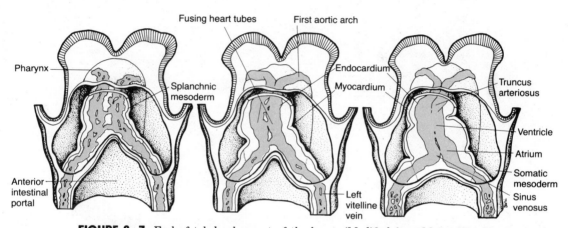

FIGURE 8-7. Early fetal development of the heart. (Modified from Moore KL. *The Developing Human,* 5th ed. Philadelphia: WB Saunders, 1993.)

allowing blood to enter the pulmonary circulation. Fetal hemoglobin has a greater capacity to bind oxygen than postnatal hemoglobin, because the oxygen saturation of blood coming to the fetus from the umbilical vein is only 70 per cent, as compared to an arterial blood oxygen saturation of 97 per cent after birth.

PULMONARY SYSTEM

The pulmonary system of the embryo arises from both endodermal and mesodermal germ cells and first appears in the 4th week of gestation. Endodermal cells from the primitive pharynx form the epithelial lining of trachea, larynx, bronchi, and lungs. Mesoderm surrounding the developing lung buds contributes to the development of smooth muscle, connective tissue, and cartilage within these structures.

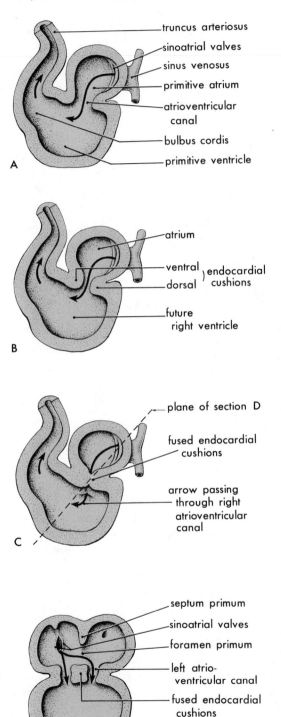

FIGURE 8–8. Fetal heart development: *A–C,* Sagittal sections of the heart during the 4th and 5th weeks, illustrating division of the atrioventricular canal. *D,* Coronal section of the heart at the plane shown in *C.* Note that the interatrial and interventricular septa have also started to develop.

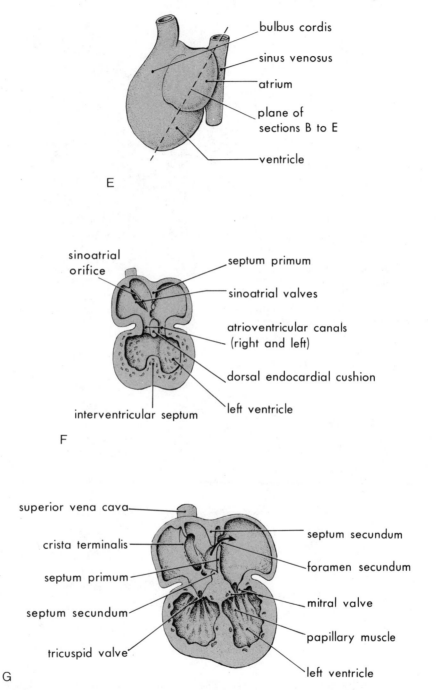

FIGURE 8–8 *Continued E,* Sketch showing the plane of the coronal section. *F,* During the 4th week (about 28 days), the septum primum, interventricular septum, and dorsal endocardial cushion first appear. *G,* At about 8 weeks, the heart is partitioned into four chambers. (From Moore KL. *The Developing Human,* 5th ed. Philadelphia: WB Saunders, 1993.)

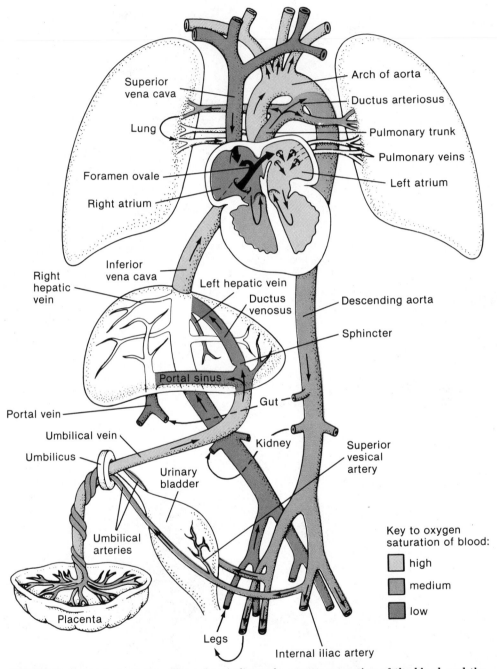

FIGURE 8–9. Fetal circulation. The colors indicate the oxygen saturation of the blood, and the arrows show the course of the fetal circulation. The organs are not drawn to scale. Three shunts permit most of the blood to bypass the liver and the lungs: the ductus venosus, the foramen ovale, and the ductus arteriosus. (From Moore KL. *The Developing Human*, 5th ed. Philadelphia: WB Saunders, 1993.)

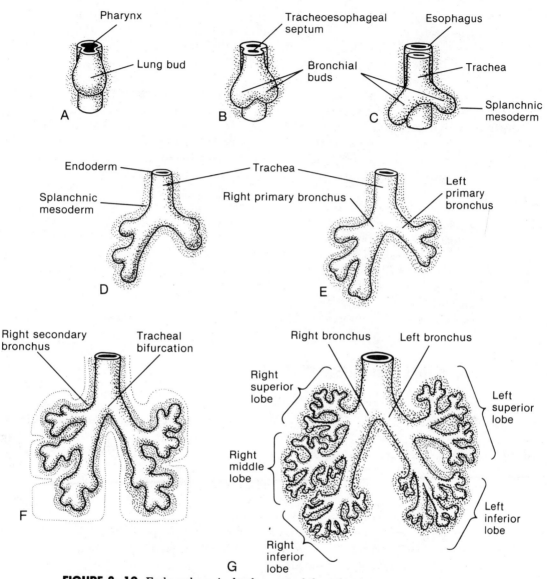

FIGURE 8–10. Early embryonic development of the pulmonary system. *A–C*, 4 weeks. *D* and *E*, 5 weeks. *F*, 6 weeks. *G*, 8 weeks. (From Moore KL. *The Developing Human*, 5th ed. Philadelphia: WB Saunders, 1993.)

Early development of the pulmonary system is shown in Figure 8–10. A single *lung bud* develops at the end of the laryngotracheal tube; the lung bud divides into the right and left lung buds and their main bronchi. By 16 weeks of gestation, all of the branches of the conducting airways are formed. Between 16 and 24 weeks of gestation, branching continues to the level of at least two respiratory bronchioles. Formation of the pulmonary arterial tree accompanies the branching of the respiratory tree. The bronchial epithelium thins and flattens, increasing the diameter of the bronchi and terminal bronchioles. Capillaries also appear in the epithelium. From 24 weeks of gestation until birth, development of *terminal respiratory units* continues. These may also be referred to as *terminal sacs* or *primitive alveoli*. Type II epithelial cells appear in the lining of the primitive alveoli, and surfactant production begins. By 26 to 28 weeks of gestation, the fetus has enough vascularized terminal sacs and surfactant to survive if born prematurely. Primitive alveoli multiply in the last few weeks of the normal gestational period. The structure of the primitive alveoli becomes more complex, and the number of alveoli increase after birth until approximately 8 to 12 years of age (Moore 1988; Murray, 1986).

The interuterine lung is not responsible for gas exchange. Weak attempts at fetal breathing appear to be in preparation for respiration after birth. Instead, the lung tissue secretes liquid that is swallowed or added to amniotic fluid. This fluid production slows shortly before birth, decreasing the amount of fluid that will need to be removed as the lungs inflate after birth. A second major function of the lung is production of surfactant, which allows maximum lung expansion after birth (Murray, 1986). Like the cardiovascular system, the pulmonary system undergoes dramatic change in the moments after birth.

Infancy and Young Childhood

CARDIOPULMONARY ADJUSTMENTS AT BIRTH

Immediately after birth, blood must be circulated to the lung tissue, and the lungs must inflate. Much of the fluid filling the lungs is pushed out during the birth process; remaining fluid can be drained by the lymphatic system. With each of the first breaths, more and more air is retained in the lungs, building up the newborn's functional residual capacity (residual volume plus expiratory reserve volume). With inspiration, alveolar expansion occurs, delivering oxygenated air to the alveoli (Murray, 1986).

After birth, blood must be shunted into the pulmonary circulation to receive oxygen from the alveoli. As the lungs expand, pulmonary vascular resistance decreases, and blood flow to the lungs increases. With the occlusion of the umbilical cord, the ductus venosus, which had delivered blood from the umbilical vein to the inferior vena cava, closes. This results in decreased pressure in the inferior vena cava and right atrium. As left atrial pressure becomes greater than right atrial pressure, the foramen ovale closes. Another circulatory change occurs as increased systemic and aortic pressure pump the blood toward the pulmonary artery, reversing the direction of blood flow through the ductus arteriosus. The ductus arteriosus constricts and eventually closes. The transition from fetal to postnatal circulation can be seen by comparing Figures 8-1 and 8-9 (Malina & Bouchard, 1991; Moore 1988).

CARDIOVASCULAR SYSTEM

The newborn heart lies horizontally in the chest cavity, but as the lungs expand and the chest cavity grows, a more vertical position is assumed. Irregularity in the electrocardiogram (ECG) of the newborn is not unusual, because stabilization of the autonomic nervous system, conductivity of cardiac muscle fibers, heart position, and hemodynamics are not yet completed (Malina & Bouchard, 1991).

Heart size increases at a rate similar to that of the increase in fat-free body weight. Heart volumes are approximately 40 ml at birth, 80 ml at 6 months, and 160 ml by 2 years of age. The ratio of heart volume to body weight remains constant at approximately 10 ml/kg body weight. Although there is no increase in the number of cardiac muscle fibers as the heart grows, the cross-sectional area of the fibers increases. The vascularization of the heart muscle increases from one vessel for six muscle fibers in the newborn to one vessel for each muscle fiber, as seen in the adult. At birth the thickness of the right and left ventricle walls is equal, but as the left ventricle starts pumping against increased pressure, the left ventricular wall increases in size and becomes approximately twice as thick as the right ventricular wall by adulthood (Sinclair, 1985).

Arteries and veins also increase in size as body weight and height increase. As increased functional demands are placed on the vessels, increased thickness of the vessel wall is seen. Development of smooth muscle within the walls of the vessels occurs more slowly. No muscle cells are present at birth in the alveolar blood vessels. Muscle cells can be seen in pulmonary vasculature at the level of the respiratory bronchiole by 4 months of age, and at the alveolar ducts by 3 years of age. Some alveolar arteries have muscle cells in their walls at 10 years, but others do not complete this process until 19 years of age (Murray, 1986).

Heart rate and stroke volume of infants and young children are very different from those of adults. Because stroke volume is related to heart size, the smaller the heart, the less blood can be pumped with each heart beat. At birth, stroke volume is only 3 to 4 ml, whereas it may be 40 ml in the preadolescent and 60 ml in the young adult. To compensate for smaller stroke volumes, children demonstrate higher heart rates. As summarized in Table 8–1, the newborn heart rate may be 120 to 140 beats per minute (bpm). This value drops to 100 bpm by 1 year of age, 80 bpm by age 6, and 70 bpm by age 10. Boys and girls younger than 10 years of age have similar heart rates (Malina & Bouchard, 1991).

Blood pressure also changes from infancy to early childhood. These changes are related to ongoing development of (1) the autonomic nervous system, (2) peripheral vascular resistance, and (3) body mass. Mean systolic blood pressure values change with age, from 40 to 75 mm Hg in the newborn, to 83 to 88 mm Hg in the 2-year-old, and to 95 mm Hg in the 5-year-old. Blood pressure continues to rise until adolescence; no difference is seen be-

	Heart Rate (bpm)	Systolic Blood Pressure (mm Hg)	Diastolic Blood Pressure	Breathing Rate (breaths per minute)
Table 8-1. MEASURES OF CARDIOPULMONARY FUNCTION IN CHILDREN				
Newborn	120–140	40–75	50–55	40
1-year-old	100	80	50–55	30
5-year-old	80	95	50–55	22

tween boys and girls. Diastolic blood pressure is reported to be relatively constant through childhood, at 50 to 55 mm Hg (Malina & Bouchard, 1991).

Blood volume also increases with body size. The total blood volume of the newborn is 300 to 400 ml, whereas the adolescent or young adult has approximately 5 L of blood. Hemoglobin levels in the blood also vary with age, affecting the oxygen-carrying capacity of the blood. In the newborn, hemoglobin levels are high (20 g/100 ml), but they fall to 10 g/100 ml by 3 to 6 months of age. Hemoglobin values then slowly increase with age to adult levels of 16 g/100 ml for men and 14 g/100 ml for women (Malina & Bouchard, 1991).

PULMONARY SYSTEM

Only a small percentage of the total number of alveoli to be developed are present at birth. Most sources agree that new alveoli develop until approximately 8 to 12 years of age, when the adult number of 300 million alveoli is attained (DeCesare & Graybill, 1990; Murray, 1986; Tecklin, 1989). The size and complexity of the alveoli increase throughout infancy and childhood, increasing the available surface area for air exchange. The growth of the alveolar surface appears to be related to the increased oxygen demand of working tissue. The pulmonary arterial and venous supplies develop concurrently with the development of alveoli.

The conducting and respiratory airways increase in length and diameter until growth of the thoracic cavity is complete. Children under age 5 years have a larger number of small airways measuring under 2 mm in diameter. For example, 50 per cent of airways in the neonate and 20 per cent of airways in the adult have diameters less than 2 mm (DeCesare & Graybill, 1990). Small airways can be problematic in two ways. First, they offer increased resistance to airflow, thereby increasing the work of breathing. Second, they are very easily obstructed by foreign objects.

The bronchioles and alveoli of infants and young children are weaker and less efficient than those of adults. Smooth muscle in the walls of the bronchioles does not develop until the child is 3 to 4 years old. As a result, the airway is more susceptible to collapse, thus trapping air. The development of elastic tissue in the alveoli may be incomplete until after adolescence; this means decreased lung compliance and distensibility for infants and young children. This makes it harder for the infant and small child to fully inflate their lungs and maintain lung volume. In children under the age of 7 years, decreased elastic recoil causes the airways to close at greater lung volume than in older children and adults. When combined with small airway size, this relative lack of recoil places young children more at risk for complications from small airway diseases such as bronchiolitis (DeCesare & Graybill, 1990).

Lung volume increases proportionally with increases in body size and also increases as the number of alveoli increases (Malina & Bouchard, 1991). Size of the conducting airways is related to stature, and the total number of alveoli an individual develops is proportional to height, which reinforces the relationship between lung volume and body size (Murray, 1986).

One other structural difference between the pulmonary systems of children and adults is the absence of collateral ventilation mechanisms in children. This decreased collateral circulation may increase the risk of respiratory infection and atelectasis in children. Pores of Kohn have not been seen in children younger than 6 years of age. Lambert's canals are not thought to develop until at least 6 to 8 years of age (Boyden, 1977; Meyrick & Reid, 1977).

From a mechanical point of view, the shape of the chest wall and limitations in posture and movement also affect the infant's breathing efficiency. At birth, the infant maintains a posture of shoulder elevation, limiting the cervical dimensions of the thorax. The ribs are also in a horizontal position, giving the lower thorax a circular dimension. This structural immaturity, combined with a lack of development and control of the abdominal muscles, prevents the infant from stabilizing the rib cage and effectively using the diaphragm to breathe. As the infant learns to move the head and upper body against gravity and to reach in the first 3 to 6 months, muscular development allows increased expansion and use of the upper chest in breathing. In the second half of the first year, the infant learns to sit, stand, and walk, systematically overcoming the force of gravity. As the upright sitting position is assumed, the force of gravity and forces from developing abdominal musculature will pull the ribs downward into a more angular position. This not only expands the thoracic cavity but also increases spacing between the ribs, allowing the intercostal muscles to work more efficiently. With growth, the diaphragm is pulled into a dome shape that improves the length-tension relationship of the muscle and improves function. Active use of the abdominal muscles stabilizes the rib cage within the thorax, providing a stable base for diaphragmatic action (Massery, 1991).

In summary, the development of the lungs into their adult form continues well into childhood. Differences between the child's and the adult's pulmonary function are seen in breathing pattern and in breathing frequency. The newborn infant undergoes dramatic changes in intrathoracic pressure, lung inflation, and pulmonary circulation. It is not unusual to observe irregular breathing patterns, including periods of apnea, during this time. Small airway size, together with the limited number of developed alveoli, leave the young infant with a small lung volume. The newborn breathes at a rate of approximately 40 breaths per minute. As seen in Table 8–1, by 1 year of age this has decreased to 30 breaths per minute, and by 5 to 6 years to 22 breaths per minute (Malina & Bouchard, 1991). In the first year of life, the infant has little pulmonary reserve and must increase breathing frequency to meet demands for increased oxygen. IRVs and ERVs sufficient to meet increased needs are evident at about age 1 year.

Adolescence

Growth and functional changes of the cardiopulmonary system continue through childhood and into adolescence. During the adolescent growth spurt, gender differences in cardiopulmonary function become apparent.

The amount of muscle in the heart increases, resulting in increased blood pressure and decreased heart rate (Sinclair, 1985). Increased blood pressure is primarily related to increased body weight. The systolic blood pressure of boys becomes slightly greater than that of girls. Gender differences in heart rate are also reported: the basal heart rate of girls is 3 to 5 bpm faster than that of boys. Heart rate stabilizes by age 16 at 57 to 60 bpm in males and 62 to 63 bpm in females (Malina & Bouchard, 1991; Porter, 1989). Stroke volume also increases but does not appear to be related only to heart size. In the year preceding the peak height velocity (PHV), stroke volume changes appear to be related to an increased arterial-venous oxygen difference. This implies that more oxygen is being extracted by the tissues, which may be due to age-related changes in muscle mass, muscle enzyme profusion, and the ratio of capillaries to muscle fiber. In the year after PHV, increased stroke volume may be related to an increased cardiac preload condition with increased venous return (Cunningham et al, 1984).

The adolescent growth spurt is also reflected in lung size and lung volume. Proximal airways and vasculature increase in size. Alveoli become larger, and greater amounts of elastic fiber can be found in the alveolar wall. The capillaries in the alveolar region also get larger, supporting increased gas exchange. By age 19, muscle is developed in the walls of the arteries found at the alveoli, increasing the efficient control of blood flow by vasodilation and vasoconstriction (Davis & Dobbings, 1981).

Adulthood and Aging

Normal function of the cardiopulmonary systems in early and middle adulthood is described in the beginning of this chapter. Heart size and weight may continue to increase in adulthood, primarily because of fat deposition (Sinclair, 1985). Some gender differences in function of the cardiopulmonary systems do exist. Stroke volume, residual lung volume, mean heart weight, and body surface area are greater in men than in women (Payne & Isaacs, 1987). Age-related changes in mean heart weight are not demonstrated in men, but in women, the mean heart weight increases between the fourth and seventh decades of life (Kitzman & Edwards, 1990). During submaximal exercise, the cardiac output of women is 5 to 10 per cent greater than that of men. This may be related to stroke volume differences and the fact that women have slightly less hemoglobin (14 g/100 ml blood) than men (15 to 16 g/100 ml blood).

With increasing age, anatomic and physiologic changes in the cardiopulmonary systems are seen. At least initially, these age-related changes do not seem to significantly interfere with function. Functional losses are more evident beginning in the seventh decade of life (Cunningham & Paterson, 1990). It is also difficult to differentiate cardiopulmonary changes related purely to aging from those due to asymptomatic disease or deconditioning (Peel, 1990). As discussed in Chapter 15, it is currently thought that physically active adults can minimize the impact of aging on cardiopulmonary function.

CARDIOVASCULAR SYSTEM

Heart. Structural changes are seen in the heart with aging. In general, the number of myocytes decreases, while their size increases. In the myocardium, increasing amounts of elastic tissue, fat, and collagen contribute to increased stiffness and decreased compliance of the ventricles. Accumulation of lipofuscin, a pigment deposit thought to be related to wear and tear, is also seen near the nuclei of the cardiac muscle cells, resulting in a darkening of the myocardium. It is not known whether increased lipofuscin has any functional significance. Thickening of the left ventricular wall is reported (Peel, 1990; Wei, 1986), but whether the thickening is really of the ventricular wall as opposed to the ventricular septum is controversial (Kitzman & Edwards, 1990). The volume of the left ventricle is slightly decreased, and the left atrium is slightly dilated. In the endocardium, thickened areas of elastic and collagen fibers can be noted, especially in the atria. Fragmentation and disorganization of elastic, collagen, and muscle fibers also occur (Peel, 1990; Wei, 1986). Increased fat is found within the epicardium, especially over the right ventricle and in the atrioventricular groove (Kitzman & Edwards, 1990).

With aging, changes are also seen in the heart valves and in the conduction system. The valves become thickened and calcified. Collagen and lipid accumulation, as well as calcification, within the aortic and mitral valves impairs the valves' ability to totally close. Collagen and fat are also laid down in the left bundle branches of the conduction system. By age 60, the number of pacemaker cells in the SA node begins to decrease; by age 75, less than 10 per cent of the number of SA node cells found in the adult heart are seen (Peel, 1990; Wei, 1986). These changes in the conduction system may contribute to the increased incidence of preventricular contractions (PVCs) and differences in the ST depression seen on the older adult's ECG.

Vasculature. The vasculature undergoes change throughout life, with vessels becoming thicker and more dilated. In general, the vascular course becomes more tortuous. Changes attributed to aging are initially seen in the coronary arteries at approximately 20 years of age and in the rest of the arterial system after 40 years of age. Dilation occurs in proximal arteries such as the aorta, whereas thickening of the arterial wall predominates in the peripheral arteries. Elastic arteries change more than muscular arteries, with irregular thickening of elastic tissue, fragmenting of elastic fibers, lipid infiltration, and calcification. These changes are seen earliest in the proximal portions of the large arteries (Wei, 1986). The older vessel is thickened and less elastic, which results in less compliance. Arteriosclerosis refers to decreased compliance of the arteries, which is a normal consequence of age-related changes in the arterial walls (Zadia, 1986). This is contrasted to atherosclerosis, a pathologic deposition of fatty plaques on the inner layer of the vessel, which also results in increased resistance to blood flow through the vessel (Peel, 1990; Shephard, 1987).

Functional Changes. The changes of the cardiovascular system associated with aging functionally affect the heart rate, blood pressure, stroke volume, and adaptability of the system to stress. These changes do not affect an individual very much at rest or during light exercise, but maximal exercise capacity decreases.

The sensitivity of regulatory mechanisms, such as the baroreceptors, is diminished in the older individual, affecting adaptability of the cardiovascular system to stressful situations such as cough, the Valsalva maneuver, and orthostasis. Increased plasma catecholamine levels and decreased end-organ responsiveness to adrenergic stimulation also affect the system's ability to increase heart rate, contractility of the heart, and vasodilation of the vessels in response to stress. Because of decreased adaptability, the heart takes longer to reach a steady state or to recover from exercise.

The resting heart rate changes minimally with aging, but maximal heart rate decreases. This decrease may be related to (1) decreased activity of the cardiac pacemaker, (2) decreased sensitivity to catecholamines, and (3) increased ventricular filling time, which results from decreased ventricular compliance. Contraction time and diastole may also be increased because of slowed calcium uptake in the sarcoplasmic reticulum of the cardiac cells. Because of poor calcium transport and storage, the heart muscle will take longer to reach peak tension and to relax.

As one ages, maximal stroke volume decreases, with elderly persons experiencing a 10 to 20 per cent decrease in stroke volume at high workload (Shephard, 1987). Factors influencing a decline in stroke volume are listed in Table 8–2 (Irwin & Zadai, 1990; Shephard, 1985). Decreased venous tone, slowed relaxation of the ventricles, thickening of the mitral valve, and left ventricular stiffness may result in a decreased preload condition. The filling rate of the 65 to 80-year-old heart has been shown to be 50 per cent that of 25 to 40-year-old subjects (Gerstenblith et al, 1977). Stiffening of the aorta and major arteries, increased systemic blood pressure, and poor perfusion of the skeletal muscle contribute to an increase in afterload (Shephard, 1987; Wei, 1986).

At rest and during exercise, blood pressure increases (systolic more so

Table 8-2. FACTORS LEADING TO DECREASED STROKE VOLUME DURING HIGH WORKLOAD IN OLDER ADULTS
Decreased cardiac compliance
Decreased cardiac contractility
Loss of cardiac muscle fibers
Increased connective tissue in myocardium
Poor myocardial perfusion
Increased peripheral resistance
Varicose veins
Decreased venous tone
Stiffening of the aorta and major arteries
Slowed ventricular relaxation
Increased systemic blood pressure
Poor perfusion of skeletal muscle
Decreased sensitivity to sympathetic input

than diastolic). This change is related to reduced compliance within the vascular system and the decreasing size of the vascular bed. If increased blood pressure can be expected with advancing age, how can this be differentiated from pathologic hypertension? What is the "normal" blood pressure of the older individual? Answers to these questions are unclear. Shephard (1987) and Peel (1990) report that blood pressure changes with aging are not seen in all populations, leaving a question about whether they are really a consequence of aging.

The efficiency of oxygen extraction from the blood at the tissue level decreases with age, narrowing the arterial-venous oxygen difference. Loss of muscle strength, decreased muscle enzyme levels, and diminished size of the capillary network that serves muscle limit oxygen extraction from the circulating blood. Obstruction of major vessels and decreased levels of hemoglobin are also factors (Shephard, 1985, 1987). With increasing age, increased obesity, and decreased efficiency of sweating, blood is shunted away from the muscles and to the skin, assisting in body cooling. This also reduces blood flow to the tissues and contributes to the decreased efficiency of oxygen extraction.

PULMONARY SYSTEM

Structural changes occur with aging and create a stiffer bony thorax, which increases the work of breathing. The thorax becomes shortened vertically and larger in the anterior-posterior dimension. Thoracic kyphosis and decreased mobility of the joints allow rib rotation. Elasticity of cartilage and collagen in the annulus fibrosus decreases, and loss of fluid from the nucleus pulposus results in a flattened, less resilient disk. Because of the resting position of the thorax, the intrathoracic pressure at end-expiration is higher, again increasing airway resistance and effort during breathing.

Elasticity and compliance are also decreased within the lung. In the conducting airways, elasticity of bronchial cartilage is diminished. Hyaline cartilage structures in the trachea may become ossified. Bronchial mucous glands increase in number, thickening the mucus layer in the airway and offering more resistance to airflow. The number and thickness of elastic fibers in the walls of smaller airways decrease, again increasing the resistance to airflow and diminishing elastic recoil of the lungs. As elastic recoil of the lungs is diminished, residual volume gets larger and vital capacity is reduced. Lungs, alveoli, and alveolar ducts get larger with age. As a result, more time is needed for inspired air to reach the alveolar area. At the alveolar level, thinning of the alveolar wall can create small openings in the wall, limiting the area available for gas exchange. Decreased elasticity of the alveoli makes them susceptible to collapse on expiration.

Respiratory muscles become less efficient with age. Structural changes in the thoracic cavity alter the length-tension relationship of the respiratory muscles, increasing the work of breathing. For example, the resting position of the diaphragm changes as the thoracic height decreases and diameter increases. Increased residual volume of the aging lung will also affect the resting position of the diaphragm. The abdominal muscles become less effective at stabilizing the diaphragm. Because of these changes, the older adult has to increase breathing rate rather than tidal volume to increase minute ventilation. This also increases the work of breathing (Frontera & Evans, 1986).

The pulmonary vasculature undergoes the same changes within the vascular wall that were discussed earlier. The capillary bed at the alveolar interface becomes smaller, which, when combined with increased alveolar size, limits the diffusing capacity of the system. Pulmonary blood flow and blood volume within the capillary bed decrease.

Functionally, the impact of these changes is reflected in lung volumes and arterial blood gas values at rest and during exercise. Although total lung capacity does not change, vital capacity decreases while functional residual capacity and residual volume increase. By 70 years of age, vital capacity is reported to decrease to 75 per cent of earlier values, and residual volume to increase by 50 per cent (Murray, 1977). Inspiratory and expiratory reserve volumes also decrease because of the decreased elasticity of the lung. The loss of elasticity causes the airways to close at a higher volume during expiration, which affects the amount of oxygenated air that is distributed to the tissue. The pulmonary system works harder to deliver less oxygen to the tissues in older adults.

FUNCTIONAL IMPLICATIONS OF CARDIOPULMONARY SYSTEM CHANGES

Because of anatomic and physiologic differences in the cardiopulmonary systems of the infant, child, adolescent, and adult, function and efficiency differ in each age group. Through childhood, most changes are related to changes in body size. Gender differences become apparent in adolescence. In adulthood and older adulthood, effects of environment and normal aging alter the cardiopulmonary efficiency and capacity.

Efficiency of the cardiopulmonary system is reflected in measures such as cardiac output, minute ventilation, and maximal aerobic capacity. Cardiac output is a measure of the efficiency of the cardiovascular system. Minute ventilation, the volume of air moved into the lungs in 1 minute, is a measure of the efficiency of the pulmonary system. These two measures, when considered with the ability of working tissue to utilize oxygen for energy production, indicate an individual's maximal aerobic capacity or level of cardiopulmonary fitness.

Cardiac output varies with an individual's age. The cardiac output of children is less than that of adults both at rest and during exercise. Small heart size limits stroke volume to such a degree that even the increased heart rate of children cannot compensate. Functionally, the lower cardiac output does not affect a child's level of activity, because even with less hemoglobin than an adult, the child efficiently extracts oxygen from the blood. In addition, the small body size of children and their ability to easily dissipate heat over their relatively large body surface area enable them to function with the smaller cardiac output (Haywood, 1986). Cardiac output increases as the body grows. In young adults, cardiac output during maximal exercise limits endurance (Shepard, 1985). With aging, both maximal heart rate and maximal stroke volume are decreased. Because cardiac output during maximal exercise is the product of these two values, it also decreases with age.

Oxygen transportation to working tissues is another important factor in determining an individual's maximal aerobic capacity. Efficient ventilation carries inspired air to a well-developed and expanded alveolar network. Efficient circulation provides enough oxygenated blood to the pulmonary capillary network and to the capillaries of working tissues. Factors such as airway resistance, compliance of the thorax, functioning of the respiratory muscles, and compliance/elasticity of the lung and airways affect efficiency. The functional volumes of air in the lungs, such as the tidal volume, vary with the demands placed on the respiratory system. As more oxygen is required during light to moderate exercise, tidal volume increases (Murray, 1986).

Changes in the functional lung volumes and decreased efficiency of the respiratory muscles reduce an older individual's ability to increase tidal volume and minute ventilation in response to exercise. During exercise, maximal oxygen uptake is decreased 25 per cent by age 65 and 50 per cent by age 75 (Shephard, 1987). The pulmonary system is less able to adapt to stress because of (1) the loss of elastic recoil and chest wall compliance, (2) changes in central nervous system control, (3) innervation of respiratory muscles, and (4) impaired perception of CO_2 levels. Breathing frequency is increased in an attempt to provide necessary oxygen transport. The pulmonary system's inability to meet needs is thought to limit exercise in the older individual (Peel, 1990; Shephard, 1985). These changes are minimized in the healthy, active, nonsmoking older adult, and endurance training is thought to improve lung function (McArdle et al, 1991; Shephard, 1987).

Cardiopulmonary efficiency contributes to an individual's level of physical fitness. Fitness is a measure of a person's functional ability. A more extensive discussion of fitness issues across the life span, including the effects of exercise and training on the body systems, can be found in Chapter 15 of this text.

SUMMARY

The structure, function, and development of the cardiovascular and pulmonary systems has been presented. These two systems work closely together to provide the food and fuel necessary for physical function. Several changes in these systems throughout the life span alter their functional ability. Some of these changes appear to be the result of normal development, but there is also evidence that regular physical activity can have a positive impact on these systems. It is currently thought that exercise at any age is important to maintain these two important systems at maximal efficiency.

References

Bacon RL, Niles NR. *Medical Histology: A Text-Atlas with Introductory Pathology.* New York: Springer-Verlag, 1983.

Boyden EA. Development and growth of the airways. In Hodson WA (ed). *Development of the Lung.* New York: Marcel Dekker, 1977, pp 3–35.

Cunningham DA, Paterson DH. Discussion: Exercise, fitness and aging. In Bouchard C, Shephard RJ, Stephens T, Sutton JP, McPherson BD (eds). *Exercise, Fitness and Health: A Consensus of Current Knowledge.* Champaign, IL: Human Kinetics, 1990, pp 699–704.

Cunningham DA, Paterson DH, Blimke CJR. The development of the cardiorespiratory system with growth and physical activity. In Boileau RA (ed). *Advances in Pediatric Sport Science, vol 1: Biological Issues.* Champaign, IL: Human Kinetics, 1984, pp 85–116.

Davis JA, Dobbing J. *Scientific Foundations of Pediatrics.* Baltimore: University Park Press, 1981.

DeCesare JA, Graybill CA. Physical therapy for the child with respiratory dysfunction. In Irwin S, Tecklin JS (eds). *Cardiopulmonary Physical Therapy,* 2nd ed. St. Louis: CV Mosby, 1990, pp 417–460.

Frontera WR, Evans WJ. Exercise performance and endurance training in the elderly. *Top Geriatr Rehabil* 2:17–32, 1986.

Gerstenblith G, Frederiksen J, Yin FCP, Fortuin NJ, Lakatta EG, Weisfeldt ML. Echocardiographic assessment of a normal adult aging population. *Circulation* 56:273–278, 1977.

Haywood KM. *Lifespan Motor Development.* Champaign, IL: Human Kinetics, 1986.

Irwin SC, Zadai CC. Cardiopulmonary rehabilitation of the geriatric patient. In Lewis CB (ed). *Aging: The Health Care Challenge,* 2nd ed. Philadelphia: FA Davis, 1990, pp 181–211.

Junqueira LC, Carneiro J, Kelley RO. *Basic Histology,* 6th ed. Norwalk, CT: Appleton & Lange, 1989.

Kitzman DW, Edwards WD. Minireview: Age-related changes in the anatomy of the normal human heart. *J Geriatr Med Sci* 45(2):33–39, 1990.

Leeson TS, Leeson CR, Paparo AA. *Text/Atlas of Histology.* Philadelphia: WB Saunders, 1988.

Malina RM, Bouchard C. *Growth, Maturation and Physical Activity.* Champaign, IL: Human Kinetics, 1991, pp 151–167.

Massery M. Chest development as a component of normal motor development: Implications for pediatric physical therapists. *Pediatr Phys Ther* 3(1):3–8, 1991.

McArdle WD, Katch FL, Katch VL. *Exercise Physiology—Energy, Nutrition and Human Performance,* 3rd ed. Philadelphia: Lea & Febiger, 1991.

Meyrick B, Reid LM. Ultrastructure of alveolar lining and its development. In Hodson WA (ed). *Development of the Lung.* New York: Marcel Dekker, 1977, pp 135–214.

Moore KL. *The Developing Human,* 5th ed. Philadelphia: WB Saunders, 1993, pp 59–62, 207–216, 286–333.

Murray JF. *The Normal Lung,* 2nd ed. Philadelphia: WB Saunders, 1986.

Payne VG, Isaacs LD. *Human Motor Development: A Life Span Approach.* Mountain View, CA: Mayfield Publishers, 1987.

Peel C. Cardiopulmonary changes with aging. In Irwin S, Tecklin JS (eds). *Cardiopulmonary Physical Therapy,* 2nd ed. St. Louis: CV Mosby, 1990, pp 477–489.

Porter RE. Normal development of movement and function: Child and adolescent. In Scully RM, Barnes MR (eds). *Physical Therapy.* Philadelphia: JB Lippincott, 1989, pp 83–98.

Shephard RJ. The cardiovascular benefits of exercise in the elderly. *Top Geriatr Rehabil* 1(1):1–10, 1985.

Shephard RJ. *Exercise Physiology.* Toronto: BC Decker, 1987.

Sinclair D. *Human Growth After Birth,* 4th ed. London: Oxford University Press, 1985.

Tecklin JS. Pulmonary disorders in infants and children and their physical therapy management. In Tecklin JS (ed). *Pediatric Physical Therapy.* Philadelphia: JB Lippincott, 1989, pp 141–172.

Wei JY. Cardiovascular anatomic and physiologic changes with age. *Top Geriatr Rehabil* 2(1):10–16, 1986.

Zadai CC. Cardiopulmonary issues in the geriatric population: Implications for rehabilitation. *Top Geriatr Rehabil* 2(1):1–9, 1986.

Chapter 9

Nervous System Changes

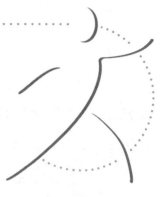

Objectives

AFTER STUDYING THIS CHAPTER, THE READER WILL BE ABLE TO:

1 Describe the roles of the nervous system.
2 Delineate components of the nervous system.
3 Describe the general organization of the nervous system.
4 Discuss changes in the nervous system over time.
5 Relate nervous system changes over time to functional differences in movement, cognition, and motivation.

ROLES OF THE NERVOUS SYSTEM

The nervous system is frequently referred to as the command center for human function. It not only receives information, but integrates all incoming messages to orchestrate fluid, appropriate responses. The nervous system truly oversees other body systems as they cooperate to perform day-to-day activities. Major functions controlled by the nervous system include moving, thinking, and feeling.

Movement is controlled when the nervous system functions as an initiator, modulator, and comparator, activating the muscular and skeletal systems. Movement is not the product of any one system, nor does one system act in isolation from the others to produce movement. Absence of movement might result from a problem in the skeletal, muscular, cardiopulmonary, or nervous system. For example, in either muscle disease (such as muscular dystrophy) or peripheral nerve injury, the end result is movement dysfunction.

A unique role of the nervous system is thought processing—that is, cognition or intelligence. Psychologic theorists such as Erikson have little to say about how the brain "thinks." Physiologists believe that the ability of the brain to form memories is a mechanism for intelligence. The frontal area of the brain has been linked to abstract thought and personality. Following head trauma, a patient's sensory, motor, and cognitive deficits can be attributed to the damaged area of the brain. In other areas of the brain, called *association areas,* sensory input is connected to meaning. For example, in the visual association areas, visual input is connected with the memory and names of shapes.

Another important aspect of nervous system control is its role in motivation and emotions. One of the oldest parts of the brain, called the *limbic system,* is responsible for attending to sensory and motor cues; monitoring basic drives for food, water, and sexual gratification; and attaching emotional meaning to actions. The nervous system's ability to react to these cues is not very well understood. Emotions can be powerful motivation for movement. The affective component of movement dysfunction is often the most difficult to deal with, as when trying to motivate a person to perform better physically.

COMPONENTS OF THE NERVOUS SYSTEM

At the cellular level, the nervous system is made up of two different types of cells: nerve cells (neurons) and glial cells (neuroglia). Both cell types are derived from embryonic ectoderm. *Neurons* allow the nervous system to communicate and to direct movement activities. *Neuroglia* provide support and protection for neurons. On a larger scale, structures such as the brain, spinal cord, and peripheral nerves make up the functional infrastructure of the nervous system.

Neurons

Neurons are complex structures that form a major communication system of the body. As shown in Figure 9–1, a neuron is made up of a *cell body,* which can be thought of as a processing center, *dendrites,* or long processes, which receive incoming stimuli, and an *axon,* which singularly conducts nerve impulses to other neurons, muscles, or glands. Each dendrite is branched to receive multiple inputs from other neurons. The pattern of branching indicates the purpose of the neuron. Each axon also is usually branched. The axon or nerve fiber terminates in an end bulb that synapses with a target cell. Neurons vary in size and shape according to their function. The structure often reflects the role the neuron plays in the communications network of the nervous system.

The neuron communicates by initiating a signal, called an *action potential.* An action potential is generated by changing the resting electric potential of the cell membrane. Normal resting membrane potential is about −70 mV and is controlled by charged ions such as K^+, Na^+, Cl^-, and HCO_3^-. The flow of positively charged sodium ions into the cell decreases the membrane potential (depolarization). Once the membrane is sufficiently depolarized, the action potential is generated. Following depolarization, there is a period during which the cell membrane is unable to react, called a *refractory period.* An axon can generate up to 1000 action potentials per second (Junqueira et al, 1989).

Myelin is a lipid and protein substance that covers axons and increases the speed of nerve impulse conduction. In the central nervous system, myelin

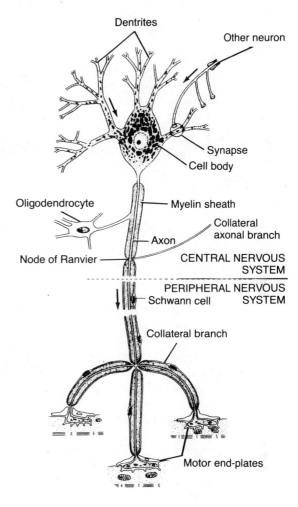

FIGURE 9–1. Schematic drawing of a motor neuron. The myelin sheath is produced by oligodendrocytes in the central nervous system and by Schwann cells in the peripheral nervous system. The arrows show the direction of the nerve impulse. (From Junqueira LC, Carneiro J, Kelley RO. *Basic Histology,* 6th ed. Norwalk, CT: Appleton & Lange, 1989.)

is produced by glial cells called *oligodendrocytes;* in the peripheral nervous system, myelin is produced by Schwann cells, as shown in Figure 9–1. The myelin laid down by the Schwann cells is interrupted at set intervals along the nerve called *nodes of Ranvier* (Fig. 9–2). At these nodes, the action potential can be boosted to keep it from fading out as it journeys along the nerve fiber. Conduction in myelinated peripheral nerves is called *leaping* (or *saltation*) because the current flow can be detected only at the nodes, as shown in Figure 9–2. How fast impulses can be conducted depends on whether the nerve is myelinated or unmyelinated and on the diameter of the nerve fiber.

Nerve fibers can be classified on the basis of their size and ability to conduct, as outlined in Table 9–1. For example, *type A fibers* are myelinated with large diameters and conduct at high speed (12 to 120 m/second). *Type B fibers* have smaller diameters and a medium rate of conduction (3 to 15 m/

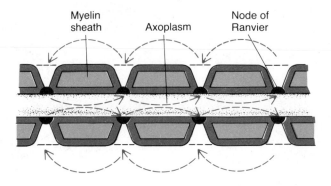

FIGURE 9-2. Saltatory conduction along a myelinated axon. (Redrawn from Guyton AC. *Textbook of Medical Physiology,* 8th ed. Philadelphia: WB Saunders, 1991.)

second). Type C fibers are smaller still and unmyelinated, with a conduction rate of only 0.5 to 2 m/second.

Neuroglia

Neuroglia provide support, nutrition, and protection to the neurons and can be thought of as the connective tissue of the nervous system. Neurons do not survive in tissue cultures unless neuroglia are present (Junqueira et al, 1989). Metabolically, neuroglia assist in regulating the concentration of sodium and potassium ions in the intracellular space; these ions affect the performance of the nerve cell. Unlike neurons, they cannot transmit electric impulses, but they do retain the ability to divide throughout the life of the organism. Injury to the central nervous system typically triggers glial cell proliferation as a means of repair. Normally, there are approximately 10 glial cells to every neuron, but because glia are smaller than neurons, they account for only half the volume of nervous tissue. Three types of neuroglia are (1) macroglia, which include astrocytes and oligodendrocytes, (2) microglia, and (3) ependymal cells.

The largest neuroglia, the *astrocytes,* provide a vascular link via foot-like projections between blood vessels, the brain, and the spinal cord. In the brain, protoplasmic astrocytes are part of the blood-brain barrier (BBB), which regulates the influx of vital nutrients and keeps out harmful substances. Preterm

Table 9-1. NERVE FIBER TYPES		
Types	**Diameter (μm)**	**Conduction Velocity (m/second)**
A	12–20	70–120
B	<3	3–15
C	0.4–1.2	0.5–2

Modified from Ganong WF. *Review of Medical Physiology,* 16th ed. Norwalk, CT: Appleton & Lange, 1993.

infants have not formed this barrier. Therefore, foreign matter such as meconium, the first stool, may be deposited in brain structures and cause movement dysfunction (Volpe, 1987).

Astrocytes are also present in the spinal cord. They lend structural support to the nervous system and may eliminate interference or cross-talk in nerve cell transmission. In injury, astrocytes and microglia clean up debris. Fibrous astrocytes fill in the space left by an injury and produce a glial scar, which can actually interfere with healing by blocking reestablishment of synaptic connections.

Oligodendrocytes produce the myelin that covers the neural processes of the central nervous system (CNS). The large number of this type of glial cell is a hallmark of the increasing evolutionary complexity of the nervous system.

Microglia are derived from mesenchyme and can be found scattered throughout the CNS. As the major scavenger cells (macrophages) they migrate to any area of injury to remove cellular debris, regardless of whether the spinal cord or brain is damaged. These small cells develop late in the fetal period after the CNS has been supplied by blood vessels.

Ependymal cells line the cavities of the brain and spinal cord and are in constant contact with cerebrospinal fluid (CSF). Because some ependymal cells have cilia, movement of the CSF is possible. A special ependymal cell, called a *tanycyte,* relays chemical information from the CSF to the capillary system surrounding the pituitary gland, which is important for regulating circulating hormones.

Central Nervous System

The brain, brain stem, and spinal cord are collectively referred to as the central nervous system. The brain consists of two cerebral hemispheres called the cerebral cortex and the cerebellum. The surface of each hemisphere is convoluted and has elevated areas called *gyri* and grooves called *sulci.* The *cortex* is divided into five lobes: frontal, parietal, temporal, occipital, and limbic (Fig. 9–3). All have different functions. The areas that are directly related to processing sensory and motor information or for coordinating movement are known as *primary* and *association sensory* (or "motor") areas, as seen in Figure 9–4.

The cortex is also organized into horizontal layers characterized by a different distribution of neurons and glial cells, depending on the part of the cortex studied. A mark of brain maturity is the establishment of these layers. Cell bodies of neurons with similar functions form groups within the central nervous system called *nuclei,* many of which are in the cerebral hemispheres.

The nervous system is topographically organized to relay signals throughout the body. This is true in the motor and sensory cortices, where the parts of the body are represented. The size of the part is directly related to the part's functional importance. For example, the sensory homunculus seen in Figure 9–5 depicts a caricature of a person with oversized lips and thumb. The same type of organizational relationship is present in the visual cortex as a

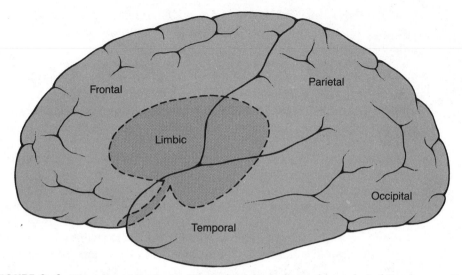

FIGURE 9–3. The lobes of the brain. The limbic lobe is depicted by a dashed line because it is internal to the other four lobes.

visuotopic map and in the auditory cortex as a tonotopic map. This type of mapping occurs at every level of the nervous system.

The concept that each side of the brain is specialized to perform certain functions has been widely accepted. In our culture, language is localized in the left hemisphere and spatial abilities in the right. While the two cerebral hemispheres appear to be mirror images of each other, gross anatomic differences have been demonstrated by Geschwind and Levitsky (1968). The differences are likely to be related to handedness, since 95 per cent of the population is left-hemisphere, or right-side, dominant (Oppenheim, 1981). The asymmetry of the two hemispheres is present even in infants (Wada et al, 1975).

The *cerebellum* is also made up of two hemispheres connected by the vermis. Despite its small size, the cerebellum contains over half of all the neurons in the brain (Ghez, 1991). The cerebellum is involved in the initiation and timing of movements and in monitoring postural tone. By receiving sensory input from the vestibular, auditory, and visual systems, as well as from the spinal cord, it compares actual to anticipated motor performance, thereby functioning as a comparator. The cerebellum influences nuclei in the thalamus and brain stem to control movement, and its circuits are modified during motor learning.

The brain stem represents a transition between the brain and the spinal cord, as depicted in Figure 9–6. Its structures include the *medulla, pons,* and *mid-brain,* moving up from the spinal cord. Loosely arranged groups of neurons in the brain stem are responsible for keeping a person alert to novel stimuli or picking up information pertinent to movement safety. This group of

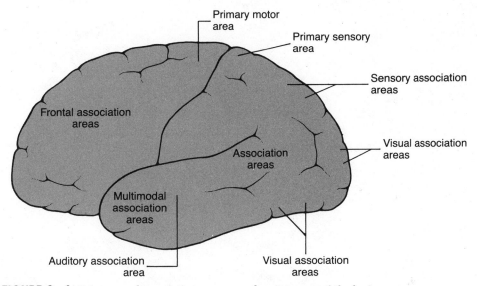

FIGURE 9-4. Primary and association sensory and motor areas of the brain.

neurons is called the *reticular activating system (RAS)*. This system regulates the level of consciousness as well as the daily cycle of arousal, which includes periods of sleep and waking. The brain stem also acts to filter sensory input, such as pain, to the cortex.

The spinal cord is made up of groups of axons, called *tracts,* which run the

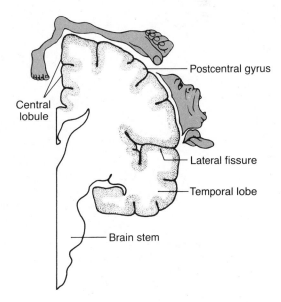

FIGURE 9-5. Sensory homunculus.

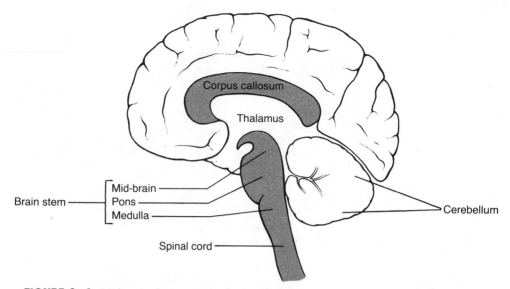

FIGURE 9–6. Mid-sagittal view of the brain. (Redrawn from Farber S. *Neurorehabilitation: A Multisensory Approach.* Philadelphia: WB Saunders, 1982.)

length of the spinal cord and relay input to and from CNS structures. Figure 9–7 depicts a cross-section through the spinal cord with representative ascending and descending tracts. The tracts surround a central *"butterfly" area* that consists of interneurons, neuronal cell bodies, dendrites, and glial cells. Cell bodies and dendrites of motor neurons are located in the anterior horn of the butterfly area; entering axons of sensory neurons are found in the poste-

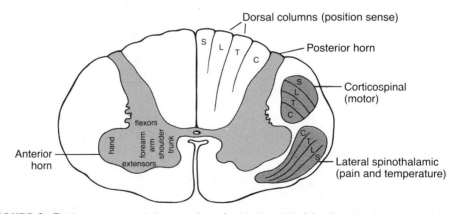

FIGURE 9–7. Cross-section of the spinal cord with functional localization (somatotopy) of ascending and descending tracts. S = sacral, L = lumbar, T = thoracic, C = cervical. (Redrawn from Romero-Sierra C. *Neuroanatomy: A Conceptual Approach.* New York: Churchill Livingstone, 1986.)

rior horn. The position of a motor neuron within the anterior horn correlates with the location of the muscle groups it innervates (Fig. 9–7).

Peripheral Nervous System

The cranial and peripheral nerves along with their accompanying nerve ganglia are referred to as the peripheral nervous system (PNS). *Ganglia* are groups of neuron cell bodies outside the CNS. Cranial nerves from the brain stem innervate head and neck muscles involved in vital functions. Some cranial nerves also connect special sensory receptors with the brain. All 31 pairs of spinal nerves are part of the peripheral nervous system and have sensory and motor components. The cell bodies of the sensory neurons are located outside the spinal cord, in the dorsal root ganglion. The peripheral process extends from the receptor to the cell body in the ganglion, and the central process (axon) goes from the ganglion into the CNS (Fig. 9–8).

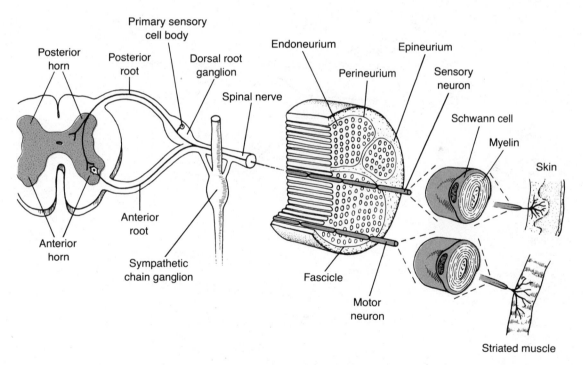

FIGURE 9–8. Schematic representation of the peripheral nervous system and the transition to the central nervous system. (Redrawn from Farber S. *Neurorehabilitation: A Multisensory Approach.* Philadelphia: WB Saunders, 1982, p 17; Junqueira LC, Carneiro J, Kelley RO. *Basic Histology,* 6th ed. Norwalk, CT: Appleton & Lange, 1989, p 177; and Ham AW. *Histology,* 6th ed. Philadelphia: JB Lippincott, 1969.)

Continuing proximally in Figure 9–8, the peripheral nerve and groups of nerve fibers are surrounded by specialized interstitial connective tissue. The *epineurium* covers the entire peripheral nerve; the *perineurium* surrounds bundles of nerve fibers called *fascicles;* and the *endoneurium* surrounds each individual nerve fiber. As seen in Figure 9–9, the bundles combine to form common nerves such as the sciatic nerve in the lower extremity, or the radial nerve in the upper extremity.

The *efferent (motor) peripheral system* can be divided into the somatic nervous system and the autonomic nervous system. The major differences are outlined in Table 9–2. The *somatic efferent system* conducts impulses to skeletal muscle; the *autonomic efferent system* conducts the impulses to smooth muscle, cardiac muscle, and glands. Both the somatic and the autonomic systems produce muscular contractions and change the rate of those contractions, but only the autonomic system causes the secretion of hormones.

The autonomic nervous system (ANS) is primarily responsible for main-

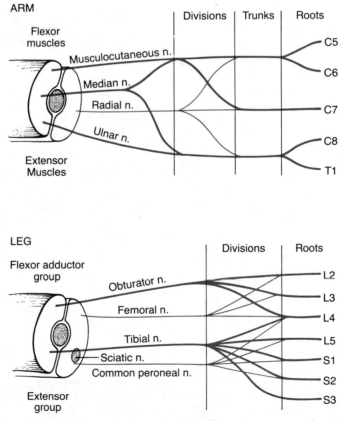

FIGURE 9–9. Relationship of common nerves to bundles of nerve roots from which they are derived. (Redrawn from Williams PL, Wendell-Smith CP, Treadgold S. *Basic Human Embryology,* 3rd ed. London: Pitman Publishing, 1984.)

Table 9-2. DIFFERENCES BETWEEN SOMATIC EFFERENT AND AUTONOMIC NERVOUS SYSTEMS

SOMATIC NERVOUS SYSTEM

1. Consists of a single neuron between the central nervous system and the effector organ
2. Innervates skeletal muscle
3. Always leads to excitation of the muscle

AUTONOMIC NERVOUS SYSTEM

1. Has a two-neuron chain (connected by a synapse) between the central nervous system and the effector organ
2. Innervates smooth or cardiac muscle or gland cells
3. Can lead to excitation or to inhibition of the effector cells

Modified from Vander A, et al. *Human Physiology: The Mechanism of Body Function,* 4th ed. New York: McGraw-Hill, 1985, p 184.

taining an internal balance of visceral functions related to the heart, smooth muscle, and glands; it consists of the *sympathetic* and *parasympathetic* divisions. Both divisions use acetylcholine as a neurotransmitter at the preganglionic synapse, as diagrammed in Figure 9–10. The parasympathetic division also uses acetylcholine at postganglionic synapses, whereas the sympathetic

PERIPHERAL NERVOUS SYSTEM

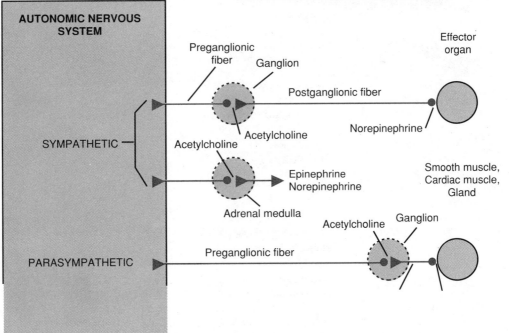

FIGURE 9–10. Neurotransmitters in the autonomic nervous system. (Redrawn from Vander AJ, Sherman JH, Luciano DS. *Human Physiology: The Mechanism of Body Function,* 4th ed. New York: McGraw-Hill, 1985.)

division uses norepinephrine to transmit nerve impulses to effector organs. The cell bodies of the sympathetic division are found in the thoracolumbar segments of the spinal cord. The sympathetic ganglia are adjacent to the thoracolumbar spinal cord in paired "sympathetic trunks," which then connect to an effector organ. The cell bodies of the parasympathetic division are in the cranial and sacral regions of the spinal cord. The parasympathetic ganglia usually lie within the effector organ. Some effects of ANS activity are outlined in Table 9–3.

Rood visualized the two divisions of the ANS on a continuum, the mid-point of which is a balance between *fight or flight* (sympathetic) responses and *vegetative* (parasympathetic) responses (Heiniger & Randolph, 1981). The mid-point is called *homeostasis* and is achieved by 1 year of age (Sullivan et al, 1982). Where an individual is functioning on the ANS continuum can influence the person's ability to process sensory input and produce motor output (Heiniger & Randolph, 1981). For example, if an individual with a head injury is easily aroused and excitable, it would help to calm the person before proceeding with any additional therapeutic intervention. Conversely, a very leth-

Table 9–3. SELECTED EFFECTS OF AUTONOMIC NERVOUS SYSTEM ACTIVITY

Organ	Effect of Sympathetic Stimulation	Effect of Parasympathetic Stimulation
Eye		
Pupil	Decrease dilation	Decrease constriction
Heart		
SA node	Increase heart rate	Decrease heart rate
Muscle	Increase rate and force	Decrease rate and force
Arterioles	Constriction	Dilation
Veins	Constriction	None
Lungs		
Bronchi	Dilation	Constriction
Gut		
Lumen	Decrease peristalsis	Increase peristalsis
Sphinchter	Increase tone (usually)	Relax tone (usually)
Liver	Release glucose	Slight glucose synthesis
Kidney	Decrease output and renin secretion	None
Bladder	Relax detrusor muscle	Contract detrusor muscle
	Contract trigone muscle	Relax trigone muscle
Glands		
Lacrimal	None/slight secretion	Copious secretion
Sweat	Copious sweat	Sweaty palms of hands
Basal		
metabolism	Increase	None

argic patient with head injury may need to be aroused in order to fully participate in any type of intervention.

COMMUNICATION IN THE NERVOUS SYSTEM

The nervous system is connected via synapses. As the system matures, more and more connections are made. A labyrinth of relay stations with an infinite number of ways to take in, disseminate, and combine information is formed (Fig. 9–11). Dendritic branching occurs after initial pathways are formed and provides a mechanism for intercommunication between brain structures. The increasing density and complexity of these structures is a mark of advanced communication seen in phylogenetically higher animals. In individuals with mental retardation, dendritic spines are more spindly and tangled (Fig. 9–12), which could decrease the level of communication.

Synapses

Neuron-to-neuron transmission of nerve impulses occurs at an interneuronal junction called a *synapse*. The direction of synaptic transmission determines where the impulses will go within the nervous system. There are two basic types of synapses, chemical and electrical. Electrical synapses are referred to as *gap junctions*. Only a very few are present in the human nervous system,

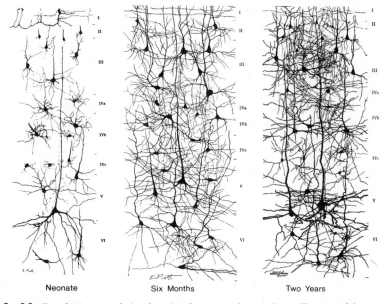

| Neonate | Six Months | Two Years |

FIGURE 9–11. Dendritic growth in the visual cortex of an infant. (Reprinted by permission of the publishers from THE POSTNATAL DEVELOPMENT OF THE HUMAN CEREBRAL CORTEX by Jesse LeRoy Conel, Cambridge, Mass.: Harvard University Press, Copyright © 1939, 1941, 1947, 1951, 1955, 1959 by the President and Fellows of Harvard College, © renewed 1967, 1969 by Jesse LeRoy Conel, renewed 1975 by the President and Fellows of Harvard College.)

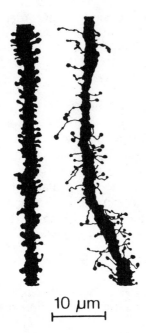

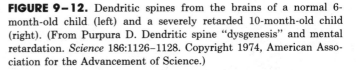

FIGURE 9–12. Dendritic spines from the brains of a normal 6-month-old child (left) and a severely retarded 10-month-old child (right). (From Purpura D. Dendritic spine "dysgenesis" and mental retardation. *Science* 186:1126–1128. Copyright 1974, American Association for the Advancement of Science.)

which uses predominantly chemical synapses that are activated by substances called *neurotransmitters.*

Over 40 different chemical substances have been classified as neurotransmitters. A few of the best known are acetylcholine, norepinephrine, serotonin, glutamate, gamma-aminobutyric acid (GABA), and dopamine. These are small-molecule, rapid-acting neurotransmitters that are manufactured by the neurons that release them. When an action potential reaches the end of an axon, it triggers the release of neurotransmitter from synaptic vesicles. Sodium ions facilitate the depolarization of the presynaptic membrane, and calcium ions facilitate the release of the neurotransmitter. The transmitter diffuses across the space between the two neurons and binds to receptors on the postsynaptic neuron membrane. At many types of synapses, surplus neurotransmitter is broken down in the cleft by enzymes and recycled by the presynaptic neuron or by glial cell uptake.

Neurons can synapse on other neurons called *interneurons,* or they can synapse on muscle or glands. Each group of axons or tract of the CNS has its own characteristic way of sending and receiving nerve signals and coding information. The intensity of a nerve signal depends on the number of nerve fibers activated. The more fibers used, the stronger the signal. This is called *spatial summation.*

Information from nerve fibers can also be varied by the pattern of neuron firing. The frequency of the firing and the time between firings is called *temporal summation,* the sum of the signals over time. Temporal summation might work like this: "dot, dot, space" means pressure, and "dot, space, dot" means light touch. The more different ways of coding information, the better the organism is able to discriminate one sensation from another, in this case pressure from light touch.

Cortical Connections

Communication within the nervous system takes place in one of three ways: by association fibers, by commissural fibers, and by projection fibers. Association areas are cortical areas responsible for horizontally linking different parts of the cortex. The parietal, temporal, and occipital association areas are involved in perception. The sensory association cortex is responsible for interfacing sensory information from the three lobes to perceive and to attach meaning to sensory input (such as identifying shapes by touch). The thalamus and other nuclei in the brain stem relay sensory information to association areas for perceptual judgments. The prefrontal and the limbic association areas are concerned with movement and motivation, respectively.

Information is communicated not only within the hemispheres, but between the right and left hemispheres. A large group of nerve fibers, called the *corpus callosum,* transmits information between similar areas of the two sides of the brain (see Fig. 9-6). For example, the anterior part of the corpus callosum transmits from the anterior cortex of one side to the anterior cortex of the opposite side.

Information is also shared vertically, up and down the neural axis, by tracts and nuclei that connect the cortex and the spinal cord. Afferent fibers bring sensory input into the spinal cord via the posterior root and connect with or continue as ascending tracts that carry information to various parts of the brain. Efferent fibers carry out commands from the motor cortex and prefrontal cortex, which travel in descending tracts to the anterior horn of the spinal cord.

ADAPTATION OF THE NERVOUS SYSTEM

Plasticity

Bishop and Craik (1982) described the nervous system's potential to adapt to change as plasticity. Hypothetically, the nervous system can adapt through the life span, but plasticity appears to be greatest when the nervous system is developing. The concept of plasticity includes the ability of the nervous system to make structural changes in response to internal or external demands. The period during which each type of nerve cell is able to change is called the *critical period* (Bishop & Craik, 1982). The critical period is also that time in developmental history when a system is most readily influenced by positive or negative environmental factors.

After birth, the nervous system continues to mature. Although most of the

10 billion neurons are already formed at birth, neurons continue to make connections with other structures through dendritic branching and by remodeling other connections. Postnatal experience plays a major role in further inducing developmental changes in the nervous system's pattern of synaptic connections. Development and experience interact to produce change.

Plasticity includes the ability to adapt to damaged neurons or nerve tracts. Adaptability within the CNS is functionally limited to reorganization, because regeneration cannot occur. The development of collateral sprouting as a recovery phenomenon is seen in the brain, spinal cord, and peripheral nervous system. Damaged axons can sprout new processes, which can lead to new synapse formation. Therapy attempts to use this reorganization for the recovery of function.

The peripheral nervous system retains the ability to regenerate, as evidenced by a return of muscle function following some types of peripheral nerve lesion. When peripheral nerve damage is severe enough to disrupt the myelin sheath and the axon, the axon will degenerate back to the node of Ranvier that is most proximal to the injury. This is called *wallerian degeneration.* After a time, the axon will regrow and try to reestablish contact. The path of nerve growth can be followed by the Tinel sign, a tingling when the nerve is tapped, as the severed nerve grows and reestablishes contact with its receptor. In the most severe peripheral nerve injury, surgical intervention is required to reestablish the connection.

Regression

Regression is an important occurrence in the development of the nervous system because the nervous system initially overproduces neurons. This overproduction ensures a sufficient number of neurons to complete the "wiring" of the organism and support optimal function. Regressive phenomena take place at the end of neuron development and can result in cell loss as high as 50 per cent. Neuron cell death is naturally programmed within the nerve cell and appears to be highly influenced by the metabolic state of the extracellular environment. The trimming of extraneous axon connections occurs without harm to the cell of origin.

Many more synapses are made than are needed to function (Evrard & Minkowski, 1989). In fact, if a neuron does not make contact with an appropriate receptor, it dies. Functionally, this allows for precise matching of neurons to their peripheral fields of innervation (Bishop & Craik, 1982), as seen in sensory dermatomes. The number of synapses present in the nervous system peaks at 6 to 12 months postnatally; regression to adult levels occurs between 5 and 10 years of age.

SUMMARY OF STRUCTURE AND FUNCTION

Neurons are the means by which the nervous system communicates. All information is received by specialized receptors and is transmitted along several distinct pathways to various regions of the brain, where it is interpreted, acted on, stored, or ignored. Structurally, neurons are produced to match their functions within the nervous system. Neurons increase their ability to communicate by the branching of dendrites. This branching can be very sophisticated and is related to the amount of information that can be processed. Complexity in dendrite formation is a mark of advanced evolution. Fewer dendritic spines are seen in individuals with mental retardation, as seen in Figure 9–11. Neurons exhibit plasticity but they do not retain the ability to divide. When a neuron dies, it is not replaced, except by glial cells.

LIFE SPAN CHANGES

Prenatal Period

The CNS develops from specialized ectoderm at 3 weeks of gestation when the neural tube is formed. The brain is created from the cranial two thirds, and the spinal cord from the caudal one third, of the neural tube by the end of the 4th week of gestation, a month before the mother feels the fetus move (Moore, 1988). When this process is disturbed, severe brain and spinal cord anomalies such as anencephaly and myelomeningocele may result. During the 4th week of gestation, the embryo develops head and tail folds because of rapid growth of the cranial region and spinal cord. The head continues to get larger during the succeeding weeks, with the brain being folded back on itself. By 8 weeks, the head of the embryo is half the size of the body. At the end of the 8th week, the fetus looks definitely human and has completed the most critical period of CNS development.

Development of the nervous system is a complicated process. By cytogenesis or cell production, the maximum number of neurons and glia are produced. Neurons of the spinal cord and brain stem are generated by the 10th week. The neurons of the forebrain, including the cerebral hemispheres, are produced by 20 weeks (Evrard & Minkowski, 1989). During histogenesis, or tissue formation, the structures of the brain and spinal cord are formed. Neurons move or migrate to their correct location within the nervous system, where they differentiate into different nerve cell types, form synaptic connections, and enlarge. Nerve cell types are genetically determined. Therefore, the size and shape of the nerve cell, the pattern of axon or dendrite branching, and even the type of neurotransmitter a neuron will use are innately determined. Nerve cell classes in the newest part of the cerebral cortex are produced in a set sequence. Cell generation order and cell position in the cortex have an inside-out relationship because of the mechanism of cell migration. The cells formed earliest occupy the deepest layer of the cortex; the cells formed later occupy progressively more superficial layers (Evrard & Minkowski, 1989).

The first endocrine gland, the thyroid, develops at 24 days (Moore, 1988). By the 11th week, it begins to secrete thyroxine, a hormone necessary for proper brain growth. This hormone triggers the cessation of nerve cell proliferation and initiates nerve cell migration (Ford & Cramer, 1977). Without thyroid hormone, axons are poorly myelinated and neurons do not completely branch. Too little hormone produces cretinism, which arrests mental and physical development.

Neuroglia form from the neuroepithelium as early as 3 weeks, although proliferation does not start until 18 weeks of gestation (Herschkowitz, 1989). Microglia appear to be derived from mesenchymal cells late in the fetal period after blood vessels have established their connections. Glial tissue provides a kind of road map for migrating neurons within the brain. The migration appears to be facilitated by some type of chemical affinity between neuronal and glial surfaces, at least in the cerebellum (Evrard & Minkowski, 1989).

Internal brain structures such as the thalamus and hypothalamus are present at 7 weeks of gestation. The internal structure of the spinal cord is achieved by 10 weeks. Over the next 5 to 15 weeks, general structural features—sulci and gyri, cervical and lumbar enlargements of the spinal cord—are attained (Moore, 1988). The 12 pairs of cranial nerves emerge during the 5th and 6th weeks of gestation.

In addition to giving rise to the neural tube, the neural plate also gives rise to neural crest cells, which are the precursors of the peripheral nervous system. The peripheral nervous system begins as paired masses of neural crest cells, one on each side of the neural tube, that differentiate into the sensory ganglia of the spinal nerves. The neural crest cells in the brain region migrate to form sensory ganglia for cranial nerves V, VII, VIII, IX, and X (Moore, 1988). Other structures also are produced from the neural crest cells: Schwann cells, meninges (the connective tissue covering of the brain), and many musculoskeletal components of the head.

Motor nerve fibers begin to appear in the spinal cord at the end of the 4th week of gestation, forming the spinal nerves. Next, the dorsal nerve root (consisting of sensory fibers) appears. It is made up of the axons of neural crest cells that have migrated to the dorsolateral part of the spinal cord, forming a spinal ganglion. The spinal nerves exit between the vertebrae, elongate, and grow into the limb buds, where they supply muscles that are differentiated from mesenchyme (Fig. 9–13). The muscles innervated by segments of the spinal nerve are referred to as *myotomes*. Skin innervation occurs in the same segmental fashion, resulting in *dermatomes*.

The relationship between the spinal roots and the vertebral column is shown in Figures 9–14 and 9–15. Any root above C8 exits above the vertebra of the corresponding number; any root below C8 exits below the vertebra of the corresponding number. This change in relationship is due to differential growth of the spinal cord and vertebral column (see Fig. 9–15).

Synapse formation occurs relatively late in the development of the nervous system, just before 6 to 7 weeks. Synapse formation is highly variable in pattern and distribution. The development of connections between the sensory neurons and the motor neurons is critical to laying the framework for spinal reflexes and for the pairing of sensory and motor information. A spinal reflex

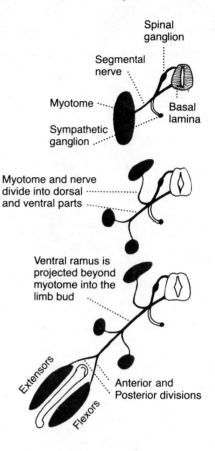

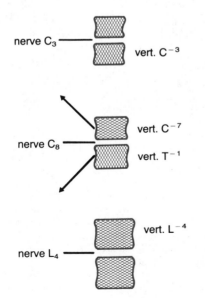

FIGURE 9–13. Spinal nerves growing into myotomes. (From Williams PL, Wendell-Smith CP, Treadgold S. *Basic Human Embryology,* 3rd ed. London: Pitman Publishing, 1984.)

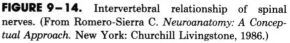

FIGURE 9–14. Intervertebral relationship of spinal nerves. (From Romero-Sierra C. *Neuroanatomy: A Conceptual Approach.* New York: Churchill Livingstone, 1986.)

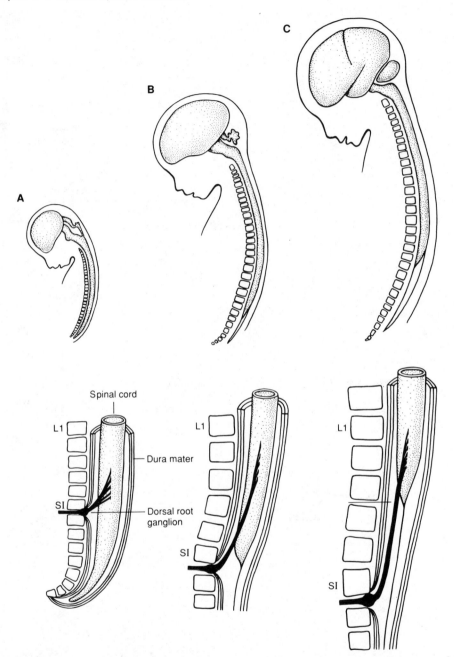

FIGURE 9–15. A side view of the lumbosacral spinal cord and vertebral column shows the changing relationship of the two structures at three stages of development. *A,* Fetus at 3 months. *B,* Fetus at the end of 5 months. *C,* Newborn. (Modified from Pansky B. *Review of Medical Embryology.* New York: McGraw-Hill, 1982; and Kandel ER, Jessell TM [eds]. *Principles of Neural Science,* 3rd ed. Norwalk, CT: Appleton & Lange, 1991, p 301.)

is the pairing of a sensory neuron and a motor neuron so that incoming stimuli produce a motor response. Once established, spinal reflexes are permanent (Sperry, 1959) and considered "hard-wired." Reflexes can be monosynaptic or polysynaptic—that is, they can involve one or more than one synapse. The establishment of reflex connections provides the fetus and eventually the infant with survival reflexes such as suck-swallow, rooting, and gag. Fetal movement begins in utero at about 6 to 7 weeks of gestation. Reflex movements in response to touch have been chronicled as early as 7 to 8 weeks of gestation. Reflex connections are established in utero in a cephalocaudal direction; arm withdrawal occurs earlier than leg withdrawal.

As another late-stage phenomenon of neural development, myelination starts after neuron formation (8 to 16 weeks of gestation) and overlaps with neuron migration (12 to 20 weeks of gestation). Myelination occurs first in those areas of the nervous system that will be used first. Myelin is initially laid down in the cervical part of the spinal medulla and in the cranial nerves related to sucking and swallowing, abilities needed for survival. The first axons to be myelinated are the anterior (motor) roots of the spinal cord at about 4 months of gestation. One month later, the posterior, or sensory, roots begin the process. Myelin is deposited as a sheath or covering in the spinal cord at the same time that functional connections (i.e., synapses) are being formed (Martinez, 1989). The vestibulocochlear system (CN VIII) is myelinated at the end of the 5th month of gestation (Almli, 1990) and is related to awareness of head and body position in space.

Rapid periods of growth such as those seen in the fetal period are critical periods when the nervous system is most vulnerable to damage. Malnutrition or trauma can have dramatic effects on the developing system. The nervous system requires adequate nutrition for cell formation and myelination to occur (Wiggins & Fuller, 1974; Wiggins et al, 1984). For example, lipids in the form of fatty acids must be available (Horrocks, 1985); because there are no endogenous fats in the brain, lipids must be transported through the blood-brain barrier (Bourre, 1989). A lack of nutrition results in a decrease in the number of synapses formed and in the amount of dendritic branching and myelination (Herschkowitz, 1989).

Infancy and Young Childhood

At birth, the brain is one quarter the weight of the adult brain while the head is already 70 per cent of its adult size. Critical periods for brain growth occur between 3 and 10 months of age (Epstein, 1979) and between 15 and 24 months of age (Rabinowicz, 1986). Brain weight doubles by 6 months of age and is half the weight of the adult brain. Malnutrition during the first 2 years of life reduces the number of glial cells formed (Dobbing, 1984), which may result in poorer vascular support for nervous system function. The relationship of brain weight and brain growth is depicted in Figure 9–16. Children who are malnourished before 3 years of age reportedly have impaired motor ability (Kretchmer, 1989).

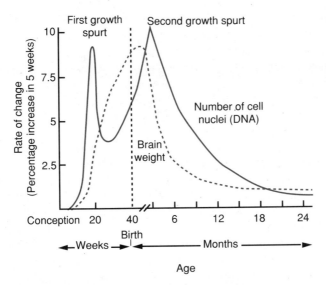

FIGURE 9–16. Relationship of brain weight (dotted line) and growth (solid line). The DNA curve has two peaks, one reflecting neuron multiplication and the other glial multiplication. (Modified from Dobbing J. Undernutrition and the developing brain. *Am J Dis Child* 120:411–415, 1970. Copyright 1970, American Medical Association. From Trevarthen CB. Neuroembryology and the development of perceptual mechanisms. In Falkner FT, Tanner JM [eds]. *Human Growth.* New York: Plenum Press, 1986.)

Myelination of the peripheral nervous system is largely complete at birth (Bishop & Craik, 1982), allowing the newborn immediate access to information about the environment through touch, motion, smell, and taste. The infant uses these sensory cues to carry out vital functions of eating, breathing, sleeping, and excreting. All cranial nerves (with the exception of the optic nerve) are completely myelinated at birth.

Within the brain, myelination continues into young adulthood. Although the peripheral nervous system is ready to function at birth, myelination has been occurring for only 2 months in the brain (assuming that the infant is born at term, 40 weeks of gestation). The primary motor cortex develops ahead of the primary sensory cortex. The rates of myelination are related to when these areas reach adult levels of function (Bronson, 1982). Figure 9–17 shows when some major structures undergo myelination. The mid-brain and spinal cord are the most advanced portions at birth in terms of myelination, which may account for early descriptions of infants as functioning only on a brain stem level. Early myelination of the brain stem supports the many vital functions controlled there and accounts for the fact that the newborn sleeps most of the time and is totally dependent on caregivers.

Brain structures are ready to support development of function during the first year of life. The major efferent (motor) tract, the corticospinal tract, begins myelination 1 month before birth and completes the process by 1 year. The sensory area of the brain catches up to the motor area by the age of 2. During the 2nd year of life, the increasing speed and complexity of movement may be related to myelination. The process slows after 2 years and is mostly complete by 10 years of age.

The first 2 months after birth are considered a period of CNS organization. During this time the infant establishes physiologic control of sleep and

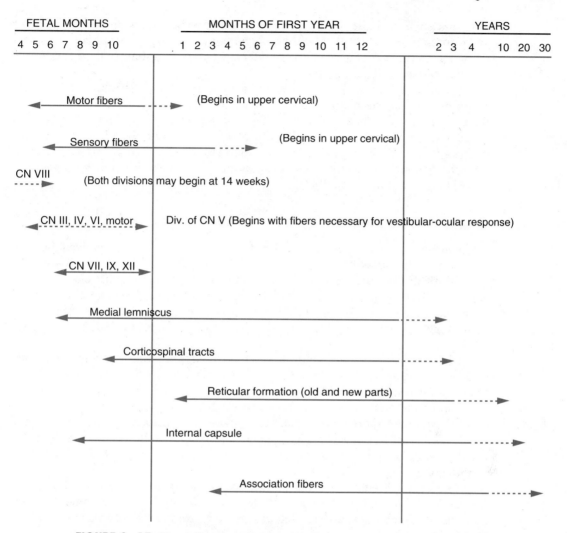

FIGURE 9–17. Timetable of myelination of selected nervous system structures. (Modified from Yakovlev PI, Lecours AR. The myelogenetic cycles of regional maturation of the brain. In Minkowski A [ed]. *Regional Development of the Brain in Early Life.* Oxford: Blackwell, 1967.)

wakefulness as evidenced by the relationship between sleep states and electroencephalograph (EEG) patterns, and by increasing the number and duration of periods of alertness. Social behavior begins around 2 months of age with the advent of the social smile. Circadian rhythm, or the 24-hour biologic cycle, is established between 2 and 4 months of age without regard for night and day (Stratton, 1982). In other words, this is a time when infants can get their days and nights mixed up.

Autonomic nervous system changes occur during the 1st year of life as the newborn responds more via the sympathetic nervous system to ever-changing stressors such as light, gravity, and air. As internal body processes (such as gastrointestinal motility) stabilize, behavioral responses gradually become more characteristic of the parasympathetic nervous system, which maintains the status quo or steady state.

Nerve conduction velocity increases over time in both skin and muscle fibers because of the change to saltatory conduction and the increase in nerve fiber diameter with age (Bishop & Craik, 1982). Values for nerve conduction speed change remarkably quickly after birth. For example, ulnar nerve conduction in infants and young children increases from 30 to 50 m/second from birth to 9 months of age and reaches adult values (60 m/second) by 3 years of age (Thomas & Lambert, 1960).

Childhood and Adolescence

To achieve its adult weight, the brain undergoes additional critical periods during growth spurts at 6 to 8 years, 10 to 12 years, and around 18 years of age. Brain growth during childhood is thought to coincide with the stages of cognitive development as described by Piaget (1952) and the development of language (Thelen & Fogel, 1989). Low-frequency EEG rhythms change to adult high-frequency rhythms by 10 to 13 years of age (Valadian & Porter, 1977).

Children develop fundamental skills such as jumping, throwing, catching, and balancing in early childhood (3 to 6 years). From 6 to 10 years of age, these skills become refined as the nervous system continues to increase the speed of conduction of nerve impulses through ongoing myelination, and motor control becomes more automatic. The adolescent may continue to improve motor skills with practice. The amount of change following adolescence is highly variable and depends more on practice, instruction, motivation, and innate ability.

The brain directs other body systems to change at puberty via hormonal influences. These changes include, but are not limited to, development of the secondary sex characteristics, changes in body composition, and the onset of menses.

Adulthood

The majority of individuals between the age of 20 and 29 years are at the peak of their ability to perform physically. Many persons involved in sports, such as recent Olympic competitors, are even younger. The nervous system begins to decline in adulthood. Brain weight and volume decline linearly with age in the average population (Duara et al, 1985). Beginning at age 20, brain weight declines (Duara et al, 1985), the cortex thins (Earnest et al, 1986), and the number of glial cells increases (Whitbourne, 1985). How much decline is necessary before functional abilities are affected is not known. We do know that age-related changes in the nervous system have far-reaching effects on all systems of the body.

Computed tomography scans confirm that atrophy of the brain occurs with aging. In addition, there is ventricular enlargement. Cerebral volume declines by 11 per cent in relation to cranial volume between the 3rd and 4th decades (Yamamura et al, 1980). The amount of these decreases is moderated by overall good health of the person and varies according to the area of the brain studied (Thomlinson et al, 1968; Frol'kis & Bezrukov, 1978).

CNS changes related to aging are not the same for every part of the brain. Aging affects the frontal and temporal lobes more than the parietal lobes (Brody & Vijayashanker, 1977; Kemper, 1984). The primary motor and sensory areas of the cortex are susceptible to neuron loss beginning at age 20. The hippocampus, a part of the limbic system associated with memory, has been reported to show a 30 per cent decrease in neurons beginning after the age of 30 (Ball, 1977; Mouritzen Dam, 1979).

In contrast to a litany of decreases in large populations of cells, the absence of significant age-related neuron cell loss has been documented in some discrete brain structures. The basal ganglia, which implement movement programs, maintain stability during adulthood (Whitbourne, 1985). Some brain stem nuclei show little or no neuron loss as a result of aging (Moatamed, 1966; Van Buskirk, 1945; Konigsmark & Murphy, 1970).

Terry et al (1987) studied 51 brains from normal individuals aged 24 to 100 years and found that the overall total number of neurons, neuron density, and percentage of cell area occupied remained unchanged. A striking reduction in neuron size, however, was noted, along with a minor degree of neuronal loss when the entire cortex was considered. Large neurons in the frontal and temporal lobes shrank while the number of smaller neurons increased (Terry et al, 1987). Haug and colleagues (1984) and Haug (1985) concluded that the total number of neurons in the cortex does not change during the aging process and that the dominant age-related change is neuronal shrinkage.

Myelination continues into adulthood in those areas responsible for integrating information for purposeful action, the association areas of the brain. Minor changes are seen in EEG patterns with aging. The oscillation frequency of the alpha wave, the EEG pattern evident during wakefulness, decreases slightly over time (Friedlander, 1958).

In the adult, nerve conduction velocity of peripheral nerves decreases (Schaumburg et al, 1983). The speed with which sensory nerves conduct impulses begins to decline after 30 years of age (Buchtal et al, 1984). Motor nerve conduction velocity, according to Schaumburg et al (1983), decreases by 1 m/second per decade after 15 to 24 years of age. Therefore, sensory information continues to come into the nervous system, albeit more slowly.

There is no conclusive proof in the literature that the total glial population changes with aging. Because of the close association of glial cells and neurons, any significant loss of neurons would be expected to cause an increase in glial cells. However, a decrease in glial cells has been reported in connection with the destruction of the myelin sheaths of some nerves. More importantly, it is thought that structural changes in several types of glial cells may have a greater effect on neuron function if, over time, such changes interfere with the transport of vital nutrients from the surrounding blood supply to the neuron (Whitbourne, 1985).

The nervous system changes that result from aging begin at age 20. Brain weight and thickness of the cortex decline while the number of glial cells increases. Whether the number of neurons increases, decreases, or stays the same with reduced neuron size is still being debated. Despite all of these occurrences, few overall changes in the structure of the brain and nervous system exceed 25 per cent of the total area, except in disease states, and only during the last few months of life (Cotman & Holets, 1985). The nervous system's built-in redundancy is such that, even if neurons are lost in one place, other connections may be gained. Most areas of the brain stem that deal with vital functions are stable throughout adulthood and show minimal change with aging.

Older Adulthood

Myriad changes happen within the nervous system during the early and middle part of adulthood, but even more significant changes are seen after 65 to 70 years of age. Decreased awareness of touch and vibration are two documented peripheral changes that occur by the age of 70 (Potvin et al, 1980). The hippocampus exhibits a number of neurofibrillary tangles (NFTs) within the neuron cell body as a result of aging (Ball, 1977; Bell & Ball, 1990). Although the incidence of NFTs increases with age in the healthy brain, an even greater incidence is seen in patients with dementia (Craik, 1993). Neuritic or senile plaques and lipofuscin accumulation are additional cellular hallmarks of aging. A senile plaque is a thickened mass of degenerating neurites (small axons, some dendrites, astrocytes) with an amyloid (starchy glycoprotein) deposit in the center (Bell & Ball, 1990). Plaques occur as a result of pathologic aging (Thomlinson et al, 1968) as in Alzheimer's disease (Katzman & Terry, 1983). They have also been observed in normal aging beginning in the 5th decade of life (Craik, 1993). The role of lipofuscin in normal aging is not clear at this time. The amount of lipofuscin has been roughly correlated to the degree of dementia in Alzheimer's disease (Finch, 1977; Brody & Vijaya-shanker, 1977).

Studies have shown that higher-order association areas lose more neurons than the primary motor or visual cortex area during aging (Ball, 1977; Brody & Vijayashanker, 1977; Kemper, 1984). Morgan (1989) considers the loss of neuron size and aging a possible explanation for forgetfulness in older adulthood. Minor to moderate neuron loss, and the loss of the ability of dendrites to produce new spines (sprouting), have been reported in many parts of the brain, but the link to a decline in function is far from apparent. Structural losses may be a result of an age-dependent decline in use, because dendrites continue to grow into old age. Synaptic remodeling and growth also occur late in adulthood (Herschkowitz, 1989).

Cerebral blood flow has been shown to decrease with age in some studies and not in others. This paradox appears to be related to a decrease in sensory function and/or the presence of arteriosclerosis. According to Duara and colleagues (1985), measures of brain metabolism done without sensory input control are skewed and therefore will show a decrease with age. If the amount of sensory input is controlled for, as in their study, no change in brain metabolism is seen. This may illustrate the adage "use it or lose it."

On a biochemical level, the loss of enzymes involved in neurotransmitter synthesis has been documented along with a moderate loss of receptor sites for certain neurotransmitters in both the CNS and the PNS (Rowe & Troen, 1980; Rogers & Bloom, 1985). A decline in motor system performance has been linked to a steady decrease in dopamine uptake sites due to age-related loss of axons in basal ganglia pathways (DeKeyser et al, 1990). Aging changes in the autonomic nervous system can be linked to changes in the sensitivity of sympathetic receptors to circulating neurotransmitters. Aging has been described as a hyperadrenergic state because of the more intense cardiac and vascular sympathetic responses seen in elderly persons (Katzman & Terry, 1983). Although increased levels of norepinephrine have been documented in older subjects (Katzman & Terry, 1983), Whitbourne (1985) postulates that the increase in circulating neurotransmitter could be an adaptive response to a decrease in receptor sensitivity, as seen in aging cardiac muscle (Kendall et al, 1982).

The concept of "use it or lose it" cannot be overlooked when assessing the competence of any body system to adapt over time. It is especially true for the nervous system. As a person ages, lifestyles and habits formed early in life will be what motivate, inspire, and provide an impetus to move. If exercise, fitness, and health are valued and the individual stays physically fit and actively participates in life, how will the outcome differ?

FUNCTIONAL IMPLICATIONS

This section discusses two aspects of nervous system function, how these aspects change over time, and the relationship between nervous system development and function. These aspects are *reaction time,* a measure of nervous system efficiency during movement, and *cognition,* which enables interaction with the environment.

Reaction Time

The batter sees the ball, swings, and hits the ball. Reaction time is defined as the amount of time between presentation of a stimulus and the motor response. It has been associated with nerve conduction velocity. Reaction time improves as the child develops more complex skills such as catching and hitting. A simple response time test measures reaction speed when only one response is required from a stimulus, such as hitting a key when a light flashes. Fast test responses are reported for subjects in their twenties, with the greatest consistency of response seen in subjects in their thirties. Responses on simple reaction tests slow with age (Stelmach & Worringham, 1985). A 20 per cent increase in reaction time is seen in 60-year-old subjects as compared to 20-year-old subjects (Birren, 1979). Whether this decline can be attributed to nervous system changes is currently being debated.

A decline in nerve conduction velocity with aging has been implicated in the slowing of reaction time and voluntary motor movements. However, Laufer and Schweitz (1968) report that only 4 per cent of the change in reaction time in aging individuals can be accounted for by the decrease in motor nerve conduction velocity, and 10 per cent by the decrease in sensory nerve conduction velocity. A recent study of simple arm movements in the elderly reports that changes in speed of movement and reaction time are due to changes in the muscle (Darling et al, 1989; Cooke et al, 1989). When the level of physical activity of the individual is considered, active older subjects have been found to have faster reaction times than sedentary older subjects (Clarkson, 1978; Spirduso, 1980). However, Panton et al (1990) conclude that exercise does not significantly improve reaction time and suggest that movement slowness is related to changes in neural pathways. Investigators using electromyography (EMG) separated premotor time (PMT) from motor time (MT). *PMT* is the time between the stimulus and EMG activity and reflects the neural component of reaction time. *MT* is the time between the EMG activity and the movement and reflects the muscular component of reaction time. Both PMT and MT are affected by aging. Simple tasks such as hand movement show more age-related effects on the PMT (Welford, 1984); jumping (Onishi, 1966) and movement against resistance (Singleton, 1954) show more age-related effects on the MT.

Complex reaction time studies involve a choice between two responses. Light and Spirduso (1990) confirm that, as the task becomes more complex, reaction time increases with the increasing age of the individual. In a complex task such as trying to recover balance, an individual's risk of falling increases with age. Both PMT and MT are related to chronologic age. Reaction times peak in young adulthood and then decline. PMT (the neural component) is slower in all older individuals regardless of task. MT (the motor component) depends more on the type of task, especially the amount of muscular force required. The more complicated the task, the more likely it is to be influenced by age-related change. After the age of 60, reaction time variability increases relative to that of younger individuals. Also, variability within older subjects increases such that on a day-to-day basis, responses are not as consistent as they are in younger individuals. Thus, results involving reaction time in the elderly must be regarded cautiously.

Cognition

Cognition is the process of knowing, and the application of that knowledge is intelligence. Cognitive processes include attending, learning, reasoning, problem solving, and decision making (Sternberg, 1986). The great developmental psychologist, Piaget (1952), attributes the origin of intelligence to the pairing of sensory and motor experiences. He views cognitive development as necessary for memory development. The nervous system controls cognition by processing thought and memory. According to Guyton (1991), a thought reflects a "pattern" of stimulation of the cortex, thalamus, limbic system, and reticular formation of the brain stem. Physiologically, memories are produced by changes in the ability of one neuron to transmit to another neuron across a synapse, producing a "memory trace." Movement of energy leaves a residue by which use of the pathway can be assessed. (Think of a thermogram, in which greater intensity of the color denotes warmth and increased blood flow.) Memories can be considered immediate, short-term, or long-term, depending on their duration. *Immediate memories* last for only a few seconds or a few minutes. *Short-term memories* can last for days or weeks but will eventually be lost if they are not converted to long-term memory. *Long-term memory* can be recalled years later and is thought to result from structural changes at the level of the synapses that influence signal conduction (Guyton, 1991).

There are two types of memory: reflexive and declarative. *Reflexive memory* includes performance of procedural skills, which include forms of perceptual and motor learning that do not require verbal expression but are exhibited by alterations in task performance. An example is matching shapes to a template. Researchers have shown that infants remember a particular motor event. Rovee-Collier (1987) experimented with connecting an infant's arm or leg to a mobile with a ribbon. The infant learned to move the mobile and even remembered which arm or leg to move after a short time had gone by. *Declarative memory* is the learning of facts and experiences that can be reported verbally—for example, naming body parts, state capitals, or muscle origins and insertions. Because relative value is placed on this type of learning, the limbic system becomes involved. Declarative learning and memory allow for categoric aspects of higher cognitive and affective (emotional) processing such as abstract thought.

The role of memory changes throughout life. Before 6 months of age, there is no conscious memory, only a learned adaptive response. After 6 months of age, an infant learns object permanence, so that he or she knows that an object does not disappear when it is out of sight. Conscious memory is demonstrated as early as 7 months, but recall of events is minimal until a child is about 3 years of age. Conscious memory may be related to the linguistic ability of the child.

Between 5 and 7 years of age, the child begins to relate past and present memories and to reason more efficiently (Mussen et al, 1974). Children no longer just monitor perceptual information, such as size, shape, and color, but correlate perceptual information (e.g., "all round objects made of rubber bounce, whereas round stones do not"). They continue to pick up and reflect on relevant perceptual cues to solve increasingly complex problems or to perform tasks after the age of 6 or 7 (Paris & Lindauer, 1982). Around the age of 9 or 10, children begin to direct their thinking. They can evaluate, plan, and refine their own thinking about how best to solve a problem. Being able to think about thinking is called *metacognition*. The ability to think about remembering is called *metamemory*. One practices metacognition when encountering a patient with an undefined movement dysfunction and thinking of ways to approach the patient's problem. One practices metamemory when planning for a test by reviewing what one does and does not know. With aging, there is a decrease in complex cognitive skills involving memory. According to some, memory loss appears to involve only recent events, leaving immediate and long-term memory intact (Flicker et al, 1984, 1985). Other researchers show a moderate decline in long-term memory with age (Fozard, 1980). Changes in memory abilities need to be considered when giving verbal direction to older patients with movement dysfunction. Written instructions that parallel the verbal instructions are often critical to provide adequate carryover in a home program.

Cognition is functionally reflected in intelligence. Horn and Donaldson (1980) describe two types of intellectual ability: fluid intelligence and crystallized intelligence. *Fluid intelligence* is the ability to form novel associations, reason logically, and solve problems. It can be measured by looking at reaction time and memory. Fluid intelligence peaks in the early twenties and declines throughout adulthood. *Crystallized intelligence* is experiential learning, education, and stored information. It is the ability to use judgment to decide on a course of action. This type of intelligence incorporates a lifetime of decision making and is postulated to improve with age (Horn & Donaldson, 1980).

According to measures of IQ, intellectual ability peaks between ages 20 and 30, and is maintained until at least 75 years of age (Katzman & Terry, 1983). Despite all we do know about the aging changes related to cognition or intelligence, we do not understand why some older individuals remain alert, sharp, and active participants in the world around them and others lose touch, disengage, or show signs of dementia. To date, there is insufficient research to relate loss of neurons from the nervous system to functional decline in cognitive function in healthy aging individuals.

SUMMARY

When looking at the function of the nervous system, the student must view it as constantly changing in response to environmental demands, both from within and from without. The degree of adaptation and accommodation varies from one person to another. Movement and change are based on the structure and function of the nervous system. How a person carries out any movement depends on the integrity of the nervous system and all other body systems needed to support and carry out the movement. The form of the movement will reflect each individual's unique nervous system characteristics across the life span.

References

Almli CR. Normal sequential behavior and physiological changes throughout the developmental arc. In Umphred DA (ed). *Neurological Rehabilitation,* 2nd ed. St. Louis: CV Mosby, 1990, pp 79–110.

Ball MJ. Neuronal loss, neurofibrillary tangles and granulovacuolar degeneration in the hippocampus with ageing and dementia. *Acta Neuropathol* 37:111–118, 1977.

Bell MA, Ball MJ. Neuritic plaques and vessels of visual cortex in aging and Alzheimer's dementia. *Neurobiol Aging* 11:359–370, 1990.

Birren JE, Woods AM, Williams MV. Speed of behavior as an indicator of age changes and the integrity of the nervous system. In Hoffmeister F, Muller C (eds). *Brain Function in Old Age.* New York: Springer-Verlag, 1979, pp 10–44.

Bishop B, Craik RL. *Neural Plasticity.* Washington, DC: American Physical Therapy Association, 1982.

Bourre JM. Developmental synthesis of myelin lipids: Origin of fatty acids—specific role of nutrition. In Evrard P, Minkowski A (eds). *Developmental Neurobiology, vol 12, Nestle Nutrition Workshop Series.* New York: Raven Press, 1989, pp 111–154.

Brody H, Vijayashanker N: Anatomical changes in the nervous system. In Finch CE, Hayflick L (eds). *Handbook of Biology and Aging.* New York: Van Nostrand Reinhold, 1977, pp 241–256.

Bronson GW. Structure, status and characteristics of the nervous system at birth. In Stratton P (ed). *Psychobiology of the Human Newborn.* New York: Wiley, 1982, pp 99–118.

Buchtal F, Rosenfalck A, Behse F. Sensory potentials of normal and diseased nerves. In Dyck PJ, Thomas PK, Lambert EH (eds). *Peripheral Neuropathy, vol 1,* 2nd ed. Philadelphia: WB Saunders, 1984, pp 981–1015.

Clarkson PM. The effect of age and activity level on simple and choice fractionated response time. *Eur J Appl Physiol* 40:17–25, 1978.

Cooke JD, Brown SH, Cunningham DA. Kinematics of arm movements in elderly humans. *Neurobiol Aging* 10:159–165, 1989.

Cotman CW, Holets VR. Structural changes at synapses with age: Plasticity and regeneration. In Finch CE, Schneider EL (eds). *Handbook of the Biology of Aging.* New York: Van Nostrand Reinhold, 1985, pp 617–644.

Craik R. Sensorimotor changes and adaptation in the older adult. In Guccione AA (ed). *Geriatric Physical Therapy.* St. Louis: CV Mosby, 1993, pp 71–97.

Darling WG, Cooke JD, Brown SH. Control of simple arm movements in elderly humans. *Neurobiol Aging* 10:149–157, 1989.

DeKeyser J, Ebinger G, Vauquelin G. Age-related changes in the human nigrostriatal dopaminergic system. *Ann Neurol* 27:157–161, 1990.

Dobbing J. Infant nutrition and later achievement. *Nutr Rev* 42:1–7, 1984.

Duara R, London ED, Rapoport SI. Changes in structure and energy metabolism of the aging brain. In Finch CE, Schneider EL (eds). *Handbook of the Biology of Aging.* New York: Van Nostrand Reinhold, 1985, pp 595–616.

Earnest MP, Heaton RK, Wilkinson WE, et al. Cortical atrophy, ventricular enlargement and intellectual impairment in the aged. *Acta Physiol Scand* 126:107–114, 1986.

Epstein HT. Correlated brain and intelligence development in humans. In Hahn ME, Jensen C, Dudek BC (eds). *Development and Evolution of Brain Size.* New York: Academic Press, 1979, pp 112–131.

Evrard P, Minkowski A (eds). *Developmental Neurobiology, vol 12, Nestle Nutrition Workshop Series.* New York: Raven Press, 1989.

Finch CE. Neuroendocrine and autonomic aspects of aging. In Finch CE, Hayflick L (eds). *Handbook of Biology of Aging.* New York: Van Nostrand Reinhold, 1977, pp 262–274.

Flicker C, Bartus RT, Crook T, Ferris SH. Effects of aging and dementia upon recent visuospatial memory. *Neurobiol Aging* 5:275–283, 1984.

Flicker C, Ferris SH, Crook T, et al. Cognitive function in normal aging and early dementia. In

Traber J, Gispen WH (eds). *Senile Dementia of the Alzheimer Type.* New York: Springer-Verlag, 1985, pp 2–17.

Ford DH, Cramer EB. Developing nervous system in relationship to thyroid hormone. In Grave GD (ed). *Thyroid Hormones and Brain Development.* New York: Raven Press, 1977, pp 1–18.

Fozard JL. The time for remembering. In Poon LW (ed). *Aging in the 1980's.* Washington, DC: American Psychological Association, 1980, pp 273–287.

Friedlander WJ. Electroencephalographic alpha rate in adults as a function of age. *Geriatrics* 13:29–31, 1958.

Frol'kis VV, Bezrukov VV. Aging of the central nervous system. *Hum Physiol* 4:478–499, 1978.

Geschwind N, Levitsky W. Human brain: Left-right asymmetries in temporal speech regions. *Science* 161:186–187, 1968.

Ghez C. The cerebellum. In Kandel ER, Schwarz JH, Jessell TM (eds). *Principles of Neural Science,* 3rd ed. New York: Elsevier, 1991, pp 626–646.

Guyton AC. *Textbook of Medical Physiology,* 8th ed. Philadelphia: WB Saunders, 1991.

Haug J. Are neurons of the human cerebral cortex really lost during aging? A morphometric examination. In Traber J, Gispen WH (eds). *Senile Dementia of the Alzheimer Type.* New York: Springer-Verlag, 1985, pp 150–163.

Haug J, Kuhl S, Mecke E, et al. The significance of morphometric procedures in the investigation of age changes in cytoarchitectonic structures of human brain. *J Hirnforsch* 25:353–374, 1984.

Heiniger MC, Randolph SL. *Neurophysiological Concepts in Human Behavior.* St. Louis: CV Mosby, 1981.

Herschkowitz N. Brain development and nutrition. In Evrard P, Minkowski A (eds). *Developmental Neurobiology, vol 12, Nestle Nutrition Workshop Series.* New York: Raven Press, 1989, pp 297–304.

Horn JL, Donaldson G. Cognitive development in adulthood. In Brim OG, Kagan J (eds). *Constancy and Change in Human Development.* Cambridge, MA: Harvard University Press, 1980, pp 445–529.

Horrocks LA. Metabolism and function of fatty acid in the brain. In Horrocks LA (ed). *Phospholipids in the Nervous System.* New York: John Wiley, 1985, pp 173–199.

Junqueira LC, Carneiro J, Kelley RO. *Basic Histology,* 6th ed. Norwalk, CT: Appleton & Lange, 1989.

Katzman R, Terry RD. Normal aging of the nervous system. In Katzman R, Terry RD (eds). *The Neurology of Aging.* Philadelphia: FA Davis, 1983, pp 15–50.

Kemper T: Neuroanatomical and neuropathological changes in normal aging and dementia. In Albert ML (ed). *Clinical Neurology of Aging.* New York: Oxford University Press, 1984.

Kendall MJ, Woods KL, Wilkins MR, et al. Responsiveness to β-adrenergic receptor stimulation: The effects of age are cardioselective. *Br J Clin Pharmacol* 14:821–826, 1982.

Konigsmark BW, Murphy EA. Neuronal population in the human brain. *Nature* 228:1335–1336, 1970.

Kretchmer N. Nutritional influences on neurological development: A contemplative essay. In Evrard P, Minkowski A (eds). *Developmental Neurobiology, vol 12, Nestle Nutrition Workshop Series.* New York: Raven Press, 1989, pp 261–264.

Laufer AC, Schweitz B. Neuromuscular response tests as predictors of sensory-motor performance in aging individuals. *Am J Phys Med* 47:250–263, 1968.

Light KE, Spirduso WW. Effects of adult aging on the movement complexity factor of response programming. *J Gerontol* 45:P107–109, 1990.

Martinez M. Biochemical changes during early myelination of the human brain. In Evrard P, Minkowski A (eds). *Developmental Neurobiology, vol 12, Nestle Nutrition Workshop Series.* New York: Raven Press, 1989, pp 185–200.

Moatamed F. Cell frequencies in the human inferior olivary complex. *J Comp Neurol* 128:109–116, 1966.

Moore KL. *The Developing Human—Clinically Oriented Embryology,* 4th ed. Philadelphia: WB Saunders, 1988.

Morgan DG. Consideration in the treatment of neurological disorders with trophic factors. *Neurobiol Aging* 10:547–549, 1989.

Mouritzen Dam A. The density of neurons in the human hippocampus. *Neuropathol Appl Neurobiol* 5:249–264, 1979.

Mussen PH, Conger JJ, Kagan J (eds). *Child Development and Personality,* 4th ed. New York: Harper & Row, 1974.

Onishi N. Changes of the jumping reaction time in relation to age. *J Sci Labour* 42:5–16, 1966.

Oppenheim RW. Ontogenetic adaptations and retrogressive processes in the development of the nervous system and behavior: A neuroembryological perspective. In Connolly K, Prechtl HFR (eds). *Maturation and Development: Biological and Psychological Perspectives.* Philadelphia: JB Lippincott, 1981, pp 73–109.

Panton LB, Graves JE, Pollock ML. Effects of aerobic and resistance training on fractionated reaction time and speed of movement. *J Gerontol* 45:M26–31, 1990.

Paris SC, Lindauer BK. The development of cognitive skills during childhood. In Wolman BB (ed). *Handbook of Developmental Psychology.* Englewood Cliffs, NJ: Prentice Hall, 1982, pp 333–349.

Piaget J. *Origins of Intelligence.* New York: WW Norton, 1952.

Potvin AR, Syndulko K, Tourtellote W. W., et al. Human neurologic function and the aging process. *J Am Geriatr Soc* 28:1–9, 1980.

Rabinowicz T. The differentiated maturation of the cerebral cortex. In Falkner F, Tanner JM (eds). *Human Growth: A Comprehensive Treatise, vol 2,* 2nd ed. New York: Plenum Press, 1986, pp 385–410.

Rogers J, Bloom FE. Neurotransmitter metabolism and function in the aging nervous system. In Finch CE, Schneider EL (eds). *Handbook of the Biology of Aging.* New York: Van Nostrand Reinhold, 1985, pp 645–691.

Rovee-Collier C. Learning and memory in children. In Osofsky JD (ed). *Handbook of Infant Development,* 2nd ed. New York: J Wiley & Sons, 1987, pp 98–148.

Rowe JW, Troen BR. Sympathetic nervous sytem and aging in man. *Endocrinol Rev* 1:167–179, 1980.

Schaumburg HH, Spencer PS, Ochoa J. The aging human peripheral nervous system. In Katzman R, Terry RD (eds). *The Neurology of Aging.* Philadelphia, FA Davis, 1983, pp 111–122.

Singleton WT. The change of movement timing with age. *Br J Psychol* 45:166–172, 1954.

Sperry R. Growth of nerve circuits. *Sci Am* 201:5–68, 1959.

Spirduso WW. Physical fitness, aging and psychomotor speed: A review. *J Gerontol* 35:850–865, 1980.

Stelmach GE, Worringham CJ. Sensorimotor deficits related to postural stability. *Clin Geriatr Med* 1:679–725, 1985.

Sternberg RJ. A framework for understanding conceptions of intelligence. In Sternberg RJ, Detterman DK (eds). *What Is Intelligence?* Norwood, NJ: Ablex, 1986, pp 3–18.

Stratton P. Rhythmic functions in the newborn. In Stratton P (ed). *Psychobiology of the Human Newborn.* New York: J Wiley & Sons, 1982, pp 119–145.

Sullivan PE, Markos PD, Minor MD. *Integrated Therapeutic Exercise.* Reston, VA: Reston Publishing, 1982.

Terry RD, De Teresa R, Hansen LA. Neocortical cell counts in normal human adult aging. *Ann Neurol* 21(6):530–539, 1987.

Thelen E, Fogel A. Toward an action based theory of infant development. In Lockman J, Hazen N (eds). *Action in Social Context.* New York: Plenum, 1989, pp 23–63.

Thomas JE, Lambert EH. Ulnar nerve conduction velocity and H-reflex in infants and children. *J Appl Phys* 15:1–9, 1960.

Thomlinson BE, Blessed B, Roth M. Observations on the brains of non-demented old people. *J Neurol Sci* 7:331–356, 1968.

Valadian I, Porter D. Physical Growth and Development from Conception to Maturity. Boston: Little, Brown & Company, 1977.

Van Buskirk C. The seventh nerve complex. *J Comp Neurol* 82:303–334, 1945.

Volpe JJ. *Neurology of the Newborn,* 2nd ed. Philadelphia: WB Saunders, 1987.

Wada JA, Clarke R, Hamm A. Cerebral asymmetry in infants. *Arch Neurol* 32:239–246, 1975.

Welford AT. Between bodily changes and performance some possible reasons for slowing with age. *Exp Aging Res* 10:73–88, 1984.

Whitbourne SK. *The Aging Body—Physiological Changes and Psychological Consequences.* New York: Springer-Verlag, 1985.

Wiggins RC, Fuller GN. Early postnatal starvation causes lasting brain hypomyelination. *J Neurochem* 30:1231–1237, 1978.

Wiggins RC, Fuller G, Enna SJ. Undernutrition and the development of brain neurotransmitter systems. *Life Sci* 35:2085–2094, 1984.

Yamamura H, Ito M, Kubota K, et al. Brain atrophy during aging: A quantitative study with computed tomography. *J Gerontol* 35:492–498, 1980.

Chapter 10

Sensory System Changes

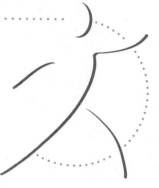

Objectives

AFTER STUDYING THIS CHAPTER, THE READER WILL BE ABLE TO:

1 Discuss the roles of sensation.
2 Describe common characteristics of sensory systems.
3 Describe age-related sensory changes across the life span.
4 Relate sensory function to state and novelty of stimulus.
5 Correlate sensory changes with function.

ROLE OF SENSATION

Our senses provide the only means of communicating with and about the world around us. The psychologist J.J. Gibson (1966) introduced the concept of *affordance* to describe the complementary effect of the environment on the developing organism. Sensation affords interaction between the infant and the environment and interaction between the environment and the infant in such a manner that both are changed. The environment includes the biologic, physical, and social surroundings that affect movement outcome, as depicted in Figure 10–1. These surroundings can also encompass people and objects. No wonder Piaget (1952) described the origins of intelligence as the sensorimotor period. An infant's initial foray into the world is guided by sensations that are paired with movement to initiate communication, motor control, and intelligence.

Because the sensory system is part of the nervous system, they have a common goal—movement production. The role of sensory input in the development and control of posture and movement is well documented (Connolly, 1977; Keshner & Cohen, 1989; Reisman, 1987; Sugden, 1986; Woollacott & Shumway-Cook, 1989). Initially, sensory input is paired with motor output, resulting in reflexes such as rooting and flexor withdrawal. Infants learn to maintain their posture and balance in response to sensory input with the development of postural reactions. Postural reactions are those that automatically occur to maintain the alignment of the head and trunk in response to a

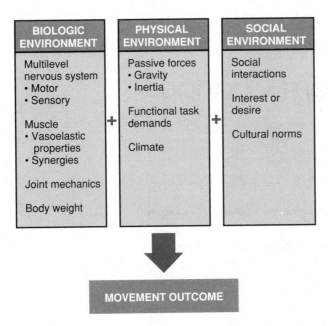

FIGURE 10–1. Environmental factors affecting movement outcome. (Redrawn from Shepard K. Theory: Criteria, importance, and impact. In Lister MJ [ed]. *Contemporary Management of Motor Control Problems.* Alexandria, VA: Foundation for Physical Therapy, 1991. Redrawn with permission of the Foundation for Physical Therapy, Inc.)

weight shift; they include protective extension, righting, and equilibrium reactions. Automatic postural reactions in response to antero-posterior body sway (postural sway) are governed by somatosensory, vestibular, and visual input.

Sensory input aids the process of learning movement by giving feedback for movement accuracy, such as in reaching for or rolling toward a desired object. Once movement is learned, sensation may not be as necessary for the movement to occur. However, as movement becomes more automatic, sensation becomes an anticipatory signal to move (e.g., gathering your things when you hear the signal that the lecture hour is up at school, or changing your walk to a run when even thinking about missing the bus). The way a movement feels can be recalled when one plays a once-forgotten piano piece, or rides a bicycle. Once you learn, you don't forget how, although execution may be impaired through nervous or muscular system deficits.

This chapter defines the sensory systems involved in functional movement. The majority of what we know about the senses comes from research with animals and infants. A second goal is to familiarize the reader with age-related changes in sensory function across the life span, including the importance of state and stimulus novelty. The normally expected changes in sensory awareness with age are just beginning to be distinguished from pathologic changes. Finally, the functional implication of sensory deficits on movement is explored.

CHARACTERISTICS OF SENSORY SYSTEMS

Sensation entails the reception of afferent stimuli from both the internal milieu of the body and the external world. To receive the input, the body must be sufficiently aroused. The state of arousal that an infant experiences will determine the level of responsivity to sensory stimuli. A patient in a coma may respond only to painful stimuli. With recovery, sensory awareness grows. Reception of sensory stimuli does not always imply that the sensation reaches conscious awareness. Each sensory system has its own unique set of receptors and pathways it travels to reach conscious awareness.

The senses monitor internal processes related to vital functions such as breathing, eating, sleeping, and excreting, as well as produce arousal in the form of general alerting, sexual responses, and fight or flight reactions. The arousal functions are choreographed by various subsystems of the nervous system (central, peripheral, and autonomic) in concert with the brain stem reticular activating, hypothalamic, and limbic systems. The interpretation of sensory stimuli is often determined by the state of the autonomic nervous system. Think of how slowly you respond to the alarm clock in the morning when you have an 8 o'clock class. Your parasympathetic system predominates during vegetative functions such as sleep. However, you animatedly respond to cold water when showering, a sympathetic response to a brief cold stimulus.

Sensory input comes in via special receptors, is conveyed by nerve fibers, and is disseminated to appropriate regions of the central nervous system (CNS). For example, your eye picks up a moving image and relays the information to the brain, which identifies a hummingbird. In the meantime, your eye muscles track the bird's movements while you safely continue your forward progression on the nature path. Different sensory receptors have sent a variety of messages to the brain that have been interpreted and have resulted in an adaptive response to allow you to enjoy a pleasurable activity while continuing a motor task.

A sensory system is basically a three-neuron system, as diagrammed in Figure 10–2. The primary sensory neuron transmits the signal along a primary

FIGURE 10–2. Three neuron nervous system. (Redrawn from Romero-Sierra C. *Neuroanatomy: A Conceptual Approach.* New York: Churchill Livingstone, 1986.)

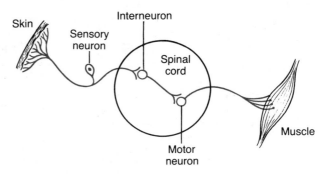

afferent axon toward the CNS. In the peripheral nervous system, cell bodies are located in the sensory ganglia. The axon of the sensory neuron enters the spinal cord and synapses with a secondary, or second-order, sensory neuron, usually in the thalamus, and then travels on to a third-order neuron along specific neural pathways, or tracts. Sensory neural pathways are made up of synaptically interconnected interneurons. Some pathways relay information from only one type of sensory receptor such as mechanoreceptors; others carry information about pain and temperature. All sensory systems have the ability to transform one type of energy (the stimulus) into an electrical signal, code for specific qualities of the stimulus, be represented topographically on many levels of the nervous system, integrate information between one or more sensory systems, and participate in motor responses.

Types of Receptors and Senses

A sensory receptor is a peripheral ending of an afferent nerve fiber or the receptor cell associated with it. Each sensory modality is served by one or more receptors that are sensitive to a particular form of physical energy such as mechanical, thermal, or chemical energy (Table 10–1). In general, there are two main categories of receptors: generalized and specialized. *Generalized receptors* are somatic receptors and motion receptors. *Specialized receptors* are those involved in the special senses of vision, hearing, taste, and smell.

Table 10-1. SENSORY SYSTEMS			
Modality	**Stimulus**	**Receptor Type**	**Receptors**
Somatic	Mechanical, thermal	Mechanoreceptors, thermoreceptors, nocioceptors	Dorsal root ganglion neurons
Propioceptive	Limb positions, muscle tension, joint angulation	Mechanoreceptors	Muscle spindles, Golgi tendon organs, joint receptors
Motion	Head movement	Mechanoreceptors	Hair cells, semicircular canals
Vision	Light	Photoreceptors	Rods, cones
Hearing	Sound	Mechanoreceptors	Hair cells (cochlea)
Taste	Chemical	Chemoreceptors	Taste buds
Smell	Chemical	Chemoreceptors	Olfactory sensory neurons

Modified from Martin JH. Coding and processing of sensory information. In Kandel ER, Jessell TM (eds). *Principles of Neural Science*, 3rd ed. Norwalk, CT: Appleton & Lange, 1991, p 334.

SOMATIC SENSES

Touch, temperature, pain and awareness of body position (proprioception) are conveyed by mechanoreceptors, thermoreceptors, and nociceptors. Touch and proprioception contribute to the development of body scheme and awareness of our relationship to the outside world. Touch defines the limits of the body and provides information about persons and objects in the environment. Temperature detection ensures survival and efficient physiologic function of the body. Pain protects the body from too much pressure, as from sitting too long in one position, and from overexposure to sun, snow, or chemicals. Somatic receptors convey pressure, vibration, temperature, pain, and some proprioceptive information about the body.

Free nerve endings found in the skin and deep tissues, pacinian corpuscles, muscle spindles, and Golgi tendon organs are examples of *mechanoreceptors*. The latter two are also classified as proprioceptors. *Proprioceptive receptors* detect the position of body parts in space and are found in the vestibular part of the ear as well as in muscles, tendons, and joints. *Pacinian corpuscles* respond to tissue vibration and rapid changes in the mechanical state of the tissues (Guyton, 1991). *Thermoreceptors* detect hot and cold by responding to changes in their own metabolic rate relative to actual temperature changes in the ambient air. Extremes of hot or cold can be detected as pain through the stimulation of pain receptors in addition to the temperature receptors. All nociceptors detect pain and are free nerve endings. As such they can respond to mechanical, thermal, and chemical stimuli, either on the skin or internally at the periosteum, arterial walls, and joint surfaces. *Muscle spindles* provide information about limb position (Matthews, 1988) whereas joint receptors relay knowledge of joint angulation, especially at end ranges. It is likely that the muscle spindle also detects rate of movement. Over half of the innervation to a muscle conveys information to and from the muscle spindles, the body's primary source of proprioceptive information (Boyd, 1985). The *Golgi tendon organ,* located in the muscle's tendon, detects tension generated by the contraction or stretch of that muscle, and it safeguards the muscle from overwork by inhibiting or stopping the muscle from contracting. Various sensory receptors are pictured in Figure 10–3.

MOTION SENSE

The vestibular system relays input about the body's relationship to gravity, head position, and head movement. Although it is considered part of proprioception in some regards, it will be discussed separately because of its intimate relationship to movement. Vestibular receptors in the inner ear provide information about head position and head movement in space, postural tone and equilibrium, and gaze stability during head movements (Fisher, 1991). Gaze stability allows the eyes to fix on an image even though the head is moving. The vestibular system resolves intersensory conflicts about balance. If the

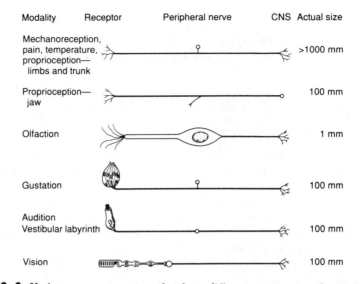

FIGURE 10–3. Various sensory receptors that have different structures and organization. (From Martin JH. Coding and processing of sensory information. In Kandel ER, Schwartz JH, Jessell TM [eds]. *Principles of Neural Science,* 3rd ed. Norwalk, CT: Appleton & Lange, 1991.)

proprioceptors think the body is not moving and the eyes think the body is moving, the vestibular system's input decides what the real situation is and relays information to appropriate motor centers.

The vestibular receptors are located within the membranous labyrinth of the inner ear. The labyrinth is made up of three fluid-filled semicircular ducts. The vestibular receptors are specialized hair cells located in the ampullae of the semicircular ducts and the maculae of the saccule and utricle (Fig. 10–4). The semicircular ducts respond to angular head movement. The saccule and utricle detect gravity; the utricle also monitors the position of the head when you are upright, and the saccule monitors it when you are lying down. Both respond to linear acceleration from the deflection of the hair cells. The three semicircular canals (or ducts) are oriented at right angles to each other and respond to angular acceleration. When these paired structures are stimulated, the hair cells (receptors) are deformed (bent). They transmit electric signals via the vestibular part of cranial nerve VIII to the vestibular ganglion and on to the vestibular nuclei in the medulla and appropriate motor centers. These nuclei also communicate with the cervical spinal cord, eye nuclei, cerebellum, vestibular nuclei of the other side of the body, brain stem reticular formation, thalamus, and hypothalamus. The vestibular system exerts a controlling influence on all other sensory systems (Ayres, 1972; Fisher, 1991).

SPECIAL SENSES

Vision, hearing, taste, and smell are considered the traditional special senses and are linked to specific cranial nerves (Table 10–2). Specialized receptors

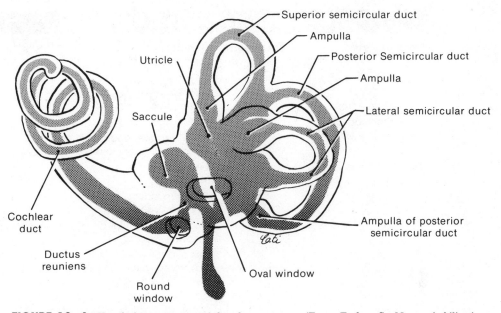

FIGURE 10–4. Vestibular system peripheral apparatus. (From Farber S. *Neurorehabilitation.* Philadelphia: WB Saunders, 1982.)

found in the eye, ear, tongue, and nose are specifically and uniquely designed to sense light, sound, taste, and odors (Junqueira et al, 1989). The distance receptors, vision and hearing, have been the most thoroughly studied.

Vision is the most complex special sense. The sharpness of vision (acuity) and the ability to focus on near and far objects (accommodation) are functions of the structure of the eye. The eye is the organ of sight, but the visual receptors are the rods and cones within the retina of the eye. After light passes through the lens of the eye, it passes over layers of cells to the back of the eye, where it is detected by the rods and cones. A very small area of the retina called the *macula* is capable of detailed and acute vision. The center of this small area, the *fovea,* consists of only cones. Pigment made by the receptors is broken down by light energy and subsequently produces a nerve impulse. The eye is innervated by cranial nerve II, the optic nerve; the eye muscles are innervated by cranial nerves III, IV, and VI. Visual recognition of objects and the interpretation of their meaning involve the occipital cortex and the limbic system.

Hearing is possible because sound waves are transformed into vibration in the ear and understood as meaningful sounds. Sound is captured by the external ear and funneled to the eardrum, or *tympanic membrane.* Three small bones (the *ossicular chain*) are linked to transmit the sound vibration from the tympanic membrane to the cochlea in the inner ear (Fig. 10–5). Remember that the *cochlea* is embedded in the temporal bone or bony labyrinth and is a set of fluid-filled coiled tubes. The sound wave travels along the *basilar* (bot-

Table 10-2. CRANIAL NERVES		
Cranial Nerve	**Component***	**Function**
I—Olfactory	S	Smell
II—Optic	S	Vision
III—Oculomotor	M	Eye muscles
IV—Trochlear	M	Eye muscle
V—Trigeminal	S	Face, tongue, and meninges
	M	Chewing, tympanic reflex
VI—Abducens	M	Eye muscle
VII—Facial	S	Taste
	M	Facial muscles
	A	Nasal and salivary glands
VIII—Vestibulocochlear	S	Linear and angular acceleration, head position in space, hearing
IX—Glossopharyngeal	S	Taste, pharyngeal sensation, chemoreception and baroreception
	M	Swallowing muscles
	A	Parotid gland
X—Vagus	S	Viceral sensation, except pain
	M	Pharyngeal and laryngeal muscles
	A	Smooth muscles in respiratory, cardiovascular, and GI tract
XI—Spinal accessory	M	Neck muscles
XII—Hypoglossal	M	Tongue muscles

*S = sensory, M = motor, A = autonomic parasympathetic.
Modified from Farber S. *Neurorehabilitation.* Philadelphia: WB Saunders, 1982, pp 53–54.

tom) *membrane* of the cochlea like a ripple of water on a pond. The hair cells of the *organ of Corti,* within the cochlea, receive the vibration of the basilar membrane and generate nerve impulses in the auditory division of cranial nerve VIII.

Taste and smell are involved in the vital functions of eating and breathing. Taste and smell are considered near and far receptors, respectively. These receptors are the only ones that are continually being replaced. Although distinct taste receptors for specific taste qualities have not been substantiated, there are generally agreed to be four primary tastes—sweet, sour, bitter, and salty. There is a continuum of tastes, with multiple receptor sites coding for sweetness. Taste buds are found in special skin structures called *papillae,* which are innervated by branches of cranial nerves VII, IX, and X. Three distinct types of papillae are present in humans and located on different parts of the tongue, soft palate, and epiglottis.

Smell is the most primitive special sense. It has a direct connection to the limbic, or emotional, system as well as to the cortex. The *olfactory receptor* is a remarkably simple structure found in the olfactory mucosa. Olfactory hairs or

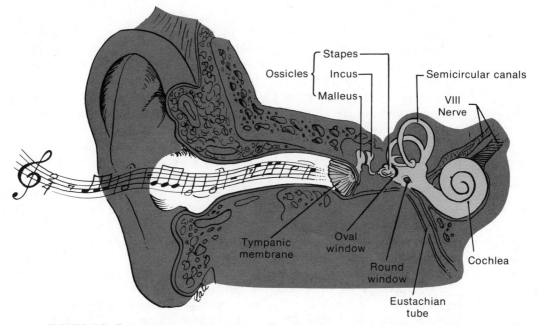

FIGURE 10–5. Schematic model of the auditory system peripheral apparatus. (From Farber S. *Neurorehabilitation.* Philadelphia: WB Saunders, 1982).

cilia project into the mucus, react to odors, and stimulate the olfactory cells. As a bipolar neuron, the olfactory receptor is the actual cell body of the sensory neuron. The receptor can be replaced if damaged and forms cranial nerve I.

Transduction and Coding

Sensory receptors transform mechanical, heat, sound, or light energy into electric signals. The process used to convert one type of energy, such as sound, into an electric signal is called *transduction.* Changing physical energy into usable neural impulses is necessary for each sensory modality (e.g., touch, pain, temperature) to be coded for intensity, duration, and location. Each sensory modality has unique features in transduction and coding and to some extent exhibits differences in anatomic and physiologic development that affect a person's perception of any given sensory stimulus. Everyone feels pain, but there are individual differences in the way each of us perceives and tolerates pain.

Receptors also have the ability to adapt to stimulation. In other words, the receptor has some way to code for the frequency of stimulation. *Rapid-adapting receptors* can detect rapid stimulation and respond with many action potentials. *Slow-adapting receptors* respond to sustained stimuli such as gravity with fewer action potentials.

Representation

Areas of the body are represented in the brain according to their relative importance to function. For example, the sensory cortex is topically arranged so that somatic information from one part of the body is transmitted to a specific part of the cortex. This is referred to as a *somatotopic* (neural) *map*. The same type of mapping is found in other sensory systems. For example, in the auditory system, high-frequency sound is detected at the base of the cochlea, and low-frequency sound is detected at the apex of the cochlea (Fig. 10–6). Each frequency is transmitted to a different part of the thalamus and then on to a specific part of the auditory cortex to be heard *(tonotopic mapping)*.

The area of the body served by a sensory receptor is called a *receptor field*. The size of the area is determined by the branching of the dendrites at the end of the afferent neuron. Think of a receptor field as the shade produced by a tree's branches—the more branches, the bigger the area shaded; the denser the branches, the darker the shade. Receptor fields are the means by which the nervous system keeps track of where on the body information is coming from.

Organization of these receptor fields provides the nervous system with a representation of the body. The map must be represented at each level of the nervous system (Coleman, 1990). For example, to detect being touched, receptors pick up the information and relay it to the thalamus and on to the appropriate part of the sensory cortex. The stimulus is identified and localized. If one is touched at two points at the same time, and the distance between the

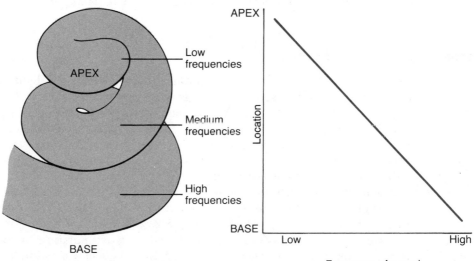

FIGURE 10–6. Tonotopic mapping in the cochlea.

two points is sufficient to be in two different receptive fields, the phenomenon of *two-point discrimination* occurs.

Specific pathways subserve specific sensory modalities. For example, the dorsal column medial lemniscal system transmits tactile, proprioceptive, and vibratory information; the lateral spinothalamic tract carries crude touch, pain, and temperature information. These pathways usually travel to the brain stem and thalamus and on to the primary sensory cortex. The dorsal columns are more discriminating in function.

Perception and Integration

When meaning is attached to sensory information, sensation becomes perception. Sensory information is shared between senses to provide for the identification and manipulation of objects and persons within the environment. Sensory input plays a major role in perceptual development. Detection, awareness, and localization come before discrimination. Sensory integration is the ability to use sensory information to move efficiently. Integration means a putting together of many sensory inputs for the purpose of adapting to the task at hand. Integration enhances the adaptiveness or effectiveness of an individual's response. An individual who has difficulty processing any one or many sensory inputs might exhibit difficulty in planning or executing certain tasks.

There are three types of sensory integration. *Intrasensory integration* occurs when information is shared within the same sensory system. Input from both eyes provides for the perception of depth. *Intersensory integration* occurs when two different sensory systems combine to impart a richer understanding than could be provided by only one sensory dimension. For example, touch and proprioception combine to provide a sense of body scheme. The last type, *sensorimotor integration,* involves the interaction of sensory and motor systems, as with the combining of vision and movement to draw or write. The combination of head turning and hearing to localize an auditory cue is another example. The linking of movement awareness and language results in the establishment of *directionality,* or the ability of the child to utilize spatial cues. Others have called this *spatial cognition.*

The role of sensation in perceptual organization was defined by Ayres (1972) as being able to make use of sensory information. A later definition explains that the sensory information from within the body and from the environment is processed to allow the individual to move effectively within the environment (Ayres, 1989). Sensory integration is an adaptive phenomenon that takes place within the context of a specific task and environment. It is one thing to maneuver a wheelchair through an obstacle course and quite another to walk on the deck of a rolling ship in a rainstorm.

Cortical and subcortical structures participate in sensory integration. Association cortices, the thalamus, and the brain stem reticular system can process, amplify or dampen, and direct sensory information to other areas of the brain. The thalamus relays the sensory stimulus to the cortex as well as to appropriate association areas to plan a response. Recognition and interpretation of the stimulus occur in the primary sensory cortex, such as the realization that you have been touched and the quality of that touch (gentle or rough). The touch is further interpreted in the higher association areas as emotionally pleasing or dangerous. In an open system, interconnected structures regulate and organize sensory input into a conceptual whole to allow a person to identify shapes by touch. This ability is called *stereognosis.* Perceptual abilities and sensory integration develop over time and reflect the increasing adaptation of the individual to the environment.

LIFE SPAN CHANGES

Prenatal Period

The senses of touch, motion (vestibular), smell, and taste are ready to function at birth, as evidenced by the complete myelination of their respective neural pathways. Vision and audition are capable of some level of function at birth but require additional time and environmental experience to complete myelination and maturation of central pathways. The sensory systems develop in utero in the following order: touch, motion, smell, hearing, vision, taste, and proprioception.

SOMATIC SENSES

The fetus develops the ability to respond to touch around the mouth as early as 7½ weeks of gestation (Hooker, 1952). The earliest response to touch is avoidance, or turning away. By 17 weeks, cutaneous sensation spreads to the entire body with the exception of the top and back of the head; these areas are subjected to the most sensory input during delivery.

Proprioceptive receptors are well developed by mid-fetal life (Lowrey, 1986). Tapping, stretching, or even a change in amniotic fluid pressure can cause a response in the fetus (Windle, 1940). Muscle spindles are known to differentiate between 11 and 12 weeks (Bergstrom & Bergstrom, 1963, cited in Wyke, 1975). Pacinian corpuscles are found in the distal parts of limbs at 20 weeks. The Golgi tendon organ does not differentiate until the 4th fetal month.

MOTION SENSE

The vestibular apparatus begins as a thickening of ectoderm, or *placode,* in the primitive ear early in the 4th week of gestation. A placode is a common precursor of most sensory organs. The semicircular canals, utricle, and saccule are completely formed at 9½ weeks of gestation (Humphrey, 1965). The fetus moves constantly in utero, and the vestibular apparatus provides information about that movement. The first sensory system to be myelinated is also the first to function. The fetus shows a generalized body response to changes in body position, including the ability to right the head. Movement in utero has been linked to later movement competence (Milani-Comparetti, 1981).

SPECIAL SENSES

Vision. The eyes also develop during the 4th week of gestation from a placode that forms a vesicle. The optic vesicle folds in on itself to produce a two-layered optic cup, from which the retina is derived. The neural cells of the retina differentiate into 10 layers containing photoreceptors (the rods and cones), cell bodies of bipolar neurons, and ganglion cells. Because of the infolding, the photoreceptors are adjacent to the pigment layer. Therefore, light must pass through the retina to reach the receptors.

Neurons in the occipital cortex are organized into their adult layers during the second half of gestation (Boothe, 1988), so they are ready to receive input after birth. Myelination begins at the optic chiasm around 13 weeks of gestation, and the rods and cones differentiate at 16 weeks. Light perception is possible in utero (Trevarthen, 1986); the fetus exhibits reflexive eye-blinking at 6 months of gestation. Thalamic connections begin to myelinate prior to term and continue until the 5th postnatal month of life. Central visual pathways develop postnally even though the neurons that constitute these pathways are formed prenatally.

Hearing. The same ectoderm that forms the membranous labyrinth of the vestibular system also forms the structures of the inner ear—the cochlear duct and the organ of Corti—during the 4th week of gestation. The remaining structures of the ear, including ligaments and muscles, come from the branchial arches. Hearing in utero is possible as early as 24 weeks and is consistently present after 28 weeks (Birnholz & Benacerraf, 1983).

Taste. The tongue is developed from the mandibular arch at 26 to 31 days of gestation. Formation is completed by the 37th day; the various types of taste buds reach maturity by 13 weeks of gestation (Bradley & Mistretta, 1988). Ingestion of amniotic fluid in utero is thought to contribute to the development of the primitive gut as well as to the regulation of amniotic fluid volume. Steiner (1979) reports that infants born at 6 to 7 months of gestation can detect citric acid.

Smell. The olfactory placode also forms during the 4th week of gestation. It is the earliest distance receptor to develop. The 5th cranial nerve innervates the walls of the nose at 5 weeks; the olfactory organ (bulb) is well developed by the 5th and 6th month of gestation. The unmyelinated nerve fibers of cranial nerve I are the olfactory nerve. It is these fibers that end in the olfactory bulb. Olfactory discrimination is possible in preterm infants beyond 29 weeks (Lowrey, 1986).

Infancy and Early Childhood

Complete maturation of sensory pathways after birth is the rule in vision, hearing, and proprioception. Physiologic changes occur after birth in all sensory systems, as evidenced by an increase in nerve conduction velocity (time to conduct) with myelination, redistribution of axon branching, and increased synaptic efficacy. Functional changes are apparant as the infant interacts more meaningfully with the world.

STATE AND NOVELTY

Behavioral state and novelty of stimulus play a role in the infant's level of interest in sensory information. A sleeping or overstimulated infant is not able to react to a new stimulus. On the other hand, a quietly alert infant looking at a mobile will generally become attentive to a new toy. Sensory awareness requires that the infant be sufficiently aroused. The concept of *state* was first described by Prechtl (1974) as levels of alertness ranging from sleep to crying. The quiet alert state has been deemed the most appropriate for testing an infant's responses to sensory stimulation. Studies show that an infant's state will affect the level of reflex and motor responsiveness (Smith et al, 1982; Casaer, 1979). The ability of the infant to change states smoothly is also an indication of the organization of the central nervous system.

Many studies of visual preference in infants have pinpointed the role of *novelty* in gaining attention and producing motor behavior. The behavior may be looking, reaching, vocalizing, or even quieting, but the common denominator is that the infant responds to a certain level of stimulus novelty. For example, when an infant is shown two pictures, the infant typically attends to the new picture (Fantz, 1966). From the earliest moment that the infant is quietly alert, there is the ability to perceive sensory stimuli and to demonstrate preferences. Learning and adaptation occur much earlier than was once believed. Perceptual abilities once reserved as the province of the older child are now being documented in infants. Sensory perception—that is, the ability to attach meaning to sensory information—occurs from the beginning of extrauterine life.

SOMATIC SENSES

Touch. The perception of touch and pain is crucial to the newborn's survival. Although the defensive movements to light touch seen in utero fade by birth, the newborn reflexively moves to clear the nose and mouth of any object that obstructs the airway. The first responses to touch are generalized diffuse responses, such as random arm and leg movements. Information from touch is initially used by the infant to locate food. Within a few days after birth, head turning in response to touching the mouth is precisely related to the part of the mouth touched. Although touch and pain are not completely differentiated in the full-term newborn, pain sensitivity has been shown to increase over the first 4 days of life (Kaye & Lipsitt, 1964). Studies of infant circumcision (Gunnar et al, 1981) show that physiologic changes in response to the procedure occur, but pain sensitivity can only be inferred from the responses. Pain sensitivity appears to increase in the 1st month of life (Reisman, 1987).

Early tactile input plays a role in parent-infant attachment, stress-coping mechanisms, sociability, and cognitive development (Gottfried, 1984). The use of tactile input to recognize differences develops gradually; a 1-month-old infant is able to distinguish between pacifier shapes (Meltzoff & Borton, 1979). Prechtl (1958) reports a refinement in the receptive field for touch-mediated reflex responses such as flexor withdrawal. Touch to any part of the leg of a newborn results in a reflexive withdrawal. Gradually, the receptive field becomes limited to the sole of the foot.

Touch sensation can be localized generally at 7 to 9 months; specific localization is demonstrated by 12 to 16 months of age (Lowrey, 1986). *General localization* is exhibited by the infant's moving the extremity; *specific localization* involves the infant's touching or looking at the area touched. A toddler can touch the place where he or she was touched and will either rub the area or push the stimulus away. The spot also will be noticed visually, which supports the possibility that intersensory association occurs between touch and vision.

The ability to use touch to identify objects is called *haptic perception* (Gibson, 1966). Haptic means "able to lay hold of" and is appropriate because the majority of information about objects comes from manipulation. Nine-month-old infants have been found to possess this ability, as determined by manual exploration (Gottfried & Rose, 1980).

Temperature. The newborn must regulate its own body temperature at birth and is sensitive to the temperature of the ambient air. Responses to changes in air temperature are often seen in common body postures assumed by the infant. Infants who are too warm may appear to be "sunbathing," decrease their calorie intake, sleep, and show peripheral vasodilation. Sweating and panting responses mature later. Conversely, the infant will wake and move about if too cool. Discrimination of hot and cold is possible early on and is characterized by more reactivity to cold. Respiratory changes, limb movement, and state changes have been documented for temperatures varying as little as 5 to 6° C (Peiper, 1963).

Proprioception. Proprioception is the foundation for purposeful movements such as imitation, reaching, and locomotion. It is used for action very early after birth when the tactile and vestibular systems are functioning. The fact that newborn infants imitate mouth opening and tongue protrusion is interpreted as a pairing of visual and proprioceptive input (Meltzoff & Moore, 1977). In the same way a child handles objects to gain haptic perception, infants move to gain proprioceptive information. Research has shown that reaching behavior in 5-month-olds depends more on the infant's motor ability and proprioception than on visual control; no difference is seen between reaching in the dark and reaching in the light (Sugden, 1986; Wishart et al,

1978). Vision becomes more important as the system matures, as evidenced by more successful reaching with vision in the 7-month-old (Lasky, 1977; Von Hofsten, 1979).

Achieving and maintaining an upright posture depends on the infant's ability to interpret and respond to information about body sway, which comes from vestibular, visual, and proprioceptive input. Multiple studies have shown that infants use vision proprioceptively in sitting and standing to maintain stable postures (Butterworth & Ciccheti, 1978; Butterworth & Hicks, 1977; Lee & Aaronson, 1974). When proprioceptive and vestibular input indicated that the body was stable, and visual input indicated movement, the majority of subjects made compensatory movements.

MOTION SENSE

The vestibular system defines the body's relationship to gravity and is completely myelinated at birth. Many of the infant's earliest activities are related to achieving and maintaining stable postures against gravity. Preterm infants have delayed vestibular responses to movement (Eviatar et al, 1974), especially preterm infants who are also small for gestational age. This delay in responding is due to immaturity, not pathology (Ornitz, 1983), and may be related to the difficulty preterm infants have in maintaining alert wakefulness.

Righting reactions of the head mediated by the labyrinths are possible from birth. The ability to move against gravity continues with the development of trunk righting and progresses to the development of equilibrium reactions. The body appears to seek the most efficient posture to support reaching, manipulation, and locomotion. Infants and children with vestibular problems demonstrate delays in motor function (Kaga et al, 1988).

Nystagmus is an alternating sequence of fast and slow horizontal eye movements normally seen in response to rotatory movement such as being spun in a swing. This *vestibular ocular reflex (VOR)* is not present until a few weeks after birth. The earliest postnatal VOR is called the *doll's eye phenomenon.* When a normal newborn is held in dorsal suspension and moved horizontally, the eyes appear to move in the opposite direction of the body motion. The eye movement corresponds to the slow component of nystagmus. Persistence of this phenomenon after the first 2 weeks of life indicates serious brain damage. The form and amount of nystagmus normally present in infants changes between birth and the first year of life (Eviatar & Eviatar, 1979).

SPECIAL SENSES

Vision. Newborns were always thought to have relatively poor, if any, visual abilities at birth. However, as technology for testing has become more sophisticated, so has our understanding of the infant's visual system. Newborns have pattern preference and can maintain attention if a stimulus is novel enough or resembles a face. To obtain visual alerting behavior, newborns need to be approached from the side, because they are unable to maintain their heads in the mid-line until 4 months of age. Visual acuity at birth varies from 20/800 to 20/200, depending on the means used to measure it (Teller & Movshon, 1986; Nelson et al, 1984), and steadily increases with age. Some authors report that adult levels of vision (20/20) are achieved as early as 1 year (Nelson, 1984), but others still use 3 years as the age at which adult resolution is possible (Coren & Ward, 1989).

The infant sees initially in black and white. As the cones (the color receptors) mature over the first several months, color vision develops. Two-month-olds see two colors, and full-color vision is present by 4 months.

Smooth tracking abilities begin by 2 months of age (Aslin, 1981) and progress over an ever-widening arc as the infant matures and head control is achieved. Accommodation is possible at 2 months but improves to adult levels by 6 months. Depth and size perception begin to develop with the ability to use the two eyes together to converge or diverge on near and far objects. This may be aided by the development of head control in the prone position as the infant practices looking down at his or her hands or up at toys.

Binocular vision depends on adequate alignment of the eyes. Most infants demonstrate good visual alignment between 3 and 6 months of age. Head control contributes to the ability of the infant to visually fix on objects. Shimojo and colleagues (1986) postulate that the change in binocular function seen at 3 months is related to the separation of the afferent input from the two eyes into eye dominance columns within the visual cortex. These bands of cells are known as *ocular dominance columns*. If the input from each eye is the same, the columns will be the same size. Two-year-olds exhibit adult-like binocular vision.

Hearing. At birth, the infant physiologically responds to sound by changing respiratory patterns or heart rate. Behaviorally, the infant may demonstrate facial grimacing, eye blinking, and crying at loud noises. The auditory system is completely myelinated 1 month after birth. By 3 months of age, head turning to localize sound is well established. In the appropriate state of wakefulness, a newborn may exhibit eye or head turning to sound. New sounds will produce searching behavior in infants over 4 months old and will encourage the infant to babble in vocal play. Vocal imitation follows, with words being produced by the first year.

The 2-year-old develops listening skills, which refine the production of speech and facilitate the rapid acquisition of language. Speech is learned by successive approximations of the correct sound. Basic auditory listening skills are mastered by 3 years of age (Lowrey, 1986). Data from auditory-evoked potentials document adult latency values by the age of 4 years, indicating the early postnatal maturation of the auditory system (Allison et al, 1984).

Ear infections that result in increased fluid in the ear are a common problem in infants and preschoolers. Because fluid in the middle ear can produce a conductive hearing loss, these infections are now treated aggressively. Prior to current practice, many children with a chronic ear infection showed delayed development of language. A recent study reports that children with chronic ear infections experience delayed gross motor development (Orlin et al, 1989).

Taste and Smell. These two chemical senses are significant to the newborn. Although obviously linked to feeding, these senses are also involved in parent-infant communication, control of respiration, and cognition (Crook, 1987). Taste may assist in modulating oral intake, as well as in coordinating breathing and eating. Smell may be related to infant attention, although this has not been adequately studied. Infants may use smell to identify familiar features of the environment, including people, before the visual system is effective in performing this function. A 5-day-old newborn can selectively orient to his or her mother's breast pad based on odor (MacFarlane, 1975). Both taste and smell are functional at birth and quickly become connected to feeding reflexes. Infants discriminate among all four primary taste sensations but prefer to ingest sweet things.

Childhood and Adolescence

Sensory changes continue during childhood and cease in adolescence. It is during childhood that the integration of sensation and movement occurs. The perceptual process, although evident in early development, is further refined by the child's increased ability to attend to more than one characteristic of a stimulus, to attach meaning to sensory stimuli, and to plan a motor response. Cognitive and language development are of paramount importance in developing and verbalizing spatial and directional concepts.

SOMATIC SENSES

Children can usually identify familiar objects by touch at 5 years of age. Two-point discrimination is possible by 7 years of age. Knowledge of where the body is in space and the sequence of movements that must be planned to perform a motor task are based on appropriate interpretation of tactile and proprioceptive input (Royeen & Lane, 1991). The ability to motor plan, or *praxis,* emerges during childhood. Tactile and proprioceptive sensation also refine the changing adolescent's body scheme and the affective view of the body.

Bigelow (1981) identified how children use proprioceptive information in visual self-recognition. Children recognized moving images of themselves sooner than they did static pictures, which supports the belief that children move their bodies purposefully to gain proprioceptive information. Proprioceptive acuity and memory for movements improve in children from 5 to 12 years of age (Bairstow & Laszlo, 1981). Examples of movement tasks from memory are a dance routine and the sequence of step-hopping that occurs in skipping.

MOTION SENSE

Vestibular responses change greatly between preadolescence and adulthood (Ornitz, 1983). The most striking maturational changes occur in preschool children (Ornitz et al, 1979). Prior to this period, children engage in repetitive self-stimulation such as rocking in a rocker or spinning themselves. With increasing maturation, these behaviors decline. Children have a stronger response to vestibular stimulation than adults, who respond less intently as the system matures. Maturation is completed between 10 and 14 years of age (Ornitz, 1983).

SPECIAL SENSES

Vision. Many aspects of visual perception develop in childhood. The child shows refinement of *size constancy,* the ability to recognize that objects remain the same size even if the distance of the viewer from the object changes. The ability to separate the figure from the background, or *figure-ground perception,* improves with age. By 8 years of age, most children are as good as adults in performing this perceptual task (Williams, 1983).

Visual perception related to object identification, movement and task performance seems to follow the same trend. By 5 years of age, children demonstrate *visual closure,* or the ability to discern a shape when seeing only part of it. Between 5 and 10 years of age, children track moving objects, such as a softball, accurately (Haywood, 1977). Perceptual judgments regarding the size of various objects at different distances become mature at the age of 11 (Collins, 1976). Adult levels of depth perception are achieved at 12 years of age.

Amblyopia. Two-and-a-half per cent of infants and children develop amblyopia. Amblyopia, or "lazy eye," is a deficit of visual acuity that cannot be corrected with glasses. Because of difficulty in producing a single image when looking with both eyes, the amblyopic person elects to see with only one eye in order to see one image. This problem may be associated with an eye that is deviated in any direction—in, out, up, or down—a condition known as *strabismus.* However, strabismus is not necessarily a cause of amblyopia. The use of only one eye may not be apparent unless screening is done. The lazy eye, if deprived of visual input for enough time, will lose sight, and the child will become functionally blind because of a lack of visual cortex development. The critical or sensitive period for amblyopia appears to be the first 8 years of life.

Adulthood and Aging

Sensory abilities present in adolescence continue to guide motor activities. Despite continued development of intersensory associations, a decline in sensory function begins in adulthood and progresses with age. Peripheral and central changes are documented in many of the sensory systems. Once again, however, these changes are not always directly related to a decline in function, nor are they universal.

SOMATIC SENSES

Some older adults show a diminished ability to detect touch, vibration, temperature, and pain (Kenshalo, 1977). Structurally, the skin changes with aging. Physiologically, the skin's growth rate, injury response, sensory perception, and thermoregulation decline (Gilchrest, 1986).

Extreme temperature changes continue to be detected by the elderly. However, small temperature changes become less distinctly perceived. Many older persons are unable to distinguish temperature differences of 5° C (Navari & Sheehy, 1986), which puts them at risk for burning themselves while cooking or for becoming chilled. Control of body temperature regulation by the hypothalamus is altered significantly with age. The ability of the sympathetic nervous system to cause vasoconstriction and impede heat loss is impaired. As a result, mild hypothermia occurs in a large number of elderly persons in cooler rooms—which is why older people accommodate by wearing sweaters, coats, and hats more often.

Effects of aging on pain perception are not clearly understood. Although deep pain perception is known to diminish with age (Katzman & Terry, 1983), conflicting reports in the literature support both a decrease and an increase in superficial sensitivity (Harkins et al, 1984). In a study (Harkins et al, 1986), age had no main effect on sensitivity, although the middle-aged and elderly participants tended to rate the stimulus lower in intensity than younger adults. Superficial pain probably diminishes with age, but the amount varies individually.

One of the most common sensory losses documented in the elderly is the loss of vibratory sensation. Awareness of vibration begins to decline at 50 (Steiness, 1957), but only in the lower extremities (Potvin et al, 1980). Although pacinian corpuscles in the skin are lost with age, Kenshalo (1977) attributes the loss of vibratory sensation to decreased nerve conduction in the lower extremities.

Joint position sense definitely declines with age (Skinner et al, 1984), especially in the lower extremities. Women exhibit an age-related decline in proprioception and static joint position sensation of the knee (Kaplan et al, 1985). Kokmen et al (1978) found no major decline in motion perception of finger movement in an aging population. Functionally, the decline in proprioception in the lower extremities could impair balance in the elderly. Additional age-related changes in somatosensation are listed in Table 10–3.

MOTION SENSE

Dizziness and vertigo are common disturbances in persons over 50 years of age. Structures of the vestibular system such as the hair cells undergo degeneration (Ochs et al, 1985; Rosenhall, 1973). Neural changes in the vestibular nerve are evident in older adults and may begin as early as 40 years. By 75 years of age, the number of myelinated vestibular nerve fibers declines almost

Table 10-3. AGE-RELATED CHANGES IN SOMATOSENSATION

Function	Nature of Change
Touch/pressure	Significant increase in thresholds after age 40 years; lower thresholds in fingers than toes
	Light touch thresholds significantly increase in hands and feet
	Men generally are less sensitive to touch than women
Vibration	Decreased sensitivity
	Greatest decline after 80 years
Proprioception (passive limb position)	Decreased sensitivity from 20 to 80 years
	Thresholds for lower extremity joints two times greater after 50 years than before 40 years
	More variability in responses
Kinesthesia (active joint motion)	No major changes across 5-year periods
	Few age-related changes generally if minimal memory involved
	Age-related changes increase with greater memory demands

Modified from Williams HG. Aging and eye-hand coordination. In Bard C, Fleury J, and Hay L (eds). *Development of Eye-Hand Coordination.* Columbia, SC: University of South Carolina Press, 1990, p 352.

40 per cent (Bergstrom, 1973). The older individual may exhibit dysequilibrium from age-related changes in the peripheral or central vestibular system.

Presbyastasis is the age-related decline in equilibrium or dynamic balance seen when no other pathology is noted (Kennedy & Clemis, 1990). Reliance on vestibular input alone may result in loss of balance and even falls in the elderly (Woollacott et al, 1986). Healthy older adults without sensory deficits show less of an increase in postural sway than those older adults who show sensory deficits. The latter group is more likely to experience falls (Ring et al, 1989).

SPECIAL SENSES

Vision. Visual acuity increases in the twenties and thirties, remains stable in the forties and fifties, and then declines (Pitts, 1982). By 85, there is an 80 per cent loss from the acuity level present at 40 years of age (Weale, 1975). Structural changes in the eye contribute to these age-related changes in function. Table 10–4 lists some age-related changes in vision.

Central vision can be impaired by cataracts, a decrease in the transparency of the lens. Cataracts begin to form in everyone over 30 years of age (Kollarits, 1986). Cotlier (1981) estimates that 60 per cent of people over 65 have some degree of reduced lens transparency. However, the rate of progression is different for everyone; total opacification of the lens occurs in relatively few people. Visual acuity of 20/50 or worse is an indication for surgical removal. Persons with diabetes have a higher incidence of cataracts than the rest of the population.

Color discrimination in the green-blue end of the spectrum becomes more

Table 10–4. AGE-RELATED CHANGES IN VISION	
Function	**Nature of Change**
General	Decreased transparency of lens
	Decreased amount of light reaching the eye
	Decrease in number of macular neurons by almost half from 20 to 80 years
Visual acuity	Usually retained throughout life
	Slight decrease from 20 to 50 years
	More rapid decrease from 60 to 80 years
	Need more light to detect objects
Light adaptation	Sharp decline in ability to quickly adapt from dark to light environments after 40 years
	Dramatic decrease after 60 years
Contrast sensitivity	Three times as much contrast needed by older individuals as younger ones to perceive a coarsely structured target
Dark adaptation	Little or no change from 20 to 40 years
	Significant increase in time to adapt after 70; an 80-year-old requires 40+ minutes
Depth perception	Little or no changes to age 60+
	Accelerated decrease from 60 to 75 years
Visual information processing	Older individuals are one third slower than younger ones
	Significant decrease in peripheral and central information between 50 and 60 years

Modified from Williams HG. Aging and eye-hand coordination. In Bard C, Fleury M, Hay L (eds). *Development of Eye-Hand Coordination.* Columbia, SC: University of South Carolina Press, 1990, p 350.

difficult as the lens of the eye yellows with aging. Pupil size declines with age, allowing less light into the eye. By 60, retinal illumination is reduced by one third, and the older adult is less able to detect low levels of light. Because of the lens changes, light may be scattered over more of the retinal surface, resulting in glare. Glare introduces extraneous light into the eye and may be particularly troublesome to the elderly. Because of retinal sensitivity loss, one's eyes are overstimulated by oncoming headlights or sudden flashes of light.

Contrast sensitivity and dark adaptation decline with age. Contrast sensitivity loss causes a loss of depth perception, which can be especially dangerous when going up or down stairs. Adaptation to dim light decreases with age, which can be hazardous when one is entering a darkened house or a less well illuminated room. A teenager needs only 6 to 7 minutes to adapt to darkness, but an 80-year-old may need more than 40 minutes (Williams, 1990).

Presbyopia is the diminished ability to focus clearly at normal reading distances. It is caused by a thickening of the lens. As the ciliary muscles become less able to adequately accommodate to distance changes, the person over 40 often complains that "my arms are not long enough to read the print of the newspaper." Accommodation difficulties may also impair the older person's ability to read the speedometer in the car because of a decreased ability of the lens size to change when switching from far to near vision. Corrective lenses such as bifocals or trifocals become necessary. By the age of 60, when the lens can no longer accommodate, presbyopia exists.

Hearing. *Presbycusis,* an age-related decline in hearing acuity, is due to a loss of sensory cells in the inner ear, or more specifically, the organ of Corti. Because the loss typically occurs at the base of the structure, hearing is initially impaired for high-frequency tones such as the whistle of a tea kettle or a doorbell. Speech perception is preserved because speech is heard at lower sound frequencies. This type of hearing loss is associated with aging and can begin as early as 30 years of age and progress until 80.

Presbycusis is more than a simple hearing loss of pure tones. It also involves speech processing and discrimination. Although speech perception is preserved, the ability to discriminate or recognize what is being said decreases. The loss of discrimination is greater than would be expected from the hearing loss alone. Seventy-five per cent of adults over 70 years of age will exhibit hearing loss of this type.

Researchers (e.g., Hinchcliff, 1962) have postulated that the losses seen in presbycusis are due not only to a decline in function of the end organ, but also to central factors. These factors include lengthier auditory processing of information in the cortex, and decreased neuron cell counts in the temporal lobes. Wingfield et al (1985) indicate that processing difficulties in the elderly might be related to a slowing of auditory decoding processes.

Taste and Smell. Taste and smell are intimately linked to the perception of the flavor of food. Age-related deficits may explain reports of flavor changes by the elderly (Weiffenbach, 1984; Murphy, 1986). Loss of taste bud function is documented (Miller, 1988), but recognition of taste, temperature, and viscosity (thickness) of stimuli have been shown to remain stable with age. Pressure detection on the tongue is the only parameter that declines with age (Weiffenbach, 1990). The loss of smell is greater than that of taste, as seen in the declining ability to detect odor intensity with age (Stevens et al, 1984). Memory distortion and/or changes in the social and emotional context in which eating occurs may also contribute to a decreased perception of the flavor and appeal of food for the elderly.

Functional Implications

Decline in function of any sensory system, whether peripheral (as in the eye with changes in lens accommodation) or central (as with the processing of sensory information), results in modification of motor behavior. Decline of visual acuity to 20/50 or less means that a person is restricted from driving. The implications of visual difficulties on the ability of the individual to drive, especially at night, or to be mobile on uneven terrain or in unfamiliar environments, are vast. The impact of the loss of mobility, both real and perceived, can substantially affect an individual's self-image.

Many changes can easily be compensated for by corrective lenses, increased ambient lighting, or use of a filter on glasses to cut down on glare and thus heighten contrast. Visual changes with age do curtail an individual's range of movement by increasing the amount of dependence on compensatory devices or strategies. In some instances, environmental modifications such as changes in lighting and floor coverings can partially reduce safety hazards (Winters, 1989). In other cases, especially when balance is concerned, assistive devices such as canes and walkers are indicated.

Impairment of any sensory system at any point in development can also lead to difficulty in function. The effects of visual deficits on the developmental course have been most thoroughly documented by Alderson and Fraiberg (1974). Visually impaired children must substitute auditory cues to direct movement; because so many movements are visually guided, their acquisition of motor milestones is delayed. Children with crossed eyes, or *strabismus,* may have difficulty in developing head control or mid-line reaching. The earlier that the visual alignment deficits are detected and corrected, the better off children are in terms of upper extremity control.

Hearing loss affects the development of motor skills and balance (Effgen, 1981; Horak et al, 1988). Many children with hearing impairments have poor vestibular function, resulting in balance deficits. Some children with primarily vestibular deficits are unsafe without protective headgear. The effects of deficits in tactile, vestibular, and proprioceptive systems on sensory integration are also well documented (Fisher et al, 1991). Deficits are linked to poor body scheme, self-image, difficulty in motor planning, or sequencing movement and balance.

SUMMARY

Sensory input plays an important role in the learning and refinement of movement. The integration of multiple sensory input and the association/coordination of sensory and motor information form the basis for cognition and perception. The autonomic nervous system and the reticular system act as gatekeepers, determining which sensory information reaches consciousness and which is dampened. The thalamus is a central relay station directing the flow of sensory information to association cortices. All sensory systems have similar characteristics: transduction and coding, representation, and integration at all levels of the nervous system. Sensory abilities change with age; deficits in any sensory system, whether from congenital absence, trauma, or decline with age, can result in functional impairment of movement. Presbyastasis, presbyopia, and presbycusis are all seen in the elderly, but not to the same degree in all individuals. Age-related changes in the sensory systems, therefore, are not uniform, nor are they universal.

References

Alderson E, Fraiberg S. Gross motor development in infants blind from birth. *Child Dev* 45:126–144, 1974.

Allison T, Hume AL, Wood CC, et al. Developmental and aging changes in somatosensory, auditory and visual evoked potentials. *Electroencephalog Clin Neurophysiol* 58:14–24, 1984.

Aslin RN. Development of smooth pursuit in human infants. In Fisher DF, Monty RA, Senders JW (eds). *Eye Movements: Cognition and Visual Perception.* Hillsdale, NJ: Erlbaum, 1981, pp 31–51.

Ayres AJ. *Sensory Integration and Learning Disorders.* Los Angeles: Western Psychological Services, 1972.

Ayres AJ. *Sensory Integration and Praxis Tests.* Los Angeles: Western Psychological Services, 1989.

Bairstow PJ, Laszlo JI. Kinaesthetic sensitivity to passive movement and its relationship to motor development and motor control. *Dev Med Child Neurol* 23:606–616, 1981.

Bergstrom B. Morphology of the vestibular nerve: III: Analysis of the myelinated vestibular nerve fibers in man at various ages. *Acta Otolaryngol* 76:331–338, 1973.

Bigelow A. The correspondence between self and image movement as a cue to self-recognition for young children. *J Genet Psychol* 139:11–26, 1981.

Birnholz JC, Benacerraf BR. The development of human fetal hearing. *Science* 222:516–518, 1983.

Boothe RG. Visual development: Central neural aspects. In Meisami E, Timiras PS (eds). *Handbook of Human Growth and Developmental Biology, vol I, part B.* Boca Raton, FL: CRC Press, 1988, pp 179–191.

Boyd IA. The isolated mammalian muscle spindle. In Evarts EV, Wise SP, Bousfield D (eds). *The Motor System in Neurobiology.* New York: Elsevier, 1985, 154–167.

Bradley RM, Mistretta CM. Development of taste. In Meisami E, Timiras PS (eds). *Handbook of Human Growth and Developmental Biology, vol I, part B.* Boca Raton, FL: CRC Press, 1988, pp 63–78.

Butterworth GE, Ciccheti D. Visual calibration of posture in normal and motor retarded Down's syndrome infants. *Perception* 7:513–525, 1978.

Butterworth GE, Hicks L. Visual proprioception and postural stability in infants: A developmental study. *Perception* 6:255–262, 1977.

Casaer P. Postural behavior in newborn infants. *Clin Dev Med* 72, 1979.

Coleman JR (ed). *Development of Sensory Systems in Mammals.* New York: Wiley & Sons, 1990.

Collins JK. Distance perception as a function of age. *Aust J Psychol* 28:109–113, 1976.

Connolly K. The nature of motor skill development. *J Hum Movement Studies* 3:128–143, 1977.

Coren S, Ward LM. *Sensation and Perception,* 3rd ed. New York: Harcourt Brace Jovanovich, 1989.

Cotlier E. The lens. In Moses RA (ed). *Adler's Physiology of the Eye.* St Louis: CV Mosby, 1981.

Crook C. Taste and Olfaction. In Salapatek P, Cohen L (eds). *Handbook of Infant Perception, vol 2: From Perception to Cognition.* Orlando: Academic Press, 1987, pp 237–264.

Effgen SK. Effect of an exercise program on the static balance of deaf children. *Phys Ther* 61:873–877, 1981.

Eviatar L, Eviatar A. The normal nystagmic response of infants to caloric and perrotatory stimulation. *Laryngoscope* 89:1036–1044, 1979.

Eviatar L, Eviatar A, Naray I. Maturation of neurovestibular responses in infants. *Dev Med Child Neurol* 16:435–446, 1974.

Fantz RL. Pattern discrimination and selective attention as determinants of perceptual development from birth. In Kidd AH, Rivoire JF (eds). *Perceptual Development in Children.* New York: International Universities Press, 1966, pp 137–143.

Fisher AG, Murray EA, Bundy AC (eds). *Sensory Integration: Theory and Practice.* Philadelphia: FA Davis, 1991.

Gibson JJ. *The Senses as Perceptual Systems.* Boston: Houghton-Mifflin, 1966.

Gilchrest BA. Skin diseases in the elderly. In Calkins E, Davis PJ, Ford AB (eds). *The Practice of Geriatrics.* Philadelphia: WB Saunders, 1986, pp 488–498.

Gottfried AW. Touch as an organizer for learning and development. In Brown CC (ed). *The Many Facets of Touch.* Skillman, NJ: Johnson & Johnson Baby Products, 1984, pp 114–122.

Gottfried AW, Rose SA. Tactile recognition in infants. *Child Dev* 51:69–74, 1980.

Gunnar M, Fisch R, Korsvik S, et al. The effects of circumcision on serum cortisol and behavior. *Psychoneuroendocrinology* 6:269–275, 1981.

Guyton AC. *Textbook of Medical Physiology,* 8th ed. Philadelphia: WB Saunders, 1991.

Harkins SW, Kwentus J, Price DD. Pain and the elderly. In Benedetti C, Chapman CR, Moricca G (eds). *Adv Pain Res Ther.* New York: Raven Press, 1984.

Harkins SW, Price DD, Martelli M. Effects of age on pain perception: Thermonociception. *J Gerontol* 41(1):58–63, 1986.

Haywood KM. Eye movements during coincidence-anticipation performance. *J Motor Behav* 9:313–318, 1977.

Hinchcliff R. The anatomical locus of presbycusis. *J Speech Hear Discord* 27:301–310, 1962.

Hooker D. *The Prenatal Origin of Behavior.* Lawrence, KS: University of Kansas Press, 1952.

Horak FB, Shumway-Cook A, Crowe TK, et al. Vestibular function and motor proficiency of children with impaired hearing or with learning disability and motor impairments. *Dev Med Child Neurol* 30:64–79, 1988.

Humphrey T. The embryologic differentiation of the vestibular nuclei in man correlated with functional development. In *International Symposium on Vestibular and Oculomotor Problems.* Tokyo, 1965, p 51.

Junqueira LC, Carneiro J, Kelley RO. *Basic Histology,* 6th ed. Norwalk, CT: Appleton & Lange, 1989.

Kaga K, Maeda H, Suzuki J. Development of righting reflexes, gross motor functions and balance in infants and labyrinth hypoactivity with or without mental retardation. *Adv Otorhinolaryngol* 41:152–161, 1988.

Kaplan FS, Nixon JE, Reitz M, et al. Age-related changes in proprioception and sensation of joint position. *Acta Orthop Scand* 56:72–74, 1985.

Katzman R, Terry RD. *The Neurology of Aging.* Philadelphia: FA Davis, 1983.

Kaye H, Lipsitt L. Relationship of electrotactual threshold to basal skin conductance. *Child Dev* 35:1307–1312, 1964.

Kennedy R, Clemis JD, The geriatric auditory and vestibular system. *Otolaryngol Clin North Am* 23:1075–1082, 1990.

Kenshalo DR. Age changes in touch, vibration, temperature, kinesthesis, and pain sensitivity. In Birren JE, Schaie KW (eds). *Handbook of Psychology of Aging.* New York: Van Nostrand Reinhold, 1977, pp 562–579.

Keshner EA, Cohen H. Current concepts of the vestibular system reviewed: 1. The role of the vestibulospinal system in postural control. *Am J Occup Ther* 43, 5:320–330.

Kokmen E, Bossemeyer RW, Williams WJ. Quantitative evaluation of joint motion sensation in an aging population. *J Gerontol* 33:62–67, 1978.

Kollarits CR. The aging eye. In Calkins E, Davis PJ, Ford AB (eds). *The Practice of Geriatrics.* Philadelphia: WB Saunders, 1986, pp 248–259.

Lasky RE. The effect of visual feedback of the hand on the reaching and retrieval behaviour of young infants. *Child Dev* 48:112–117, 1977.

Lee DN, Aaronson E. Visual proprioceptive control of standing in infants. *Percep Psychophys* 15:529–532, 1974.

Lowrey GH. *Growth and Development of Children,* 8th ed. Chicago: Year Book, 1986.

MacFarlanc A. Olfaction in the development of social preferences in the human neonate. *Ciba Found Symp* 33:103–113, 1975.

Matthews PBC. Proprioceptors and their contribution to somatosensory mapping: Complex messages require complex processing. *Can J Physiol Pharmacol* 66:430–438, 1988.

Meltzoff AN, Borton R. Intermodal matching by human neonates. *Nature* 282:403–404, 1979.

Meltzoff AN, Moore MK. Imitation of facial and manual gestures by human neonates. *Science* 198:75–78, 1977.

Milani-Camparetti A. The neurophysiological and clinical implications of studies on fetal motor behavior. *Semin Perinatol* 5:183–189, 1981.

Miller IJ. Human taste bud density across adult age groups. *J Gerontol Biol Sci* 43(1):26–30, 1988.

Murphy C. Taste and smell in the elderly. In Meiselman H, Rivillin R (eds). *Clinical Measurement of Taste and Smell.* New York: Macmillan, 1986, pp 343–371.

Navari RM, Sheehy TW. Hypothermia. In Calkins E, Davis PJ, Ford AB (eds). *The Practice of Geriatrics.* Philadelphia: WB Saunders, 1986, pp 291–301.

Nelson LB, Rubin SE, Wagner RS, et al. Developmental aspects in the assessment of visual function in young children. *Pediatrics* 73:375–381, 1984.

Ochs A, Newberry J, Lenhardt M, et al. Neural and vestibular aging associated with falls. In Birren JE, Schaie KW (eds). *Handbook of the Psychology of Aging,* 2nd ed. New York: Van Nostrand Reinhold, 1985, pp 378–399.

Orlin MN, Effgen SK, Handler SD, et al. Effect of otitis media with effusion on the development of gross motor skills in the preschool aged child. *Pediatr Phys Ther* 1(4):185, 1989.

Ornitz EM. Normal and pathological maturation of vestibular function in the human child. In Romand R (ed). *Development of Auditory and Vestibular Systems.* New York: Academic Press, 1983, pp 479–536.

Ornitz EM, Atwell CW, Walter DO, et al. The maturation of vestibular nystagmus in infancy and childhood. *Acta Otolaryngol* 88:244–256, 1979.

Piaget J. *Origins of Intelligence.* New York: International University Press, 1952.

Pitts DG. Visual acuity as a function of age. *J Am Optometr Assoc* 53:117–124, 1982.

Potvin AR, Syndulko K, Tourtellotte WW, et al. Human neurologic function and the aging process. *J Am Geriatr Soc* 28:1–9, 1980.

Prechtl HFR. The directed head turning response and allied movements of the human baby. *Behavior* 13:212–242, 1958.

Prechtl HFR. Behavioral states of the newborn infant (a review). *Brain Res* 76:185–212, 1974.

Reisman JE. Touch, motion, and proprioception. In Salapatek P, Cohen L (eds). *Handbook of Infant Perception, vol 1: From Sensation to Perception.* Orlando: Academic Press, 1987, pp 265–303.

Ring C, Nayak USL, Isaacs B. The effect of visual deprivation and proprioceptive change on postural sway in healthy adults. *J Am Geriatr Soc* 37:745–749, 1989.

Rosenhall U. Degenerative changes in the aging human vestibular neuroepithelia. *Acta Otolaryngol* 76:208–220, 1973.

Royeen CB, Lane SJ. In Fisher AG, Murray EA, Bundy AC (eds). *Sensory Integration: Theory and Practice.* Philadelphia: FA Davis, 1991, pp 108–136.

Shimojo SJ, Bauer J, O'Connell KM, Held R. Pre-stereoptic binocular vision in infants. *Vision Res* 26:501–510, 1986.

Skinner HB, Barrack RL, Cook SD. Age-related decline in proprioception. *Clin Orthop Rel Res* 184:208–211, 1984.

Smith SL, Gossman M, Canan BC. Selected primitive reflexes in children with cerebral palsy: Consistency of response. *Phys Ther* 62:1115–1120, 1982.

Steiner JE. Human facial expression in response to taste and smell stimulation. *Adv Child Dev* 13:257–295, 1979.

Steiness I. Vibratory perception in normal subjects. *Acta Med Scand* 158:315–325, 1957.

Stevens JC, Bartoshuk LM, Cain WS. Chemical senses and aging: Taste versus smell. *Chem Senses* 9:167–179, 1984.

Sugden DA. The development of proprioceptive control. In Whiting HTA, Wade MG (eds). *Themes in Motor Development.* Boston: Nijhoff, 1986, pp 21–39.

Teller DY, Movshon JA. Visual development. *Vision Res* 26:1483–1506, 1986.

Trevarthen CB. Neuroembryological development of perceptual mechanisms. In Falkner F, Tanner JM (eds). *Human Growth, A Comprehensive Treatise, vol 2,* 2nd ed. New York: Plenum, 1985, pp 301–383.

Von Hofsten C. Development of visually directed reaching: The approach phase. *J Hum Movement Studies* 5:160–178, 1979.

Weale RA. Senile changes in visual acuity. *Trans Ophthalmol Soc UK* 95:36–38, 1975.

Weiffenbach JM. Taste and smell perception in aging. *Gerontology* 3(2):137–146, 1984.

Weiffenbach JM, Tylenda CA, Baum BJ. Oral sensory changes in aging. *J Gerontol* 45:M121–125, 1990.

Williams HG. *Perceptual and Motor Development.* Englewood Cliffs, NJ: Prentice Hall, 1983.

Williams HG. Aging and eye-hand coordination. In Bard C, Fleury M, Hay L (eds). *Development of Eye-Hand Coordination.* Columbia, SC: University of South Carolina Press, 1990, pp 327–357.

Windle WF. *Physiology of the Fetus.* Philadelphia: WB Saunders, 1940.

Wingfield A, Poon LW, Lombardi L, et al. Speed of processing in normal aging: Effects of speech rate, linguistic structure and processing time. *J Gerontol* 40(5):579–585, 1985.

Winters RK. Adapting the environment to age-related sensory losses. *J Am Acad Nurse Practitioners* 4:106–111, 1989.

Wishart JG, Bower TGR, Dunkeld J. Reaching in the dark. *Perception* 7:507–512, 1978.

Woollacott MH, Shumway-Cook A (eds). *Development of Posture and Gait Across the Life Span.* Columbia, SC: University of South Carolina Press, 1989.

Woollacott MH, Shumway-Cook A, Nashner L. Aging and postural control. *Int J Aging Hum Dev* 23:97–114, 1986.

Wyke B. The neurological basis of movement: A developmental review. In Holt KS (ed). *Movement and Child Development.* Philadelphia: JB Lippincott, 1975, pp 19–33.

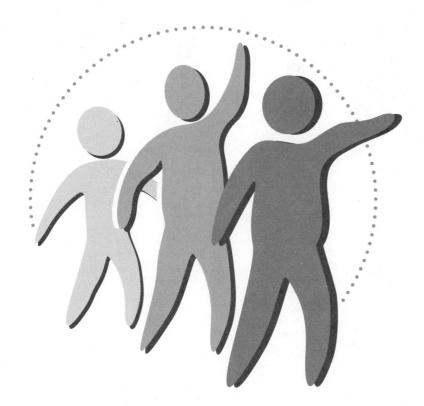

Unit Three

Functional Movement
Outcomes

Chapter 11

Vital Functions

Objectives

AFTER STUDYING THIS CHAPTER, THE READER WILL BE ABLE TO:

1   Describe vital human functions.
2   Identify the systems involved in vital functions.
3   Discuss changes in vital functions across the life span.
4   Understand the interactions between vital functions.

Vital functions are defined as those functions necessary for survival. In human beings, vital functions are breathing, sleeping, eating, and eliminating. All of these functions involve multiple systems of the body. The systems interact to produce functions that support an organism's ability to explore the environment and experience life. The four vital functions can be broken down into the following processes: respiration, sleep-wake, ingestion, digestion, absorption, and excretion. All processes must occur for life to be sustained.

These processes and the functions they are part of are cyclic. Each process has a rhythm or occurs in a cycle. Breathing brings air in and lets carbon dioxide (CO_2) out; wakefulness and sleep occur in patterns that generally correspond to day and night; food and water are taken in and wastes are eliminated. Biologically, the cycles of change seen in the vital functions make it easier to adapt to different environments.

The cyclic nature of the vital functions provides a clue to their control and a way to explain behavior. Hormonal control of cyclic vital functions is mediated by the autonomic nervous system and the endocrine system, which together maintain the body's internal homeostasis. In this chapter, the balance attained by the release of specific hormones is discussed generally; for a more in-depth discussion, the reader is referred to any physiology text.

BREATHING

Oxygen is needed by the body to convert organic carbon compounds into usable energy. Oxygen, however, cannot be stored in the body. The cardiopulmonary, musculoskeletal, and nervous systems work together to take in oxygen and expel carbon dioxide in breathing. Respiration is the process of gas exchange at the cellular level. Breathing and respiration involve the lungs, heart, thorax, diaphragm, central nervous system breathing centers, and central and peripheral chemoreceptors.

Control Mechanisms

Control of breathing is achieved by two interacting systems, each with a specific purpose and affected by different stimuli. One system is neural and the other is chemical. Both systems are automatic but can be overriden by the need to talk, swallow, or perform other functions such as swimming underwater.

NEURAL SYSTEM

At least three brain stem centers coordinate the rhythmic breathing cycle and maintain the depth of breathing. It is generally thought that there are groups of cells, called *pattern generators,* at these sites that pace the breathing rhythm (Remmers, 1990). These neurons require adequate input to continue to pace. Figure 11–1 shows this arrangement schematically. Voluntary control of breathing occurs through the corticospinal tract and spinal neurons that drive the muscles of respiration.

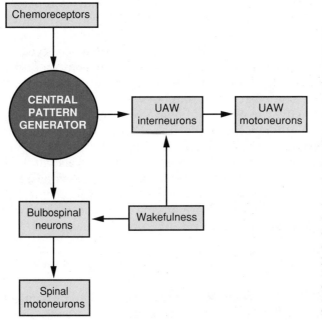

FIGURE 11–1. Schematic diagram of the functional relationships of neural components that control breathing. A central pattern generator produces rhythmic output when activated by adequate chemoreceptor input. The output of this pattern generator is processed by interneurons and ultimately reaches upper airway and spinal respiratory motor neurons to cause rhythmic bursts of action potentials, which in turn cause contractions of the respiratory muscles. Wakefulness conveys an excitatory influence that compensates for mechanical or neuromuscular abnormalities. (Redrawn from Remmers JE. Sleeping and breathing. *Chest* 97[3]:77S, 1990.)

FIGURE 11–2. Cheyne-Stokes breathing showing the changing P_{CO_2} in the pulmonary blood (solid line) and the delayed changes in P_{CO_2} of the fluids of the respiratory center (dashed line). (From Guyton AC. *Textbook of Medical Physiology,* 8th ed. Philadelphia: WB Saunders, 1991.)

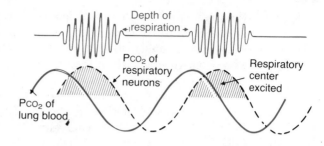

The dorsal group of neurons in the medulla sends out repetitive bursts of inspiratory signals. The pneumotaxic center in the pons continuously sends signals to the dorsal region of the medulla to affect the rate of breathing by limiting inspiration. The ventral group of neurons sends signals only when greater pulmonary ventilation is needed.

A possible fourth center in the lower pons, the apneustic center, can turn off the inspiratory center and thus additionally control inspiration (Guyton, 1991).

CHEMICAL SYSTEM

The chemical system regulates alveolar ventilation and monitors the blood gases. Central chemoreceptors located in the medulla respond to the composition of the extracellular fluid—specifically, to the hydrogen ion concentration. Although hydrogen ions cannot pass the blood-brain barrier, CO_2 in the extracellular fluid reacts with water to form hydrogen ions. Input to this chemically sensitive area must be adequate before it can generate a rhythm.

The peripheral chemoreceptors, the aortic and carotid bodies, are directly influenced by the oxygen content of the arterial blood to which they are exposed. A decrease in oxygen content excites the receptors to cause an increase in breathing. Peripheral receptors provide an accessory mechanism for controlling breathing activity. The breathing pattern can also be modified by sensory input from the lungs and chest wall, as in the case of a person who hyperventilates. Another example is when a person blows off too much carbon dioxide too quickly. The delay in the detection of the change in blood chemistry by the respiratory centers causes periodic breathing (Fig. 11–2). This type of breathing is seen in patients with brain damage and in chronic or severe cardiac failure.

Function Across the Life Span

PRENATAL

The lungs develop early in gestation, but it is not until a pulmonary blood supply is established and adequate amounts of surfactant are produced that the lungs are capable of efficient gas exchange. The heart, although not a part of the respiratory system per se, is needed to perfuse the lungs with blood to allow gas exchange to take place. For the fetus to receive an adequate supply of oxygen through the placenta, the fetal heart must pump a large volume of blood.

Once surfactant is produced at 24 weeks of gestation, the amniotic fluid begins to contain lecithin, a phospholipid. The ratio of two types of phospholipids, lecithin and sphingomyelin (or the *L/S ratio*), is used as an index of lung maturity. A ratio of 2:1 or greater indicates that the lungs are "mature" and that the fetus' risk of developing hyaline membrane disease is less than 5 per cent (Burgess & Chernick, 1986). In this disease, the lungs collapse easily because of a lack of surfactant. Giving steroids to a mother at risk of delivering prematurely has been shown to promote fetal lung maturity (Burgess & Chernick, 1986). Premature infants cannot survive without an adequate pulmonary blood supply and sufficient surfactant (Moore, 1988). Fetuses born at 24 weeks may survive, but those born at 26 to 28 weeks weighing about 1000 g have a better chance because of the lungs' ability to provide adequate gas exchange.

Although respiration cannot occur during fetal life, respiratory movements do occur in utero. Respiratory movements are possible at the end of the first trimester, but because the amniotic fluid is very thick, the fetus "breathes" only a small amount. Burgess and Chernick (1986) think that this "breathing" trains the respiratory muscles and is important for lung development. Fox and colleagues (1978) note that fetal breathing ceases for up to 1 hour after maternal ingestion of alcohol, which may relate to the developmental problems seen as a result of fetal alcohol syndrome.

During the last trimester, fetal respiratory movements appear to be inhibited (Guyton, 1991). This may prevent the lungs from filling with debris from the gastrointestinal tract. Because at birth the lungs are half filled with fluid, the first breath is possible only if the fluid is cleared from the lungs. This process is assisted by the compression of the thorax during vaginal delivery.

CHILDHOOD

The infant's lungs are not miniatures of the adult's and will undergo many age-related changes. At birth, the ribs are horizontal to the vertebral column. The infant relies on the diaphragm to breathe and is therefore a "belly" breather. Around the age of 6 months, or when the infant is placed more consistently in a sitting position, the relationship of the ribs to the vertebral column changes because of the effects of gravity. The ribs move down and out to achieve an adult configuration and establish a normal sternal angle. These changes in the skeletal system (Fig. 11–3) result in improved efficiency of the diaphragm, increased size of the thoracic cavity, and increased vital capacity of the lungs. Furthermore, the structural changes allow the abdominal musculature to participate more effectively in active expiration. Rib flaring and inefficient breathing movements can result if this change does not occur, as in children with developmental delay.

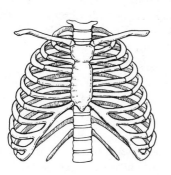
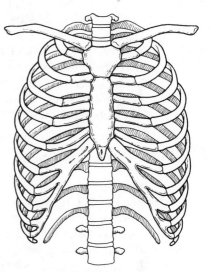

FIGURE 11–3. Comparison of the infant (left) with the mature (right) thorax. A major difference between the infant and mature adult thorax, besides the size, is the orientation of the ribs. The ribs are oriented horizontally in the infant thorax, whereas they are angled downward in the mature thorax.

The depth and rate of breathing change in relationship to the activity or work to be performed. The diaphragm is the major muscle of breathing until around 5 to 7 years of age, after which the thoracic muscles play a larger role (Valadian & Porter, 1977). Adult breathing patterns, according to Adkins (1986), are usually an equal combination of diaphragm and chest movements (2–diaphragm, 2–chest), according to a 4-point scale that measures the four possible components of breathing—diaphragm, chest, neck accessory muscles, and abdominal muscles. Pathologic changes in the musculoskeletal and cardiovascular systems can have a significant effect on the breathing pattern, as in scoliosis, spinal cord injury, or congenital heart defect. Major changes in lung volumes occur in childhood and correlate best with the height of the child. The relationship between work capacity, ventilation, and oxygen consumption is the same for a child as for an adult.

OLDER ADULTHOOD

With normal aging, functional changes are seen in the volume of air moved, the rate of the airflow, and the amount of oxygen exchanged. Although the overall total lung volume remains constant, individual lung volumes change. For example, the residual volume increases and the vital capacity decreases (Block, 1979). Compliance of the lung and chest wall decreases with normal aging. Possible reasons for this decline are an increase in calcification of the ribs, stiffening of connective tissue, and disproportionate growth of the chest wall relative to the lungs (Burgess & Chernick, 1986). Measures of airflow decrease with age. Total lung capacity remains the same because the stiffness of the chest wall is balanced by the loss of elastic recoil of the lungs (Stark & Lipscomb, 1983). Arterial oxygen tension (Pao_2) is the most often used measure of the amount of oxygen in the blood. King and Schwarz (1982) showed that there is a 4 mm Hg drop in Pao_2 per decade. In addition, the amount of hemoglobin available for oxygen transport diminishes with age (Wahbe, 1983). Despite these documented age-related changes in the cardiopulmonary system, function can be improved with progressive endurance exercise (Shephard, 1985).

SLEEPING

Sleeping is a large part of our lives, but the exact benefits or purposes of sleep are not yet fully understood. For most of us, sleep is a rhythmic, predictable process that occurs at night. It has always been said that a good night's sleep repairs the mind and the body. Anyone who has had difficulty sleeping knows the far-reaching effects of a lack of sleep. The purpose of sleep is probably to allow the nervous system time to reorganize or possibly to promote memory and learning (Guyton, 1991; Vander et al, 1985). Most of us have had the experience of going to bed trying to solve a problem, and awaking in the morning to find the solution.

The sleep-wake cycle consists of periods of sleep lasting from 6 to 10 hours and periods of wakefulness lasting from 14 to 18 hours a day. This 24-hour cycle is the *circadian cycle,* from *circa* meaning "about" and *dies* meaning "day" (Klivington, 1989). Physiologically, sleep is a state of unconsciousness from which a person can be aroused (Guyton, 1991). Human beings alternate between three states: wakefulness, nonrapid eye movement (NREM) sleep, and rapid eye movement (REM) sleep.

Wakefulness is associated with an increase in most physiologic parameters from sleep levels; further increases in blood pressure and rate of breathing are associated with sympathetic nervous system activation. In a person who is awake, the brain wave pattern seen on an electroencephalogram (EEG) is desynchronized (Fig. 11–4). There are two types of sleep: NREM sleep and REM sleep. Each involves the brain, lungs, heart, and specific brain stem centers. NREM sleep has four stages, with the fourth stage also known as slow-wave sleep. All four stages of NREM sleep and REM sleep exhibit characteristic physiologic functions and are further distinguished by different brain wave patterns (see Fig. 11–4).

NREM sleep occurs when decreased activity in the reticular activating system (RAS) in the brain stem causes the brain waves to slow down. Slow-wave sleep is associated with a 10 to 30 per cent decrease in blood pressure, rate of breathing, and basal metabolic rate (Guyton, 1991). A sleeping person goes through the four stages of NREM sleep, each stage showing a slower EEG wave pattern. Stage 1 is the lightest sleep, with stages 2, 3, and 4 being increasingly deeper.

NREM sleep occurs when the brain waves do not slow down but the person is asleep and exhibits REM and muscle atonia. These incongruent characteristics explain why REM sleep is also called paxadoxic sleep. Dreaming occurs in REM sleep, but the atonia prevents acting out the dreams. An

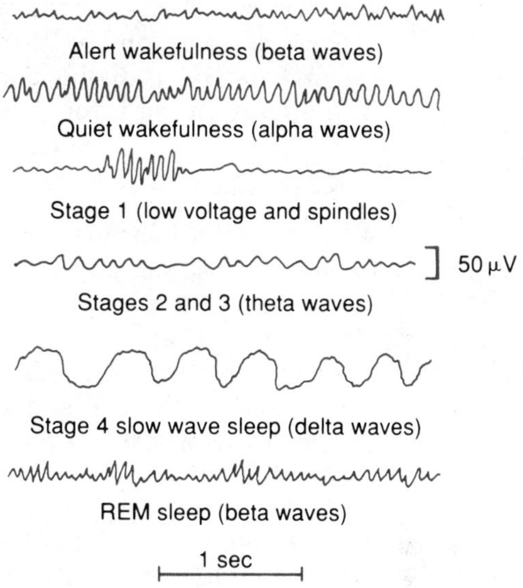

Alert wakefulness (beta waves)

Quiet wakefulness (alpha waves)

Stage 1 (low voltage and spindles)

] 50 μV

Stages 2 and 3 (theta waves)

Stage 4 slow wave sleep (delta waves)

REM sleep (beta waves)

⊢———— 1 sec ————⊣

FIGURE 11–4. Progressive change in the characteristics of the brain waves during different stages of wakefulness and sleep. Stages of slow-wave sleep and corresponding EEG patterns. Stage 1: Very light sleep, low-voltage synchronized waves with sleep spindles. Stages 2 and 3: Light sleep characterized by low-voltage theta waves. Stage 4: Deep sleep characterized by high-voltage waves. (From Guyton AC. *Textbook of Medical Physiology,* 8th ed. Philadelphia: WB Saunders, 1991.)

irregular heart rate and breathing rate and increased brain metabolism are characteristic of paradoxic sleep. Periods of paradoxic, or REM, sleep are interspersed between periods of NREM sleep and are characterized by low-voltage, asynchronous brain waves. An episode of REM sleep in adults can last from 5 to 40 minutes and usually happens every 90 minutes of sleep. Depending on how long you sleep, you may experience four to five episodes of REM sleep. Persons awakened while in REM sleep recall their dreams.

Control Mechanisms

At least three endogenous pattern generators are responsible for the sleep-wake cycle. These centers are located in the brain stem. One group of mid-line nuclei, known as the *raphe nuclei,* secrete serotonin and are thought to produce NREM or slow-wave sleep. Another collection of cells in the brain stem, called the *locus ceruleus,* secrete norepinephrine and may produce REM sleep. A less well-defined group of cells, the RAS, is responsible for arousing the cortex. If the RAS is not inhibited by the sleep centers, the reticular nuclei become active spontaneously and continue to be aroused by the positive feedback from the cortex and the peripheral nervous system. When the RAS tires or is inhibited, sleep occurs. Despite the research done to isolate additional transmitter substances and sleep factors, there is no complete explanation for the reciprocal, cyclic operation of the sleep-wake cycle (Guyton, 1991).

Function Across the Life Span

PRENATAL

Dawes and colleagues (1972) documented the presence of both NREM and REM sleep in fetal lambs. The sleep states were connected to fetal breathing. Patrick et al (1980) confirmed that the human fetus exhibits a circadian rhythm, although the situation was complicated by changes in maternal glucose levels. Milani-Comparetti (1981) also noted that the fetus had alternating periods of sleep and wakefulness at 29 weeks of gestation. Rosen and co-researchers (1973) distinguished REM, NREM, and wakefulness EEG patterns in the fetus during labor.

CHILDHOOD

A newborn's 4-hour sleep-wake cycles appear to be related to cyclic variation in gastrointestinal physiology and can be altered by changing the infant's feeding schedule. Newborns may spend as much as 16 hours sleeping each day. Half of that sleep will be REM sleep, which may lend credence to its speculated role in nervous system organization. A stable circadian rhythm is established between the 2nd and 4th month after birth. At that time, wakefulness is recognized as a stable state necessary for the infant to learn about the environment. Gradually, the "naps" between wakeful periods at night lengthen until the infant sleeps through the night, at about 28 weeks after birth. The 3-month-old spends only 40 per cent of sleeping time in REM sleep (Coons & Guilleminault, 1984); after the age of 5 years, children engage in the same amount of REM sleep as an average adult (Short-DeGraff, 1988).

An infant's sleep begins with REM sleep and progresses to NREM, whereas an adult begins with NREM sleep. The quality of sleep states, changes in EEG activity, and the percentage of time spent in different states of sleep and wakefulness change during the first 2 years of life. NREM sleep is especially enhanced during early childhood and has been linked to an increase in protein synthesis and release of growth hormone. The ability of the nervous system to inhibit REM sleep, thus allowing more NREM sleep, may be a result of central nervous system maturation (Challamel, 1988).

OLDER ADULTHOOD

As one grows older, the length of time spent in deep, slow-wave (stage 4) sleep decreases (Ancoli-Isreal & Kripke, 1986), the quality of the sleep decreases (Woodruff, 1985), and the amount and relative proportion of REM to NREM sleep decreases (Ancoli-Israel & Kripke, 1986) (Fig. 11–5). Older persons take longer to fall asleep and may wake up more frequently (Dement et al, 1985). Daily average sleep time decreases from a little over 7 hours at 25 years of age to less than 5 hours at 75 years of age (Atchley, 1991). The temporary cessation of breathing during sleep, or *sleep apnea,* increases with age. Subclinical levels of sleep-disordered breathing occur in up to 80 per cent of elderly persons (Berry et al, 1990). Research has shown that the quality of sleep in persons over 50 years of age can be improved by relying less on medication (sleep aids) and by spending less time in bed (Woodruff, 1985).

EATING AND DIGESTION

Eating involves taking in food to provide needed nutritional substrates that foster growth, maturation, and repair of all the body's systems. Specific nutri-

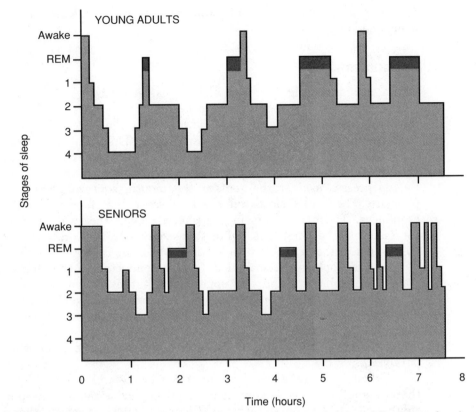

FIGURE 11–5. Normal sleep cycles. As we get older, it takes us longer to fall asleep and we have less deep sleep, more awakenings, and less REM. (Redrawn from Ancoli-Israel, Kripke. Sleep and aging. In Calkins et al [eds]. *The Practice of Geriatrics.* Philadelphia: WB Saunders, 1986.)

tional requirements for each system will not be discussed here, but can be found in any basic nutrition text. Eating, although a pleasurable experience for some, is seen by others as merely something that must be done to keep the body fueled for movement. The initial act of ingesting food or taking in liquid continues in the acts of digestion, absorption, and elimination. Digestion and elimination are crucial to the smooth running of the human body and the maintenance of the internal chemical balance needed for homeostasis. The digestive and excretory systems function together to process all nutrients, except oxygen. The useful components of ingested food and liquids are extracted during the process of digestion and absorption. Waste products are removed and excreted via the gastrointestinal (GI) or the genitourinary tract during elimination.

The act of eating is a skeletal motor activity that demands close coordination with breathing. Eating also requires neuromuscular coordination for mastication (chewing) and deglutition (swallowing), as well as the use of sensory input for motivation and feedback. The process of ingestion involves the mouth, teeth, tongue, pharynx, and esophagus. The process of digestion and absorption requires also the stomach, intestines, salivary glands, pancreas, liver, and gallbladder.

Control Mechanisms

The oral phase of digestion and chewing is caused by a reflex (Guyton, 1991). The presence of a bolus of food prevents the muscles of mastication from closing the jaw, allowing the lower jaw to drop, thus stretching the muscles of mastication, which in turn causes jaw closure. This chain of reflexes produces chewing. Although swallowing is also thought to be reflexive, the initial tongue tip elevation that occurs prior to the swallow is voluntary. The body of the tongue presses against the roof of the mouth, squeezing the food into the pharynx. The glottis closes off the trachea so that food is directed into the esophagus. Touch receptors in the pharynx elicit the swallow, which propels the food into the esophagus. All of this occurs within seconds and is controlled by an area in the brain stem called the *swallowing center.*

In the esophagus, the food is further conducted to the stomach by peristalsis. The pharynx and the upper part of the esophagus are made up of striated muscle that is innervated by the glossopharyngeal and vagus nerves. The remaining part of the esophagus is made up of smooth muscle that is controlled by the myenteric plexus via the vagus nerve; thus, there is a backup system for food to reach the stomach even if the swallowing reflex is paralyzed.

Although the reflex explanation for chewing and swallowing is plausible, there is another possible control mechanism that is more in keeping with the rhythmicity of this vital function. Campbell (1981) suggests that if chewing were strictly reflexive, the movement previously described would occur too quickly. The timing of the reflexes does not fit with the observed rhythm of chewing. She postulates a brain stem pattern generator for the rhythmic and repetitive movements of chewing, drinking, and swallowing. In fact, chewing is controlled by nuclei in the brain stem, which when stimulated near the center for taste produce continual, rhythmic chewing movements (Guyton, 1991).

The regulation and control of digestion take place within the GI tract itself. GI reflexes cause changes in muscle wall contractility and the secretion of digestive enzymes. Two major nerve plexuses control these reflexes: the *myenteric plexus* and the *submucosal plexus.* Together they are called the *enteric nervous system.* The myenteric plexus lies within the intestinal wall, controls the motor activity of the wall and the sphincters that separate the parts of the digestive tract, and is needed for effective peristalsis. The submucosal plexus controls the local segmental responses such as secretion, absorption, and contraction.

Receptors for the two plexuses, along with the parasympathetic and sympathetic innervation, provide the neural support for the GI reflexes, which respond to the following conditions: stretch of the wall, concentration of the chyme, acidity of the chyme, and presence of specific organic digestive by-products (Guyton, 1991). Secretions within the GI tract are therefore under hormonal, central, and local nervous system control and can be divided into three phases: cephalic, gastric, and intestinal. The first phase begins even before the food reaches the stomach, when the sight, smell, taste, and texture of the food and the emotional state of the person eating trigger the secretion of *pepsinogen,* the precursor of *pepsin,* an enzyme that digests protein. Next, gastrin is released in response to local vagal reflexes, which stimulates gastric acid secretion. Finally, secretin and cholecystokinin (CCK) are secreted during the intestinal phase.

Function Across the Life Span

PRENATAL

The earliest oral reflex in utero is the gag reflex, present at 16½ weeks of gestation. Other oral reflexes such as rooting and suck-swallow are present by 28 weeks of gestation. The fetus has been shown to suck its thumb in utero as well as to take in amniotic fluid. The oral reflexes are elicited by touch or pressure and can be considered "survival" reflexes because their purpose is to obtain nutrition and protect the fetus from swallowing unwanted material.

Buchan and colleagues (1981) demonstrated the presence of regulatory gut peptides or hormones as early as 8 to 10 weeks after conception. These protein complexes regulate the activity of the digestive system (Junqueira et al, 1989). Aynsley-Green (1985) documented a large number of gut hormones and metabolites in the fetal and maternal circulations at 18 to 21 weeks of gestation and postulated that these circulating peptides facilitate the development of the fetal lung and GI tract. By the 5th month of gestation, the fetus shows peristaltic movements within the GI tract, and the liver is secreting bile. GI tract function approaches that of a normal newborn by 6 to 7 months of gestation (Guyton, 1991). Meconium, from the unabsorbed amniotic fluid and excretory byproducts, is continually formed and excreted in small amounts. All of these developments appear necessary to prepare the fetus to independently seek, find, and assimilate food efficiently after birth.

CHILDHOOD

The fetus uses glucose, which is primarily obtained from the mother's blood. Once the umbilical cord is cut, the infant must regulate his or her own blood glucose level. Because the infant has a very limited amount of stored glucose, the supply is quickly depleted. Because the infant's liver is not functionally adequate at birth, stored fats and proteins must be used as energy sources until feeding can begin.

The introduction of food produces changes in not only the digestive system but also the endocrine system to allow efficient utilization of food. With the first enteral (or by-mouth) feeding, blood glucose and plasma insulin increase. Within days, the secretion of gut hormones brought on by feeding has fostered growth of the gastric mucosa and development of gastric motility

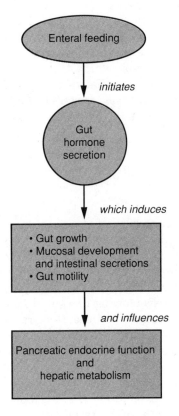

FIGURE 11–6. Hypothesis to explain regulation of postnatal nutritional adaptation. (Redrawn from Aynsley-Green A. Metabolic and endocrine interrelations in the human fetus and neonate. *Am J Clin Nutr* 41:399–417, 1985. © Am. J. Clin. Nutr., American Society for Clinical Nutrition.)

and secretion, pancreatic endocrine function, and liver metabolism. Regulation of postnatal nutritional adaptation is schematically represented in Figure 11–6.

Eating. Eating progresses from being reflexive at birth to being voluntary at 2 to 5 months of age. At this time, a voluntary sucking pattern is established that allows the tongue to stroke the food source. In the process of obtaining food, the tongue's shape is modified. This change prepares it for articulating specific speech sounds and is an example of feeding as prespeech. Solid food is introduced at about 6 months of age, as is cup drinking. As oral control improves, the lips can close around a spoon to remove food and the infant learns to drink liquids from a cup. Again, this oral motor skill carries over into the ability to produce closed mouth sounds such as "p," "b," and "m." Table 11–1 presents a brief developmental history of oral motor skills. For a more in-depth discussion, the reader is referred to Morris & Klein (1987).

Dental Development. Dental development begins in utero and continues through adolescence (Junqueira et al, 1989). The tooth buds of the deciduous or "baby" teeth form at 6 weeks of gestation. Some tooth buds of permanent teeth are formed before birth, whereas others are not developed until after

Table 11-1. ORAL MOTOR DEVELOPMENT

Age	Oral Motor Behavior
Prenatal	Oral reflexes present by 28 weeks of gestation Suck-swallow reflex allows ingestion of small amounts of amniotic fluid
Birth	Suck-swallow reflex, good lip closure
1 month	Reflex sucking changes to suckling Tongue strokes nipple
2–4 months	Oral reflexes except gag fade
4 months	Separate and voluntary suck and swallow Tongue becomes more pointed, variable movement
5 months	Teething Voluntary bite replaces bite reflex
6 months	Tongue thrust decreases Begins cup drinking Munches finger foods Top lip begins to clean spoon
8 months	Slurp-swallows liquids from cup Rotary chewing Tongue lateralizes
9 months	Drooling may occur when infant pulls to stand Eats a cracker Complete lip closure around spoon
10 months	Self-feeds
15 months	Independent with a spoon but messy
24 months	Able to supinate spoon
36 months	Chews with mouth closed

birth. Healthy teeth are important for a person's nutrition, general health, and appearance. The timing of tooth eruption varies greatly among infants, although there is a set sequence (Valadian & Porter, 1977). The average infant's first tooth appears at about 7 months; the rest of the 20 baby teeth are in place by 2½ years of age. Typically, the first permanent tooth erupts at 6 years, with the third molars or "wisdom" teeth appearing last at 17 years. The replacement of the baby teeth by the 32 permanent ones is gradual and can span up to 11 years.

Digestion. Digestion begins in the mouth, where the food is chewed and first exposed to saliva. After swallowing, digestion continues in the stomach, where chyme is produced. *Chyme* is partially digested food that is made highly acidic by the addition of gastric acid. The final stage of digestion occurs in the small intestine, where food is maximally digested and absorbed. The pancreas and gallbladder supply organically specific digestive enzymes and bile to aid this process. The small intestine absorbs the nutrients, so that by the time material reaches the large intestine, the volume has been significantly reduced.

Waste is stored temporarily until its bulk is sufficient for it to be moved on to the last segment of the GI tract, the rectum, where (following distension) defecation is initiated.

Children are usually ready to control defecation around the age of 2 years. However, as with other things, the age is highly variable. The following cues are helpful to determine a child's readiness to be potty trained: regular bowel movements, the ability to sit alone well, the ability to recognize the need for a bowel movement, and the desire to cooperate with an adult, as in releasing an object on request (Valadian & Porter, 1977).

OLDER ADULTHOOD

Dentition. With good oral hygiene and a regular schedule of preventive care, adults should be able to keep their teeth for their entire life span. However, oral tissues undergo substantial changes with age. Teeth can be lost because of deterioration in periodontal structures such as the gums, bones of the jaw, and membranes around the teeth. Many older adults do not take proper care of their teeth, which can result in tooth loss. It is not uncommon for people to lose all their teeth by the age of 50 (Winkler & Massler, 1986), either from progressive tissue atrophy or from periodontal infection. Close to 2 million older adults wear dentures. Although dentures can provide a more positive self-image, nutritional concerns should be of paramount importance.

Digestion. Physiologic changes in the digestive system due to aging are less marked than in other systems (Whitbourne, 1985). Although it is true that changes occur in all phases of digestion, these appear to have a relatively small impact on function. A decrease in the amount of saliva produced in later adulthood translates into an increase in the symptom of dry mouth. Protein is less easily digested because of a decline in gastric acid production, such that there is a 25 per cent loss by the age of 60 (Whitbourne, 1985). Carbohydrates are also not as well metabolized as one ages. In fact, blood glucose levels may rise to the point at which the older adult develops diabetes. Studies of age-related diabetes show no change in the number of insulin receptors available, but a decrease in the body's sensitivity to insulin with age (Minaker et al, 1985).

Despite some structural changes in the small intestines with age, absorption remains functional. Researchers have tried to link lack of absorption of iron, folic acid (a B vitamin), and B_{12} to anemia in the elderly. Although the reports of impaired absorption of vitamins B_6 and B_{12}, folic acid, and vitamin C with age have some basis (Sklar, 1986; Whitbourne, 1985), functional consequences are debatable. Fat is digested within the small intestines through the action of bile secreted by the liver. The liver shows definite anatomic changes with age, but because of its large margin of safety, none of these structural changes affects the production and secretion of bile; therefore, intestinal function, with regard to the digestion of fat, remains essentially unchanged.

Despite what television commercials imply about the elderly person's need for laxatives, there is no evidence for decreased motility in the large intestine. Autonomic nervous system responses to stress can aggravate GI function by decreasing salivary and gastric secretions. However, other factors such as decreased physical activity, decreased fluid or fiber intake, and living alone often lead to, or compound, functional constipation. Unsound dietary practice and habitual use of laxatives are far more likely than any structural or physiologic age-related change to create constipation (Whitbourne, 1985).

ELIMINATION

The last vital function to be discussed is elimination. In the case of solid waste, elimination is an extension of digestion. Spinal level reflexes coordinate contraction of the colon and rectum to expel feces. These autonomic reflexes are mediated by the parasympathetic system and involve sacral cord segments.

The elimination of liquid waste is more complex. The urinary system is made up of two kidneys, two ureters, a bladder, and a urethra. The kidneys have been described as a million functional units held together by connective tissue. Normal function depends on circulatory, endocrine, and nervous system interaction. The kidneys are the filtering system for the body, and they produce urine as the byproduct of filtering the plasma. The purpose of the kidneys is to maintain water and electrolyte balance within the body and to regulate plasma concentration. Maintenance of the internal environment is accomplished by the multiple processes of filtration, absorption, and secretion.

Control Mechanisms

Arterial blood pressure is controlled by the kidneys' regulation of the body's fluid system, which is relatively simple. If there is too much fluid in the system, the pressure rises; if there is not enough, the pressure drops. The two determinants of arterial blood pressure are the volume of renal output and the amount of salt and water in the system. The kidneys control renal output by changing the extracellular fluid volume. An increase in extracellular fluid increases blood volume and ultimately cardiac output, which increases arterial pressure. This increase in arterial pressure is accomplished by controlling the amount of salt in the system, which is the main determinant of the amount of extracellular fluid.

Because the kidneys are also a part of the endocrine system, they have an additional means of controlling pressure: the renin-angiotensin system. This system is a more powerful mechanism than that already described for controlling arterial pressure, but it is also much more complex. Following a drop in blood pressure, the kidneys release renin, which enzymatically causes the release of angiotensin I. Within seconds, angiotensin I is converted by an enzyme in the lungs to angiotensin II. The latter produces systemic vasoconstriction and decreased excretion of salt and water by the kidney. Angiotensin can secondarily cause fluid retention by stimulating the adrenal gland to

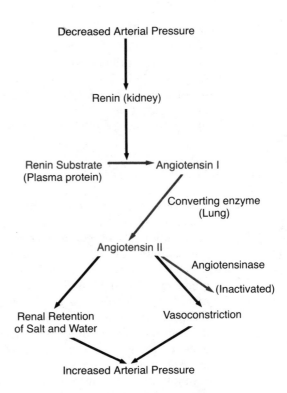

FIGURE 11-7. Renin-angiotensin-vasoconstrictor mechanism for arterial pressure control. (From Guyton AC. *Medical Physiology*. Philadelphia: WB Saunders, 1991.)

secrete aldosterone (Fig. 11-7). The renin-angiotensin vasoconstriction system is important for maintenance of normal arterial blood pressure despite wide fluctuations in salt intake. The system takes about 20 minutes to become fully active.

Function Across the Life Span

PRENATAL

The human embryo develops three different sets of kidneys from mesoderm (Moore, 1988). The first set is rudimentary and nonfunctional. The second set does function for a short time in utero, but is replaced by a third and final set of permanent kidneys, which develop in the early part of the 5th week of gestation and are capable of producing urine 6 weeks later. The collecting tubules and ducts are of endodermal origin, as is the urinary bladder (Junqueira et al, 1989). Urine formation continues throughout fetal life and makes up a large part of the amniotic fluid. Because the placenta removes the waste products from the fetus, the kidneys do not need to function until after birth. However, because the mature fetus swallows amniotic fluid daily and it is absorbed by the fetal intestines, the fetal kidneys do play a role in regulating amniotic fluid volume. The permanent kidneys ascend to their adult position around the 9th week of gestation (Moore, 1988).

CHILDHOOD

The infant's kidney function is adequate but immature for the first few weeks of life. The rate of fluid intake and output in the infant is seven times that of the adult. The infant cannot readily adjust to large changes in fluid loads; any undue loss of water and solutes from fever, vomiting, and diarrhea can be life-threatening. Renal function changes rapidly in response to increased blood flow at birth and steadily increasing metabolic demands. Renal function improves greatly by 6 months; mature function is possible at 2 to 3 years of age. The kidneys enlarge after birth because of hypertrophy of the nephrons. In infants and children, the bladder occupies space within the abdomen. At 6 years, the bladder is still not fully contained in the pelvis; only after puberty is the bladder considered a pelvic organ.

Maturation of bladder function, or voiding, occurs between 1 and 4½ years of age (Meullner, 1960). During infancy, the bladder wall responds to a small amount of urine, contracting to expel its contents. Expulsion is automatic. From 1½ to 2½ years of age, the child develops an awareness of having to void and can retain urine for short periods before voiding. The daily urine volume gradually increases, and as a child gains control over the diaphragm and the abdominal and perineal muscles, he or she learns to initiate voiding. Bladder control continues to improve as the child retains larger volumes of urine for longer periods. Mature bladder control is finally achieved between 2½ and 4½ years of age. A child may first sleep through the night dry when the bladder can retain about 10 to 12 ounces (300 to 360 ml) of urine (Muellner, 1960). This is not quite double the amount normally voided during the day.

The kidneys contribute to homeostasis by expelling waste products in the form of urine and by regulating the balance of fluid and electrolytes in the body. One measure of kidney function and health status is how quickly certain substances, such as creatinine, are cleared from the body. Normal creatinine clearance averages 124 ml/minute in men (Byrne et al, 1981). Another function of the kidneys is to secrete substances that are part of hormonal systems such as erythropoietin, renin, and active forms of vitamin D (Guyton, 1991). Renin is synthesized and stored in the kidneys and is important in controlling blood pressure.

OLDER ADULTHOOD

Renal function declines with age, such that an elderly person has 40 per cent of normal adult capacity to clear creatinine from the body (Rowe et al, 1976). Gross anatomic changes occur, with loss of nephrons and renal mass, and thickening of membranes. Physiologically, the surface area for filtration decreases. Renal blood flow decreases with age, as does the glomerular filtration rate (GFR) (Rowe, 1986). The kidney's endocrine functions change with age. The amount of renin declines, which may be why the ability to conserve salt and water diminishes with age. A decrease in erythropoietin, the hormone secreted by the kidney to stimulate red blood cell production, may contribute to anemia (Bichet & Schrier, 1982). The ability to concentrate urine is less-ened (Whitbourne, 1985), and the diurnal (daytime) rhythm of urine produc-tion is lost (Brundage, 1988) because of age-related changes in the renal tubules. These tubular changes may significantly affect the ability of elderly persons to benefit from medication. An adult dose may have an adverse rather than beneficial effect because of the lower excretion rate in the aged individual (Whitbourne, 1985).

The bladder's smooth muscular wall and elastic tissue are replaced by noncontractile connective tissue as a result of aging. Weakening of the bladder and pelvic floor muscles prevents complete emptying and may lead to stress incontinence, defined as a loss of urine associated with laughing, coughing, or lifting; stress incontinence is primarily a problem with reduced urethral resist-ance. Bladder capacity decreases over time, and frequency of urination in-creases. The loss of self-esteem related to bladder dysfunction in the elderly is significant (Diokno, 1986). The prevalence of urinary incontinence has been estimated at 15 to 30 per cent (Diokno, 1986). Many older women seem to expect some degree of incontinence to occur as a result of aging. Therefore, it is important to teach Kegel exercises to prevent stress incontinence.

INTERRELATIONSHIPS OF FUNCTIONS

Breathing and Sleeping

The control of breathing becomes automatic while the body is asleep. Commu-nication between the sleep-wake and breathing brain stem centers would be expected, although this appears to occur more easily during non-REM sleep than during REM sleep. During non-REM sleep, the respiratory centers con-tinue to regulate breathing in response to chemical feedback from chemore-ceptors and to input from upper airway receptors. However, during REM sleep, most respiratory muscles are inactivated, and the ability of the respira-tory system to respond to chemical changes is significantly decreased (Rem-mers, 1990). The control of breathing must then rely on higher centers such as the locus ceruleus. Remmers' (1990) research with patients who experience sleep-disordered breathing confirms this fact.

Breathing and Eating

The relationship of breathing and eating is also one of coordination and by necessity is established early in development. For the first 6 months of life, the infant is protected from choking by the anatomic proportions of the oral structures and their relationship during swallowing (Valadian & Porter, 1977). The tongue's movements allow the mouth to be separated from the trachea so that sucking and breathing can occur simultaneously. The infant loses this ability as the oral cavity grows. At 3 months, swallowing follows sucking with no pauses. Poor coordination is indicated by choking or coughing. If the infant does not take breaks for breathing, the caregiver must impose them. During this time, it is not unusual for the infant to take air into the stomach, which necessitates burping. Once voluntary control of oral motor function is established at 6 to 8 months, the infant interrupts sucking and swallowing to breathe. Breathing has to be coordinated with the oral motor skills of sucking, chewing, and swallowing. Airflow is also controlled when the infant emits sounds and is modified by mouth and tongue movements to produce recognizable sounds and words.

SUMMARY

All of the vital functions depend on an adequate blood supply to provide the necessary nutrients for the organs involved. The skeletal system provides the frame from which the muscles of mastication, respiration, digestion, and elimination work. The nervous system, especially the autonomic nervous system, plays a significant role in maintaining homeostasis. Breathing, sleeping, and eating are cyclic activities that conform to neural control mechanisms based on oscillations. Vital functions that do not appear to have such neural control, such as digestion and elimination, do exhibit cyclic function. The ability to maintain a fixed level of performance allows the organism to adapt to a fluctuating environment. A built-in pacemaker for repetitive functions, as is present in breathing, "buys time" until other systems mature (Stratton, 1982).

The environment can and does influence the adaptation of vital functions to changing internal and external demands. Possibly because these functions are vital, the age-related changes in them do not often result in significant or life-threatening effects. No one system of the body works entirely without the other. If one system malfunctions, it will affect all the others in some way at some time and eventually lead to either adaptation or failure.

References

Adkins HV. Improvement of breathing ability in children with respiratory muscle paralysis. *Phys Ther* 48:577–581, 1968.

Ancoli-Israel S, Kripke DF. Sleep and aging. In Calkins E, Davis PJ, Ford AB (eds). *The Practice of Geriatrics*. Philadelphia: WB Saunders, 1986, pp 240–247.

Atchley RC. Physical aging. In Atchley RC. *Social Forces and Aging*. Belmont, CA: Wadsworth, 1991, pp 69–81.

Aynsley-Green A. Metabolic and endocrine interrelations in the human fetus and neonate. *Am J Clin Nutr* February, 41:399–417, 1985.

Berry DTR, Phillips BA, Cook YR, et al. Geriatric sleep apnea syndrome: A preliminary description. *J Gerontol* 45(5):M169–174, 1990.

Bichet DB, Schrier RW. Renal function and diseases in the aged. In Schrier RS (ed). *Clinical Internal Medicine in the Aged*. Philadelphia: WB Saunders, 1982, pp 211–221.

Block ER. Pitfalls in diagnosing and managing pulmonary diseases. *Geriatrics* 34(2):70–79, 1979.

Brundage DJ. Age-related changes in the genitourinary system. In Matteson MA, McConnell ES (eds). *Gerontological Nursing*. Philadelphia: WB Saunders, 1988, pp 279–290.

Buchan AMF, Bryant MG, Polak JM, et al. Development of regulatory peptides in the human fetal intestine. In Bloom SR, Polak JM (eds). *Gut Hormones.* London: Churchill Livingstone, 1981, pp 119–26.

Burgess WE, Chernick V. *Respiratory Therapy in Newborn Infants and Children,* 2nd ed. New York: Thieme, 1986.

Byrne CJ, Saxton, DF, Pelikan PK, et al. *Laboratory Tests: Implications for Nurses and Allied Health Professionals.* Menlo Park, CA: Addison-Wesley, 1981.

Campbell SK. Neural control of oral somatic motor function. *Phys Ther* 61:16–22, 1981.

Challamel M-J. Development of sleep and wakefulness. In Meisami E, Timiras PS (eds). *Handbook of Human Growth and Developmental Biology, vol I, part B.* Boca Raton, FL: CRC Press, 1988, pp 269–84.

Coons S, Guilleminault C. Development of consolidated sleep and wakeful periods in relation to the day/night cycle in infancy. *Dev Med Child Neurol* 26:169–176, 1984.

Dawes GS, Fox HE, Leduc MG, et al. Respiratory movements and rapid eye movement sleep in the fetal lamb. *J Physiol (London)* 220:119–143, 1972.

Dement W, Richardson G, Prinz P, et al. Changes of sleep and wakefulness with age. In Finch CE, Schneider EL (eds). *Handbook of the Biology of Aging.* New York: Van Nostrand Reinhold, 1985, pp 692–711.

Diokno AC. Urinary incontinence in the elderly. In Calkins E, Davis PJ, Ford AB (eds). *The Practice of Geriatrics.* Philadelphia: WB Saunders, 1986, pp 358–369.

Fox HE, Steinbrecher M, Pessel D, et al. Maternal ethanol ingestion and the occurrence of human fetal breathing movements. *Am J Obstet Gynecol* 132:354–358, 1978.

Guyton AC, *Textbook of Medical Physiology,* 8th ed. Philadelphia: WB Saunders, 1991.

Junqueira LC, Carneiro J, Kelley RO. *Basic Histology,* 6th ed. Norwalk, CT: Appleton & Lange, 1989.

King TE, Schwarz ME. Pulmonary function and disease in the elderly. In Schrier RS (ed). *Clinical Internal Medicine in the Aged.* Philadelphia: WB Saunders, 1982, pp 124–148.

Klivington KA (ed). *The Science of Mind.* Cambridge, MA: MIT Press, 1989.

Meullner SR. Development of urinary control in children: Some causes and treatment of primary enuresis. *JAMA* 172:1256, 1960.

Minaker KL, Meneilly GS, Rowe JW. Endocrine systems. In Finch CE, Schneider EL (eds). *Handbook of the Biology of Aging.* New York: Van Nostrand Reinhold, 1985, pp 433–456.

Milani-Comparetti A. The neurophysiological and clinical implications of studies on fetal motor behavior. *Semin Perinatol* 5:183–189, 1981.

Moore KL. *The Developing Human—Clinically Oriented Embryology,* 4th ed. Philadelphia: WB Saunders, 1988.

Morris SE, Klein MD. Pre-feeding Skills. Tuscon: Therapy Skill Builders, 1987.

Patrick JK, Campbell K, Carmichael L, et al. Patterns of human fetal breathing during the last 10 weeks of pregnancy. *Obstet Gynecol* 58:24–30, 1980.

Remmers JE. Sleeping and breathing. *Chest* March, 97(3):77S–80, 1990.

Rosen MG, Scibetta JJ, Chik L, Borgstedt AD. An approach to the study of brain damage: The principles of fetal EEG. *Am J Obstet Gynecol* 115:37–47, 1973.

Rowe JW, Tobin JD, Andres RA, et al. The effect of age on creatinine clearance in man. *J Gerontol* 31:155–163, 1976.

Rowe JW. Renal and lower urinary tract diseases in the elderly. In Calkins E, Davis PJ, Ford AB (eds). *The Practice of Geriatrics.* Philadelphia: WB Saunders, 1986, pp 339–349.

Shephard RF. The cardiovascular benefits of exercise in the elderly. *Top Geriatr Rehabil* 1(1):1–10, 1985.

Short-DeGraff M. Sensory and perceptual development and behavioral organization. In Short-Degraff M (ed). *Human Development for Occupational and Physical Therapists.* Baltimore: Williams & Wilkins, 1988, pp 337–410.

Sklar M. Gastrointestinal disease. In Calkins E, Davis PJ, Ford AB (eds). *The Practice of Geriatrics.* Philadelphia: WB Saunders, 1986, pp 555–575.

Stark JE, Lipscomb DJ. Physiological and pathological aspects of the respiratory system. In Platt D (ed). *Geriatrics,* 2nd ed. New York: Springer-Verlag, 1983, pp 294–314.

Stratton P. Rhythmic functions in the newborn. In Stratton P (ed). *Psychobiology of the Human Newborn.* New York: J Wiley & Sons, 1982, pp 119–145.

Valadian I, Porter D. *Physical Growth and Development from Conception to Maturity.* Boston: Little Brown, 1977.

Vander AF, Sherman JH, Luciano DS. *Human Psychology: The Mechanisms of Body Function,* 4th ed. New York: McGraw-Hill, 1985.

Wahbe WM. Influence of aging on lung function—Clinical significance of changes from age twenty. *Anesth Analg* 62:764–776, 1983.

Whitbourne SK. *The Aging Body—Physiological Changes and Psychological Consequences.* New York: Springer-Verlag, 1985.

Winkler S, Massler M. Oral aspects of aging. In Calkins E, Davis PJ, Ford AB (eds). *The Practice of Geriatrics.* Philadelphia: WB Saunders, 1986, pp 477–487.

Woodruff DS. Arousal, sleep and aging. In Birren JE, Schaie KW (eds). *Handbook of the Psychology of Aging,* 2nd ed. New York: Van Nostrand Reinhold, 1985, pp 261–291.

Chapter 12

Development of Posture

by ANN F. VANSANT

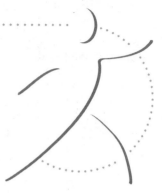

Objectives

AFTER STUDYING THIS CHAPTER, THE READER WILL BE ABLE TO:

1 Define posture, balance, and righting.
2 Discuss and differentiate theoretic approaches of the study of posture.
3 Discuss acquisition of posture and characteristics of posture at different stages of development.

The term *posture* refers to the alignment of the body—specifically, the alignment of body segments with respect to each other and with respect to the outside world. Posture suggests the idea of maintenance or preservation of body alignment. The functions that maintain or preserve alignment have been called "equilibrium" or "balance." The idea of maintaining alignment is the basis of the classic distinction between posture and movement. Posture is more than just maintaining a position of the body, however. Posture is also the act of bringing or moving body segments into alignment with one another. This latter postural function has traditionally been referred to as *righting* the body.

Righting means to bring the body into "normal" alignment. For human beings, normal alignment is considered erect bipedal stance. Newborn infants cannot stand up by themselves or balance. During the 1st year of life, infants acquire righting and balance abilities that enable them to move from lying to standing position and to balance in the transitional postures they might assume while rising: sitting, quadruped, and kneeling. Righting functions enable an individual to move from one stable posture, such as lying supine, to another stable posture, such as lying prone. The essence of righting is movement from one stable posture to another while seeking a more upright posture. When one can stand without assistance, one moves out of the period of infancy and enters childhood. Thus, the postural function of rising is so important to our development that it has been used as a marker of transition to childhood.

In summary, the common concept of posture has two facets: the idea of balance, or preserving alignment, and the function of righting, or moving from one posture to another to attain erect standing posture.

Posture is a complex neuromuscular function that has been heavily researched. The idea that balance maintains a stable posture has evolved to distinguish two facets of balance: *static* and *dynamic*. When an individual sits still, without engaging in any functional activity, static balance is demonstrated. When the individual begins to reach out and to move within the postural pattern of sitting while engaging in purposeful activity, dynamic balance is exhibited.

Our characteristic standing posture has both practical and symbolic meaning. Practically, supporting weight on the feet frees the upper limbs for other activities, including feeding, grooming, and work using our hands. Symbolically, the vertical posture has indicated our ascendancy over other animals. Part of our dignity as human beings is rooted in our ability to assume the upright posture. Temple Fay (1955), an eminent neurologist of the mid 20th century, pointed out that the loss of postural control is akin to being knocked down and out, a physical and psychologic blow.

For physical therapists, the study of posture development is an integral part of the study of motor development. Posture, like movement, varies characteristically with age. In this chapter, the specific changes in human postural function are examined from a life span perspective. A real constraint to a broad and systematic study of posture is the lack of information about posture during large periods of the human life span. Typically, research and collections of literature regarding posture, even when claiming a life span perspective, skip important life periods. We know most about the very young infant and child and the elderly individual. Less is known about postural development in later childhood, adolescence, and young and middle adulthood. Thus, this chapter reflects what is known, and it is only as comprehensive as the supporting literature will allow.

This chapter first presents two theoretic approaches to the study of posture: one classic and one contemporary perspective. Typical postural patterns of individuals at different points in the life span, including both righting and balance, are reviewed. Finally, the systems that interact in support of posture are outlined and discussed.

THEORETIC APPROACHES TO THE STUDY OF POSTURE

Reed (1989) distinguished between two theoretic approaches to the study of posture: a traditional reflex hierarchy approach and an "action systems" approach.

A reflex represents the relationship between sensory input, or a stimulus, and a motor output, or a response. According to the reflex hierarchy theory, posture is a reflexive response that results from the algebraic summation of the various sensory inputs to the motor centers of the central nervous system. Reed suggests that the traditional reflex hierarchy approach to the study of posture is no longer justifiable because its main theoretic assumption—that the central nervous system is a simple sensory-motor input-output mechanism — is no longer valid.

The action systems approach, in contrast, is one of several contemporary theoretic perspectives rooted in systems theory. The action systems approach suggests that posture is a dynamic process, an ongoing resolution of forces that supports a task (Reed, 1989). The action systems approach is concerned not with physiologic systems but with the perceptual systems deemed relevant to postural control. Both the traditional theory of reflexive control of posture and the more contemporary action systems approach are outlined below in more detail.

Postural Development Based on Reflexes

In Chapter 3 of this text, the basic framework of the traditional reflex hierarchy is reviewed. Figure 3–2 depicts specific reflexes associated with each anatomic level of that hierarchy: the spinal cord, the brain stem, the midbrain, and the cortex. With the exception of the spinal cord, which is concerned with movement responses only theoretically, all levels of the reflex hierarchy are involved in mediating postural reflexes. The brain stem, midbrain, and cortex are all engaged in the production and maintenance of posture. According to the developmental theory that rests on this hierarchic model, the infant gains progressive control over reflexive behavior as higher centers of the nervous system mature and exert an integrating and controlling influence over the physiologic processes of lower levels of the nervous system.

The brain stem, the lowest level of the nervous system proposed to be involved in postural control, was believed to mediate the "tonic" reflexes, which were maintained postural responses as defined and described by Magnus (1926a, b). To clarify the sensory and motor components of postural responses, Magnus surgically transected the nervous system of quadrupedal animals at various levels of the neuraxis. Following each transection, he carefully noted the posture of the animal and the animal's response to any change in spatial position or change in the relative position of body parts. When the neuraxis was transected just above the caudal portion of medulla oblongata in the brain stem, the animal demonstrated contraction in antigravity extensor muscles, even when at rest. This posture was known as *decerebrate rigidity*. Decerebrate animals also demonstrated the classic tonic or postural reflexes: the tonic neck reflex, the positive supporting reaction, and the tonic labyrinthine reflex. The tonic neck reflex was brought about by changes in the position of the head with respect to the body. The tonic labyrinthine reflex was evoked when the position of the head was changed with respect to gravity. The labyrinths of the inner ear were found to house the sensory receptors, specifically the otolith organs, that were responsible for detecting the stimulus for the tonic labyrinthine reflex. The positive supporting reaction was demonstrated when stretch or pressure was applied to the soles of the animal's feet. It is important to understand that the animal would demonstrate extensor postures at rest but would not be able to assume the upright posture. The capacity to assume a normal posture was exhibited only in animals whose mid-brains were left intact.

When higher centers of the central nervous system were left intact, the tonic reflexes of the brain stem came under their influence and were "integrated" and mediated by these higher centers. The mid-brain region, an area considered higher than the brain stem, was regarded as the mediating center for the righting reflexes. "Righting" was the term used to describe those postural responses that allowed the animal to attain normal posture. For a quadrupedal animal, "normal posture" is on all fours.

If a transection was made through the foremost half of the superior colliculi, the animal was able to right the body into a quadrupedal posture from any abnormal position that might be imposed. Through observation of "mid-brain" animals, Magnus described four types of righting reflexes: labyrinthine righting, body-righting acting on the head, neck-righting reflexes, and body-righting acting on the body.

The labyrinthine-righting reflex enabled alignment of the head in space. Gravity was the stimulus, and the response was orientation of the head so that the eyes were in a horizontal relationship with respect to gravity. The body-righting reflex was evoked by asymmetric pressure on the body surface. The response was alignment of the head with respect to gravity. The animals seemed most susceptible to the stimuli when engaged in climbing activities. Further, stimuli appeared most effective if they arose from the trunk or the plantar surfaces of the forelimbs and hind limbs.

Neck-righting reflexes assured alignment of the head with respect to the body. If an animal was restrained in an abnormal posture such as lying on its side, the labyrinthine and body-righting reflexes described above kept the head in a normal position with respect to gravity. When the animal was released from restraint, the body would untwist to achieve a normal head-body posture. This untwisting action was attributed to the neck-righting reflex. The stimulus was rotation of the head with respect to the body, and the response was untwisting to achieve normal alignment of the body and head.

If the labyrinths were removed from a mid-brain animal and the animal was not provided with surface cues such as asymmetric contact on the body, no righting was seen. However, if the animal's nervous system was left intact, but the labyrinths were removed and the animal was deprived of surface contact information, righting did occur. This observation prompted Magnus to define the fifth type of righting reflex: optical righting. If surface sensation and labyrinthine information were absent, Magnus concluded that the only source of useful information for righting would be vision. He confirmed his observation by blindfolding the animal and noting that righting no longer took place.

Magnus' findings not only influenced our concepts of posture but also strongly affected medical neurology and, ultimately, our concepts of motor development.

Schaltenbrand (1928), a German neurologist working in the 1920s, attempted to replicate Magnus' work by studying the righting reflexes of infants. Schaltenbrand believed that infants' motor behavior reflected the dominance of righting responses, and that through the developmental process, these righting reflexes were ultimately brought under the control of higher centers of the nervous system. He attempted to test this theory but could not replicate Magnus' work because, of course, the infants' nervous systems were intact. He could not separate the effects of each of Magnus' reflexes.

Magnus' work on righting also influenced McGraw's (1945) classic studies of motor development in the 1930s and 1940s. McGraw, like Schaltenbrand, worked under the assumption that the newborn infant demonstrated behaviors dominated by reflexes controlled through lower centers of the central nervous system. As the cortex of the brain matured, it influenced the subcortical regions, inhibiting the reflexes and allowing volitional control of motor behavior. McGraw charted the development of several righting behaviors in infants and young children, including rolling, sitting, and assuming the upright posture. For each of these behaviors, she described a period of subcortical reflexive control over the posture and a later period of "integration" and volitional control.

Equilibrium responses were elaborated from a developmental perspective by Weisz (1938) at about the same time that Schaltenbrand and McGraw were completing their research. Weisz, like Schaltenbrand and McGraw, based his work on previous studies of animal behavior. According to Weisz, Rademaker had described equilibrium responses in animals. These responses were evoked by changing the position of the body in space, altering the position of the support surface, or changing the position of the extremities with respect to the body. Weisz maintained that equilibrium responses developed in an orderly sequence. They were noted to lag behind development of the ability to sustain a new antigravity posture. For example, an infant might be capable of sitting, but when tested for equilibrium in this position, the infant could show negative responses. Equilibrium responses took time to develop into reliable responses in each position. Weisz (1938) stated that children preferred postures and "postural changes" in which balance or equilibrium was secure. Body action used in righting responses were a result of sufficiently developed equilibrium. Weisz pointed out that righting reflexes fade in the course of motor development, while a parallel process involved the appearance and breaking in of equilibrium reactions. He felt that righting and equilibrium were synergic, alternating in their overt expression in the infant and child.

Schaltenbrand (1928) was the first to suggest that neurologic dysfunction in children could manifest itself as a lack of development of righting responses. Schaltenbrand defined two syndromes: the *decerebrate syndrome,* in which righting behaviors were completely absent, and the *quadrupedal syndrome,* characterized by a primitive form of rising and an inability to assume the upright stance using a mature form of body action.

This idea was later championed by Bobath (1965) and was a basic tenet of her theory of abnormal motor development. Physical therapists came to understand the abnormal motor behavior of children with neurologic dysfunction as evidence of an *abnormal postural reflex mechanism,* one in which the tonic reflexes dominated and the righting reflexes were absent. The *normal postural reflex mechanism* as defined by Bobath was composed not only of righting behaviors but also of equilibrium responses.

The literature describing righting and equilibrium responses struggles with stringently defining a reflex. Righting and equilibrium responses are often referred to as "reactions," quite different from reflexes because of their variable form. Even the stereotypic tonic reflexes described in animals do not fit the strict definition of a reflex, for these are evoked by "multimodal" stimuli and involve an entire limb, if not the entire body. For example, the tonic neck reflex may be brought about by proprioceptive stimuli arising in joint or muscle receptors, and it results in extensor activity on one side of the body and a release of extension on the opposite side. Reed (1989) pointed out that confusion pervades the literature on posture. He confines the definition of a reflex to meaning a localized peripheral-central arc, rather than a system-wide action.

In summary, the concept of posture as a set of reflexes was founded in studies of animal behavior under unnatural conditions. The discovery of tonic-postural and righting reflexes in brain stem and mid-brain animals spurred several studies of the sequential development of postural responses in infants and young children. The hierarchic model of postural control remained popular, was well understood, and was well accepted until relatively recently. A renewed interest in human posture has arisen from theories grounded in a systems approach.

Postural Development Based on the Concepts of Action Systems

Reed (1989) suggests that a more functional perspective leads one to consider posture a component of volitional behavior. Posture should therefore be studied with regard to its role in supporting volitional actions. Postures vary with the context of the tasks they support. The standing posture one would assume while stirring a pot on the stove is different from the standing posture one would assume while playing tennis. Within this new perspective on posture, the flexibility of the postural systems needs to be explored, and the range of postures used to support daily activities needs to be identified.

A fundamental concept in the action systems perspective is that *posture is anticipatory to most functional actions.* That is, the postural adjustments needed to perform a task occur prior to the onset of the overt movement component of the action. The evidence for this comes from Cordo and Nashner (1982), who demonstrated that the postural activity that precedes action prepares the body to counterbalance the forces that will be generated within the movement task. This postural activity prevents one's equilibrium from being perturbed by self-generated movements. This characteristic of postural activity is a relatively recent concept. Traditionally, postural adjustments were thought to be primarily triggered by movements—thus the adage, "posture follows movement like a shadow." Our understanding of posture is expanding to encompass action before, during, and following movement. Posture is integral to motor behavior.

Another characteristic of posture that is receiving attention as a result of the action systems perspective is that of *variability*. For physical therapists, the terms "posture," "postural evaluation," and "postural training" most often evoke images of a standard, normal, or ideal body alignment, typically defined solely for upright stance. Three types of variability are missing from this perspective: one is the other habitual postural configurations such as sitting, leaning, and lying; a second is the number of variations within the general limits of a defined postural configuration such as standing, sitting, and lying; and a third is the systematic variation of posture across the human life span.

Reed (1989) pointed out that we need studies of the dynamic limits of postures. Most studies to date have focused on the static maintenance of standing, in which case—as Reed indicated—no real task is being accomplished. Reed also suggested that we need studies of dynamic standing across the human life span. Studies of other common postures are needed as well. We know little about other habitual postures assumed while sitting or lying beyond infancy. We know neither the most common postures nor the common motor patterns within these postures. Without definition of these common postural patterns, the study of the systems that support posture is severely limited.

One of the most basic premises of the action systems perspective is that *flexibility of behavior is achieved through practice and repetition.* With repetition, a movement pattern becomes more adaptable, not consistent or stereotypic. Practice and experience allow the organization of action systems to accomplish a functional end. Reed (1989) suggests that, rather than acquiring a motor program, the individual develops a skill. This skill is the ability to use information to coordinate movements and postures flexibly in the context of a task.

According to the action systems perspective, all perceptual systems are capable of contributing useful information to the control of posture. Infants are capable of using multimodal perceptual information after 6 months of age. This capacity is important in the development of action, and postural control is an indicator of this ability. The intimate relationship between postural accomplishments and movement skills is clearly evident in the examples gathered in support of the action systems theory perspective. Reed points to a series of research reports from the early 1980s that indicate the role of posture in producing so-called mature movements. The work of Amiel-Tison and Grenier (1980) shows that head support enables infants of 1 and 2 months of age to produce relatively mature reaching patterns; the work of Fentress (1981) indicates that young mice, when provided postural support, produce adult-like grooming movements of their forepaws.

The framework suggested by Reed is but one of several contemporary approaches to the more general study of the motor behavior development that rely on tenets of systems theory. Another related approach can be found in the work of Woollacott and colleagues (1986; 1987; 1988; 1989a, b), who have focused on the role of sensory systems in the control of posture of individuals of different ages.

AGE DIFFERENCES IN POSTURE

If we think of the newborn infant, and then consider the healthy young child, the young adult, and the elderly individual, each brings to mind a different posture. Human posture varies with age in an orderly way. The movement patterns used to acquire posture and typical postures across the life span are reviewed below. This approach is in keeping with the definition of posture: the action of aligning body segments with respect to each other and with respect to the outside world to accomplish a functional task.

Prenatal Period

Motor development during the prenatal period has become a subject of increased interest as a result of the development of ultrasound imaging. We now know that early in the fetal period, the fetus routinely changes posture within the uterus. These movements were described as thrusting, jumping, and creeping by Milani-Comparetti (1981). He believed that the actions were used early in the fetal period to change from one resting posture to another. Prechtl (1986) described early fetal movements as somersaults and axial rotations and noted that such positional changes occur frequently. Later, closer to the end of pregnancy, fetal movements are used to move into a head-down position in the birth canal.

As the time of birth approaches, the fetus demonstrates less movement and an increasing tendency to assume a posture of full flexion of the axial region and extremities. This posture is a necessity given the physical constraints of the uterus and the increasing size of the fetus.

Infancy

POSTURE DURING THE 1st TRIMESTER AFTER BIRTH

The fully flexed posture of the newborn infant is well known. This configuration of the body is seen in prone and supine positions and when the infant is held in sitting position. The typical postural pattern of the newborn shows symmetry of the limbs early in the 1st postnatal trimester. Both upper and lower limbs are held up off the support surface and close to the body when the infant is lying in the supine position. In the prone position, the flexion of the hips and trunk keep the anterior iliac spines up off the supporting surface. The head, in contrast, is more commonly turned to the side, with a cheek resting on the supporting surface, when the infant is in either the prone or supine position.

When the infant is held in sitting position, the head is typically oriented forward of the vertical plane but the chin is up off the chest. The back is rounded, and the arms are held close to the chest in flexion. The baby cannot balance in sitting position and requires support to maintain this posture.

When held standing, the infant accepts weight and straightens the lower limbs, trunk, and head. The infant cannot control the standing posture alone, however. External support also is needed to balance in this posture. Toward the end of the 1st trimester, this first standing posture wanes and there is a period during which the infant does not accept weight. This period of *astasia,* which means "without stance," gradually gives way to a secondary standing posture that typically appears during the 2nd trimester.

Toward the end of the 1st trimester, when the infant is observed in the supine position, the upper limbs more commonly demonstrate postural asymmetry. Frequently, one limb is abducted and flexed, while the other is positioned in extension and abduction. Although the hips and knees are flexed, the feet commonly rest on the support surface. In the prone position, the infant will gradually straighten the lower limbs. Increasingly, the head is lifted up off the support surface, and the arms are brought under the chest, elevating the upper trunk from the support surface. This posture, known as *prone on elbows,* becomes more common as the infant approaches the 2nd trimester.

POSTURE DURING THE 2nd TRIMESTER AFTER BIRTH

In the prone position during the 2nd trimester, the on-elbows posture is gradually replaced by an up-on-hands posture, and then by a hands-and-knees posture. The infant actively pushes with the upper limbs, elevating the chest off the support surface. There is sustained extension of the cervical and thoracic spine, and the infant may maintain the chest-up position for relatively long periods. As spinal extension begins to include the lumbar region, the lumbar lordosis brings the anterior iliac spines to rest in contact with the supporting surface. This gradual appearance of spinal extension from the cervical to the lumbar region is one of the hallmarks of normal postural development. It is characteristic of the gradual acquisition of an increasingly vertical posture. First the head is lifted up and aligned, with the face vertical and mouth horizontal; then the chest is elevated off the support surface with increasing frequency. The hips will be drawn into flexion, bringing the thighs up under the body, and the infant's abdomen and iliac crests are elevated off the supporting surface. Balance in the hands-and-knees position is learned gradually, with the infant frequently falling back into the prone position. It is not until the 3rd trimester that the infant consistently can attain and maintain the hands-and-knees posture. With time, however, the child learns to control the body's position, eventually engaging in vigorous rocking back and forth on hands and knees.

During the 2nd trimester, the infant begins to establish independence in the sitting posture. Placed in sitting position by parents or caretakers, the baby's first sitting posture involves leaning the trunk forward of the vertical plane. The caretaker provides support, commonly on the anterior aspect of the chest of the infant. The cervical spine and upper back are maintained in extension. The arms, held initially in a high guard posture of abduction and lateral rotation, gradually move to approximate the support surface in wide abduction and extension, with the wrists dorsiflexed and the fingers spread. The first independent sitting posture is one in which the baby props body weight forward on the hands.

Intimately linked with the ability to sustain this posture is the development of reliable "parachute reactions." When the infant of 6 to 8 months of age loses balance in sitting position and falls forward, the arms are quickly moved into abduction and extension to catch and break the fall. This is a *parachute reaction.* Parachute responses reportedly develop between the ages of 6 and 12 months to protect the child from falling out of the sitting position (Schaltenbrand, 1928). Described as appearing initially in response to forward displacement of the trunk, the parachute responses later appear as a result of rapid loss of balance sideward, and finally as a result of the infant's being displaced backward.

Coupled with the development of these protective extension responses is an increasingly erect posture while sitting. Extension of the spine, initially involving the cervical and upper thoracic regions, gradually spreads to the lower thoracic and lumbar spine. The infant will typically sit erect, with a normal lumbar curve, by the end of the 2nd trimester.

Standing posture during the 2nd trimester evolves from the previous period of astasia. The standing posture of the 2nd trimester is characterized by an alignment of the upper trunk and shoulder girdle well behind the feet. Repeated movements of the legs into extension gradually bring the child to an increasingly erect stance, which can be maintained for longer and longer periods. Babies typically enjoy standing during this period and will actively support the body weight and attempt to move into an increasingly vertical alignment. This secondary standing posture is characterized by the feet being spread in a more abducted and laterally rotated posture than was seen during the 1st trimester. Incipient stepping may be seen, but this is often relatively uncoordinated and staccato.

It is important to remember that at this young age, the infant is unable to move into sitting or standing position independently. Rather, the child is placed in these postures by parents or caretakers. But the ability to "right" the body, or to move into the upright posture, is beginning to evolve during these early months. The seeds of this ability are in initial rolling movements from back or stomach lying to a side-lying position, and in the actions that lift the chest and pelvis up off the support surface in the prone position. Gradually these movements will be used in the process of rising from a supine or prone position to standing, but this ability is not developed until after the child has gained the ability to maintain the vertical stance, a static balance task, and is capable of walking, a dynamic balance task. Probably because in our culture caretakers and parents place infants in sitting and standing positions, static balance abilities are gained in the vertical postures before the child is able to independently sit or stand.

POSTURE DURING THE 3rd TRIMESTER AFTER BIRTH

Between 6 and 9 months following birth, several postural milestones are accomplished. The child begins to roll out of the supine position into the prone position and then moves to the quadruped or sitting posture, and finally pulls up to standing.

Rolling is used by the infant ·to move from the supine to the prone position. The movement patterns used to accomplish this task are variable during the 3rd trimester. It is as though the infant is trying out various strategies for rolling; only later in the trimester does a rolling pattern appear that is common among infants of similar age. That relatively common pattern involves block rotation of the trunk with flexion patterns of the upper and lower limbs.

Another feature of rolling during this period is a tendency for the infant to roll to side-lying position and to pause there for a time before continuing into the prone position. The infants seem to spend time lying on their sides to develop balance abilities. One characteristic pattern used by infants who pause in the side-lying position is trunk action involving a rapid rotation of the pelvis, which moves them from their sides to the prone position.

The initial rolling movements are eventually used purposefully by infants to attain the prone position and to move about, through either crawling or creeping patterns. Descriptions of early prone locomotion speak strongly to the integral role of balance in early locomotor attempts (Schaltenbrand, 1928). McGraw (1945) described this "incipient propulsion" as follows: an infant supporting weight on the arms, dropping into the prone position and reaching forward with the arms or pulling on the support surface, or swaying from side to side when supporting weight up on the hands, or pushing on the extended arms and propelling the body backward. Incipient propulsion with the arms gradually begins to include the lower limbs. Initially, as the child attains the hands-and-knees posture, the urge to locomote seems to be abated. Sometimes the infant rises up on hands and knees, falls forward, and again rises up, resulting in some forward progression. But the driving effort seems to be more directed toward elevating the abdomen than moving forward. As with rolling, the infant seems to pause in the hands-and-knees posture and to spend time gaining static balance before this postural pattern becomes the substrate for more dynamic locomotor efforts. Initial attempts at creeping often result in a loss of balance and a fall from the hands-and-knees posture back down into the prone position, but the infant perseveres.

As the infant learns to creep, he or she also learns to independently move to a sitting position. Prior to this time, infants are helped with sitting by the parents or caretakers, who grasp the child's hands and pull the baby from a supine to a sitting position. Infants progress within this content of assisted sitting when they can align the head with the body while being pulled up to sit. This ability typically has become a stable part of the child's motor capacity at the end of the 1st trimester. During the 2nd trimester, the baby begins to use active flexion, first of the head and then of the trunk, to assist in the process of rising. Finally, during the 3rd trimester, the baby reaches out to the caretaker in anticipation of being pulled up and actively flexes the upper limbs to assist in the rising movement.

Sometimes the early successful independent acquisition of the sitting position is a result of falling from a somewhat wobbly hands-and-knees posture, or of a strong push backward from the hands-and-knees position that causes the child to sit on the heels. But with time, the goal of sitting seems to help form the movements that begin in the supine position. The infant will push up on both hands and one knee, abduct the other leg and lower the buttocks to a side-sitting posture. Ultimately, the child will be able to move more directly from supine to sitting position by flexing and rotating the trunk to the side, accepting weight on just one extending arm and the lateral aspect of one thigh. In this form of moving up to sitting position, the abdomen never contacts the support surface. Later, the form of movement changes to a pattern that brings the body more directly forward from supine to sitting position with less and less rotation of the trunk. McGraw (1945) pointed out that one of the characteristics of more advanced forms of rising to sitting is the smoothness of the movements. Early attempts at rising to sitting position are characterized by staccato and incoordinate movements (McGraw, 1945). In addition, the number of intermediate postures from supine to sitting position is reduced. Rather than rolling to prone position, possibly with a pause in the side-lying position, then rising up on the hands and knees and then lowering the buttocks to the support surface to sit, the child moves directly forward from supine to sitting position by using a pattern of trunk flexion. With continued development, the number of transitional postures assumed during the process of rising to sitting position declines. Rather than using a circuitous route through prone position, the child is able to sit up directly from supine.

With time, a pattern of hitching or scooting in the sitting position will appear as a form of locomotion in some babies. This pattern involves using the arms and feet to push and slide the buttocks across the floor while maintaining a sitting posture. It seems to appear, as does creeping, after the attainment of static balance abilities in the substrate posture—in this case, after the baby can maintain static equilibrium while sitting.

It is during the 4th trimester that the infant will first pull to standing position using furniture or parents' legs for support. The desire to stand upright appears to drive the infant's rapid acquisition of increasingly vertical postures. To pull up to stand is to achieve the postural pattern uniquely characteristic of human function. Being close to furniture, the child reaches out and grasps for support, spreads the feet, and brings them closer to the buttocks for support, gradually pushing with both legs toward the vertical position. If two hands are used for support (e.g., on a crib post), the baby may soon let go with one hand and reach up higher as if climbing up the post. Balance in standing position during these initial attempts is precarious at best. The child often assumes a pike position, with the buttocks stuck out behind the feet and shoulders. Falling backward, or dropping down to the side, is not uncommon. But the child keeps at the activity and within days is adept at rising while using furniture for support. Despite early falls, the baby cannot move back down to sitting position, and will often cry when "caught" in this new posture without recourse to the more familiar and supported position of sitting.

POSTURE DURING THE 4th TRIMESTER AFTER BIRTH

The standing position is becoming the infant's preferred posture for developing balance. Hanging on to furniture or with parental support, the child begins to exercise stepping movements that challenge dynamic balance development in the upright position. The child's widely based standing posture also is characterized by seemingly flat feet, lordosis, and a protruding abdomen. The arms assume an abducted, laterally rotated posture with elbow flexion (termed a "high guard" posture of the upper limbs). With experience in the standing position, the infant gradually lowers the hands to a position beside the hips. The quadruped posture is still a very secure and comfortable posture during this period. Children will frequently drop to hands and knees when they need to move quickly. Balance in quadruped position typically correlates with advanced development in standing balance.

At the end of the 4th trimester, the child begins to control the upright posture and to walk. The arms move back up to high guard during early attempts at walking; the gradual lowering of the hands to a position beside the hips indicates the increasing experience of the new walker. Eventually, during the 2nd or 3rd year of life, the child will begin to demonstrate the alternating arm-swing action characteristic of a more mature use of the upper limbs for balance during walking.

Commonly during the 4th or 5th trimester, the baby begins to come to standing from supine without pulling up. A child who can stand without outside assistance has accomplished a major milestone in physical independence. The initial form of rising typically involves rolling into the prone position, pushing up with both arms, elevating the pelvis by extending both lower limbs, walking forward toward the hands, lowering the buttocks to a squat position, then letting go with the hands, and rising from squatting to standing position.

Thus the 1st year of life culminates in standing and walking and finally in the ability to rise to standing from supine position without assistance. The child has moved during the first year from a position of full support to one of independent upright posture.

Childhood

STANDING POSTURE DURING EARLY CHILDHOOD

A study of the development of standing posture among British children concluded that the characteristic lordosis of the 2nd and 3rd years of life ranges between 30 and 40 degrees (Asher, 1975). Children are able to vary the degree of lordosis exhibited while standing by altering the posture of the lumbar spine. This is accomplished by leaning forward and bending the knees. Gradually, the abducted broad-based stance of the toddler begins to narrow. Typically, the knees approach each other, maintaining a slight degree of spreading of the feet through tibial torsion. The abdomen becomes less prominent during this period, and the feet begin to show a longitudinal arch as the fat pad that obscured the arch during infancy begins to diminish.

TRANSITIONAL MOVEMENTS USED TO RISE TO STANDING POSITION DURING EARLY CHILDHOOD

The decrease in transitional postures with development of the ability to stand from supine position is similar to that seen in the gradually acquired direct approach to sitting. In the early part of the 20th century, Schaltenbrand noted that infantile forms of rising to standing position involved rolling to prone position, attaining hands-and-knees posture, then moving to squatting and finally standing. According to Schaltenbrand (1928), "mature form" in rising is demonstrated at about 4 or 5 years of age, when the child can rise by coming directly forward from supine position to sit, then squat, and then stand. This advanced rising action is characterized by symmetric body action involving flexion, followed by extension of the head, trunk, and upper and lower limbs.

A more recent study demonstrates that mature symmetric rising does not occur during early childhood (VanSant, 1988). Although children rise by coming predominantly forward from supine position, they tend to rotate the trunk from side to side on the way to sitting position, to push with one arm while reaching with the other, and to assume a relatively wide-based and asymmetric squat pattern. The wide-based squat seems to reduce the amount of freedom that must be controlled at the hips. This strategy is a simple way to assure balance while elevating the center of mass of the body. When the young child assumes a wide-based squat, the hips are typically flexed and medially rotated, bringing the feet back beside the pelvis. After the feet are positioned, a simple thrust of extension of the hips and knees elevates the trunk; the lower limbs end in a wide-based stance with the hips extended and medially rotated in a "close-pack" position.

STANDING POSTURE DURING MIDDLE CHILDHOOD

Two standing postural patterns have been described for children during the elementary school years. These patterns are related to body type: one for the ectomorph and one for the mesomorph. The ectomorphic pattern has been described as a passive posture, with very little effort directed toward resisting the force of gravity. The pelvis is tilted anteriorly, with a slight protrusion of the abdomen. The knees are hyperextended. The scapulae are in a winged posture with the shoulders and head forward.

The child with a more mesomorphic build demonstrates a more active posture. The pelvis is tilted forward with accompanying lordosis; the knees are hyperextended; the scapulae are held back by action of the trapezius; and the spine is described as sloping backward so that the curve of the upper back and scapulae is directly above or behind the curve of the buttocks. The head is held erect with the neck in a straight posture.

TRANSITIONAL MOVEMENTS DEMONSTRATED DURING MIDDLE CHILDHOOD

Symmetry in movements tends to become more frequent during the middle childhood years in the process of rising from supine position. The lower limbs are more likely to demonstrate asymmetry than are the trunk or upper limbs. Lower limb asymmetry during rising may result in part from slight variations in force production during the process of rising. If too much force is generated during rising, the center of mass may be carried outside the initial base of support established by the feet, and the child may have to move the feet into an asymmetric posture to prevent loss of balance. It appears that with repeated trials, the child anticipates the variations in force production and establishes a larger base of support from the outset by assuming an asymmetric foot posture.

Brown and collegues' (1993) study of children's rising movements demonstrated a relationship between the child's body build and the movement patterns used to stand up. Specifically, children who are very large for their age are more likely to demonstrate asymmetric and primitive rising patterns. These children's development within this task appears to be delayed with respect to their peers.

Adolescence

STANDING POSTURE DURING ADOLESCENCE

The postural alignments of childhood—increased lordosis and a protruding abdomen—stabilize during adolescence (Asher, 1975). In standing position, the pelvic inclination lessens to approximately 20 degrees, the buttocks are less likely to protrude, and the knees are less commonly hyperextended. The head is aligned over the shoulders, hips, and ankles. This balanced posture is sometimes referred to as *ideal posture*. It has been suggested that ideal posture, typically achieved during adolescence and young adulthood, looks pleasing, resists disability, and serves function well (Appleton, 1964). Further, ideal posture does not lead to pain. It is important to realize, however, that posture varies with body build and an individual's neuromuscular and musculoskeletal development, activity level, and habits. As individuals approach adulthood, their postural individuality becomes increasingly apparent.

TRANSITIONAL MOVEMENTS DEMONSTRATED DURING ADOLESCENCE

A study of rising movements in teenagers revealed what appears to be a peak in incidence of symmetric movement patterns around the age of 15 years (Sabourin, 1989). Younger and older teens were found to exhibit more asymmetry while rising than did middle teens. This is particularly true for lower limb movements. It may be that peak performance in a task occurs when most individuals demonstrate the greatest ability to control force within this task. Whereas children seem to have difficulty controlling force production in this task, and as a result demonstrate asymmetry in their rising actions, teens exhibit a refined competence in simultaneously controlling the upper limb, trunk, and lower limb movements. They move from recumbency by flexing the trunk and moving the feet directly in front of their buttocks while balancing in sitting position, and then transfer weight from buttocks to feet with ease. Control of the force and direction of movement in the righting task is impressive at this age.

Adulthood

STANDING POSTURE DURING ADULTHOOD

Standing posture is typically defined with reference to the young adult. This age group serves as the model for the ideal posture discussed above. Typically, symmetry is apparent in the standing posture from a frontal view. In the sagittal plane, a plumb bob is often used as a reference for normal alignment. The line created by the suspended plumb bob transects the mastoid process, the acromion process, the greater trochanter, and the lateral epicondyle, and passes just anterior to the lateral malleolus. This "plumb" posture is a standard used to identify postural abnormalities, but it is far from an expression of dynamic standing posture, which serves as a basis for locomotion and a variety of work-related tasks performed by young adults. The healthy adult is highly flexible in choosing postural patterns for a functional task. During adulthood, the vertical posture has reached its supremacy.

TRANSITIONAL MOVEMENTS DEMONSTRATED DURING ADULTHOOD

The mid-teen peak in symmetric performance is diminished slightly during the late-teen period and in the early twenties. Although symmetric performance is the most common form of rising, it is the mode of action of approximately one fourth of young adults. The remainder demonstrate asymmetry in at least one component of body action, be it the upper limbs, the trunk, or the lower limbs. This is when individuals are making the transition from high school to college or the work force. Compared to the high school years, young adulthood presents fewer formalized opportunities to participate in physical activity. Green and Williams (1992) found that activity level is related to performance in the rising task during the middle adult years. More active adults are more likely to use symmetric patterns. Another study demonstrated that body size is also a significant factor among adult women performing the righting task (VanSant et al, 1989). Taller and more slender women are more likely to demonstrate symmetric patterns than shorter and heavier women.

Older Adulthood

STANDING POSTURE DURING LATER ADULTHOOD

The stooped posture of the older adult is a well-known stereotype. Yet the posture of the older adult is related to a variety of factors, including activity level, health, and mental status (Moncur, 1993). If variability is a characteristic of adult posture beginning in the later teen years, that variability reaches its peak among older adults. Even so, the standing posture of the older adult can be characterized by reference to common features. These features include a widened base of support, slightly flexed knees and hips, inclination of the trunk forward of the vertical plane, a flattened lumbar spine, increased thoracic kyphosis, and a forward head posture.

Age-related changes in the musculoskeletal system account for some postural changes in older individuals. Specifically, bones lose density, the intervertebral disks may degenerate, and the ligaments of the spine lose tensile strength. All of these changes can lead to shortened stature and forward head posture. The widened base of support is often attributed to decreased balance that may result from the sensory and nervous system changes of aging. Mental status is also a factor expressed in posture. The depressed individual may more commonly exhibit a stooped posture (Moncur, 1993).

TRANSITIONAL MOVEMENTS DEMONSTRATED DURING LATER ADULTHOOD

The effects of inactivity are noticeable in the task of standing from supine position. Over 8 years, a group of approximately 30 elderly persons who were engaged in a program of rigorous physical activity were studied at yearly intervals performing the righting task. Their performance was initially similar to that of individuals in their fifties, although the mean age of the group was approximately 70 years. Their performance gradually regressed, characterized by increasing asymmetry of movement and a tendency to return to several intermediate, transitional postures. Typically, the oldest subjects, who by then were nearly 80 years old, turned from supine to side-lying position, raised up into side sitting position, got onto their hands and knees, moved to half kneeling, and then stood. Like young children, the oldest individuals tend to pause in each transitional posture, as though gaining balance before moving on to a less stable posture characterized by an increasingly elevated center of mass, and a smaller base of support. It appears that decreased balance, ability to generate force, flexibility, and confidence all contribute to the change in movement patterns in the righting task. There has been a concomitant decrease in physical activity among this group of elders that goes hand in hand with the decline in performance. The relationship of these factors is likely a more powerful explanation of the change in righting abilities than a single isolated influence.

SUMMARY

This discussion of postural development has referred to the various factors that influence age-related change in posture. Among these are the neurophysiologic systems, both sensory and motor, used to explain postural control. The contributions of sensory systems to the control and development of posture have received increasing attention in recent years, spearheaded by the initial work of Nashner (1977) and more recently by Woollacott and her colleagues (1986, 1987, 1988, 1989a, b). As a result of their research, we now appreciate the role of the somatosensory (proprioceptive and tactile), visual, and vestibular systems in organizing responses to external disturbances of posture. We also recognize the important contribution of anticipatory postural adjustments generated prior to the onset of overt movement that protect us from falls as a result of our own movements. Changes in cellular structures within the nervous system occur at a relatively rapid rate early and later in the human life span. These changes contribute to both the acquisition of postural abilities and their decline. The neural control of posture varies with age.

As Reed (1989) has pointed out, perceptual systems also influence the development of posture. Rather than focusing on neurophysiologic systems, he suggests redirecting attention to perceptual motor tasks carried out in natural functional contexts. Reed suggests that the goals of a task and the environmental contexts in which tasks are accomplished profoundly influence the organization of postural support for volitional action. The movement tasks of infancy, childhood, adolescence, and adulthood differ. Naturally occurring age-related tasks are likely to strongly influence postural development.

Another factor that influences age-related change in posture is the musculoskeletal system. Individuals grow when they are young. They get bigger and taller, and their body proportions change. The effects of these physical changes challenge the postural systems across the growing years. The anatomic structure of bone and muscle also change with age. These changes contribute to one's ability to generate force, capacity for flexibility, and overall stature.

During adulthood, activity level influences one's weight and body dimensions, which influence postural alignment and righting abilities. Physical dimensions vary with age, not only because of internally mediated growth processes, but also because of psychosocial factors related to work, lifestyle, mental status, and activity level.

The factors that contribute to age-related change in posture are widely and richly varied. Understanding these various factors and their relationships leads to increased understanding not only of postural development, but also of all motor development throughout the human life span.

References

Amiel-Tison C, Grenier A. *Neurological/Evaluation of the Human Infant.* New York: Masson, 1980.

Appleton AB. Posture. *Practitioner* 156:5–7, 1964.

Asher C. *Postural Variations in Childhood.* Boston: Butterworths, 1975.

Bobath B. *Abnormal Postural Reflex Activity Caused by Brain Lesions.* London: Heinemann, 1965.

Brown L, Maracheski R, Phillips B, Tobin C, VanSant A. "The relationship during later childhood between body build and movement patterns used to rise to standing." Poster Presentation at the 68th Annual Conference of the American Physical Therapy Association, Cincinnati, June 14, 1993.

Cordo P, Nashner L. Properties of postural adjustments associated with rapid arm movements. *J Neurophys* 47:287–302, 1982.

Fay T. The origin of human movement. *Am J Psychiatry* 111:644–652, 1955.

Fentress J. Sensorimotor development. In Aslin R, Alberts J, Peterson M (eds). Development of Perception, Vol 11 Audition, Somatic Perception, and the Chemical Senses. New York: Academic Press, 1981.

Green LN, Williams K. Differences in developmental movement patterns used by active versus sedentary middle aged adults coming from a supine position to erect stance. *Phys Ther* 72:560–568, 1992.

Magnus R. Some results of studies in the physiology of posture. Cameron Prize Lectures Part I. *Lancet* 211(2):531–535, 1926a.

Magnus R. Some results of studies in the physiology of posture. Cameron Prize Lectures Part II. *Lancet* 211(2):585–588, 1926b.

McGraw M. *Neuromuscular Maturation of the Human Infant.* New York: Hafner, 1945.

Milani-Comparetti A. The neurophysiologic and clinical implications of studies on fetal motor behavior. *Semin Perinatol* 5:183–189, 1981.

Moncur C. Posture in the older adult. In Guccione AA (ed). *Geriatric Physical Therapy.* Philadelphia: Mosby, 1993, pp 219–236.

Nashner LM. Fixed patterns of rapid postural responses among leg muscles during stance. *Experimental Brain Research* 30:13–24, 1977.

Prechtl HFR. Prenatal motor development. In Wade M, Whiting H (eds). *Motor Development of Children: Aspects of Coordination and Control.* Boston: Martinus Nijhoff, 1986, pp 53–64.

Reed ES. Changing theories of postural development. In Woollacott MJ, Shumway-Cook A. (eds). *Development of Posture and Gait Across the Life Span.* Columbia, SC: University of South Carolina Press, 1989, pp 3–24.

Sabourin P. "Rising from supine to standing: A study of adolescents." Thesis, Virginia Commonwealth University, 1989.

Schaltenbrand G. The development of human motility and motor disturbances. *Arch Neurol Psychiatry* 20:720–730, 1928.

VanSant AF. Age differences in movement patterns used by children to rise from a supine position to erect stance. *Phys Ther* 68:1130–1138, 1988.

VanSant AF, Cromwell S, Deo A, et al. Relationships among body dimensions, age, gender, and movement patterns in a righting task. Poster Presentation at the 64th Annual Conference of the American Physical Therapy Association, Nashville, June 12, 1989.

Weisz S. Studies in equilibrium reactions. *J Nerv Ment Dis* 88:150–162, 1938.

Woollacott MH, Shumway Cook A, Nashner LM. Aging and posture control: Changes in sensory organization and muscular coordination. *Int J Aging Hum Dev* 23:97–114, 1986.

Woollacott M, Debu B, Mowatt M. Neuromuscular control of posture in the infant and child. *J Motor Behav* 19:167–186, 1987.

Woollacott MH, Inglin B, Manchester D. Response preparation and posture control in the older adult. In Joseph J (ed). *Central Determinants of Age-Related Declines in Motor Function.* New York: New York Academy of Sciences, 1988.

Woollacott MH, Shumway-Cook A, Williams HG. The development of posture and balance control in children. In Woollacott MH, Shumway-Cook A (eds). *Development of Posture and Gait Across the Life Span.* Columbia, SC: University of South Carolina Press, 1989a, pp 77–96.

Woollacott MH. Aging, posture control and movement preparation. In Woollacott MH, Shumway-Cook A (eds). *Development of Posture and Gait Across the Life Span.* Columbia, SC: University of South Carolina Press, 1989b, pp 155–175.

Chapter 13

Development of Locomotion

by PATRICIA A. WILDER

Objectives

AFTER STUDYING THIS CHAPTER, THE READER WILL BE ABLE TO:

1   Describe how motor development has been studied across the life span.
2   Define several locomotion patterns and how each pattern has evolved across the life span, including rolling, crawling and creeping, erect walking, running, galloping, hopping, and skipping.
3   Explain how the bodily systems of the individual, the environment, and the exact task to be done interact to produce the desired result, locomotion from one point to another.

The term *locomotion* is defined as the process of moving from one place to another. Exactly how an individual accomplishes the task of getting from point A to point B depends on many factors: the exact task to be done, the interaction of the bodily systems that will perform the task, and the environment in which the task will take place. This chapter discusses (1) the development of locomotion across the life span and (2) how the bodily systems of the organism, the environment, and the specific task interact to accomplish the desired result.

STUDY METHODS

The task of independently moving from one place to another can be accomplished using any one of a variety of motor patterns: rolling, crawling, creeping, erect ambulation, running, galloping, hopping, and skipping. The work of Shirley (1931), McGraw (1945), and Whitall (1989) reveals that the development of independent locomotion progresses from birth to childhood from rolling to crawling to creeping to erect ambulation. After erect ambulation, the locomotion patterns that develop are the upright patterns of running, galloping, hopping, and skipping.

Researchers such as McGraw (1945) studied motor development by dividing the development of a particular pattern into phases (i.e., the four phases of rolling, the nine phases of prone progression, and the seven phases of erect locomotion). McGraw also studied transitional patterns—patterns used to move between postures—such as moving from supine to sitting position or moving from sitting to standing position. McGraw's phases for locomotion development are completely described later in this chapter.

Another way in which researchers of motor development used descriptive analysis to study locomotion patterns was to divide a particular pattern into its "component" parts—that is, movement of the head and neck, the trunk, the upper extremities, and the lower extremities. The research of Roberton and Halverson (1984, 1988) was instrumental in this concept. These researchers identified a developmental progression for the hopping patterns of children.

Exactly how a researcher investigating motor pattern development decided to study a particular motor pattern depended most often on the underlying theory. As has been explained in more detail in Chapters 2 and 4, McGraw (1945) was guided in her thinking by the neuromaturational theory (i.e., the motor patterns of infants and young children are the results of the developing central nervous system). Roberton and Halverson thought that the changes in motor patterns over time were partly due to physical development (Getchell & Roberton, 1989).

Another way of studying developing motor patterns has been to describe the pattern and the changes that occur over time by using some type of biomechanical analysis. Inman et al (1981), Winter (1991), Murray (1967), and Sutherland et al (1988) have given the most comprehensive biomechanical analyses of the locomotion patterns for upright walking, or ambulation. There is little biomechanical information in the literature on most other locomotion patterns, except for running.

A biomechanical analysis of a movement pattern usually includes a description of the kinematics and the kinetics of the movement pattern—the dynamics of the movement pattern. *Kinematics* refers to the relationships between the segments that produce the motion: displacements, velocities, and accelerations in translational or rotational motion. *Kinetics* refers to the moving bodies and the forces that produce the motion. Forces involved include both internal and external forces: internal forces are referred to as the *stresses* that are needed to produce the motion or that result from the motion (i.e., joint forces); external forces are referred to as the *loads* that are necessary to produce the motion or that result from the motion (i.e., ground reaction forces).

Many variables are used in a biomechanical analysis of a locomotion pattern. Walking, the most common of locomotion patterns, is usually described by the variables of step length, step width, stride length, cycle time, velocity, and cadence—variables that involve distance or time.

Most forms of locomotion involve some aspect of reciprocal movements of the extremities. Reciprocal movements of the extremities were once linked conceptually by describing stance time and swing time of a particular limb.

Now the extremities are linked through the ideas of interlimb and intralimb phasing. Phasing relationships are used to describe the coordination of the movement pattern (Clark et al, 1988). *Temporal phasing* refers to the proportion of time of one limb's stride before the contralateral limb starts its stride. *Distance* or *amplitude phasing* is defined as the proportion of the distance covered in one limb's stride when the contralateral limb starts its stride. A *stride* is defined as the time or distance from the heel strike of one foot to the next heel strike of that same foot. In the locomotion pattern of erect walking, temporal and distance phasing are considered to be at 50 per cent—that is, the contralateral limb starts its cycle when the other limb has completed 50 per cent of its cycle.

In summary, the traditional method used to describe the development of locomotion patterns has been to divide the particular pattern into specific phases or component parts. Although the descriptive method of analysis has been beneficial, biomechanical analysis has provided a more in-depth and objective method for analyzing movements.

LOCOMOTION PATTERNS ACROSS THE LIFE SPAN

Rolling

Rolling is the earliest pattern used for locomotion. *Rolling* is defined as moving from supine to prone or from prone to supine position, and it involves some aspect of axial rotation.

Rotation has been described as a righting reaction because, as the head rotates, the rest of the body twists or rotates to become realigned with the head. The earliest spontaneous axial rotation is seen in the fetus at about 10 weeks of gestation (deVries et al, 1984). Rotation around the longitudinal axis can result from rotation of the head followed by trunk rotation or from rotation of the leg (lower extremity) followed by trunk rotation. In either instance, one part of the body initiates the movement and the other parts of the body follow, which is called *segmental rotation*. Researchers believe that the functional significance of these movements is for the fetus to become repositioned from time to time to prevent adhesions and stasis (Prechtl, 1986).

McGraw provided the most detailed account of how rolling progresses from infancy to the toddler stage. Figure 13–1 provides a modified version of the four phases of rolling according to McGraw. The first phase is the *newborn phase, phase A*. In this phase the newborn infant is predominantly in a posture of flexion and is unable to produce the movements that would create the activity of rolling. Infants first begin to roll spontaneously. The first pattern of rolling is from sidelying posture to supine position; this pattern, *phase B, spinal extension,* is seen at about 1 to 2 months of age. Rolling from sidelying to prone position is observed at about 4 to 5 months of age. These movements are initially performed with the body moving as a unit; the movement is described as "log rolling," a movement performed without segmental rotation.

Why is the infant unable to roll segmentally at 1 to 2 months of age when

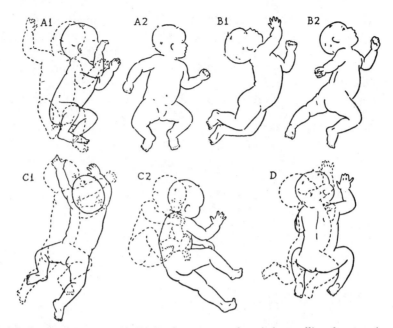

FIGURE 13–1. Four positions (A–D) in the pattern of an infant rolling from supine to prone position. (From McGraw MB. *The Neuromuscular Maturation of the Human Infant.* 1945, © Columbia University Press, New York. Reprinted with permission of the publisher.)

the infant was capable of segmental rotations in utero? The answer to this question is best sought from a biomechanical perspective. The infant at 1 to 2 months of age does not have the necessary strength to overcome gravity for rolling supine to prone or for rolling segmentally. Muscle strength was not as critical in utero to produce movement, because gravity for the most part was eliminated in the fluid-filled environment. According to McGraw, infantile rolling is complete but has no purpose—that is, the movement is not performed to accomplish some other function, such as to obtain a toy or to achieve a sitting posture.

At about 4 months of age infants begin to roll from prone to supine position more deliberately; by 6 to 8 months such deliberate action involves segmental rotations of the body. This pattern is referred to as *phase C,* or *automatic rolling.* It is most often initiated by the upper extremities, followed by the trunk and lower extremities; the pattern can also be initiated by the lower extremities, followed by the trunk and the upper extremities. Performance of the movement with more segmentation and with more deliberation is described by McGraw as *phase D, deliberation.*

Adult rolling patterns have been described by Richter et al (1989), who studied young adults, aged 20 to 29. The most important finding was that normal adults used a variety of movement patterns to roll. Most likely the variety of the patterns was related to flexibility and muscle strength of the individual performing the movement. Figures 13–2 and 13–3 illustrate some examples of adult rolling patterns identified by Richter and colleagues.

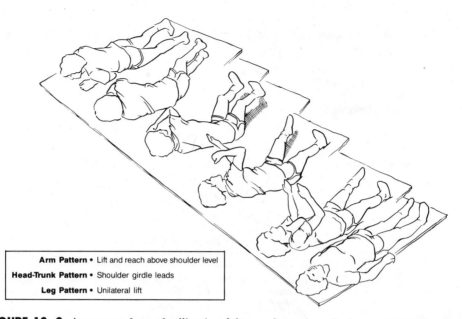

Arm Pattern ●	Lift and reach above shoulder level
Head-Trunk Pattern ●	Shoulder girdle leads
Leg Pattern ●	Unilateral lift

FIGURE 13–2. A common form of rolling in adults, as shown from the lower right-hand corner to the left-hand corner. (From Richter RR, VanSant AF, Newton RA. Description of adult rolling movements and hypotheses of developmental sequence. *Phys Ther* 69[1]:67, 1989.) Reprinted from PHYSICAL THERAPY with the permission of the American Physical Therapy Association.

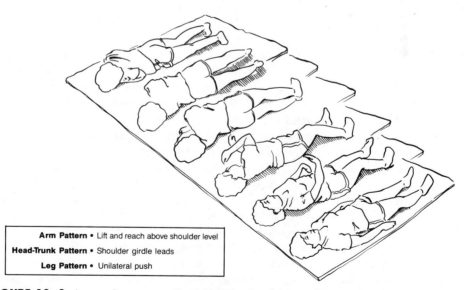

Arm Pattern ●	Lift and reach above shoulder level
Head-Trunk Pattern ●	Shoulder girdle leads
Leg Pattern ●	Unilateral push

FIGURE 13–3. A second common pattern of rolling in adults, as shown from the lower right-hand corner to the left-hand corner. (From Richter RR, VanSant AF, Newton RA. Description of adult rolling movements and hypotheses of developmental sequence. *Phys Ther* 69[1]:67, 1989.) Reprinted from PHYSICAL THERAPY with the permission of the American Physical Therapy Association.

Table 13-1. THE THREE COMPONENTS OF THE BODY INVOLVED IN ADULT ROLLING AND THE VARIATIONS WITHIN EACH REGION		
Body Region	**Sequence Order**	**Pattern**
Upper extremity	1	Lift and reach below shoulder level
	2	Lift and reach above shoulder level
	3	Push and reach
	4	Push
Head-trunk	1	Aligned pelvis and shoulder girdle
	2	Pelvis leads
	3	Relationship between pelvis and shoulder girdle changes
	4	Shoulder girdle leads
Lower extremity	1	Bilateral lift
	2	Unilateral lift
	3	Unilateral push
	4	Bilateral push

Adapted from Richter RR, Van Sant AF, Newton RA. Description of adult rolling movements and hypothesis of developmental sequences. *Phys Ther* 69(1):63–71, 1989. Reprinted from PHYSICAL THERAPY with the permission of the American Physical Therapy Association.

Table 13–1 identifies the three body components involved in adult rolling patterns and the variations within each region. These variations of "normal" adult rolling contrast with those of brain-injured adults, who tend to use only a few patterns, or to use stereotyped patterns for rolling, according to Richter et al.

Crawling and Creeping

Crawling is defined as prone progression in which the belly remains on the supporting surface as the arms and legs move in a reciprocal pattern to propel the body forward or backward. *Creeping* is defined as a prone progression in which the abdomen is lifted off the supporting surface while the arms and legs move reciprocally to propel the body forward or backward.

According to McGraw, the prone progression of crawling and creeping is a nine-phase sequence (Fig. 13–4). McGraw indicated that she had not observed a movement sequence with more individual variation than this progression. The majority of infants are able to perform a reciprocal creeping pattern (belly off the floor) by 10 months of age.

McGraw attributed the progression to cortical maturation, which results in effective inhibition of earlier components of reflexive control of the movement. From a biomechanical perspective, muscle strength is important in getting the belly up off the ground and propelling the body forward or backward. Most likely the truth behind this or any motor pattern progression is a combination of cortical development, musculoskeletal development, and the environment in which the progression is taking place.

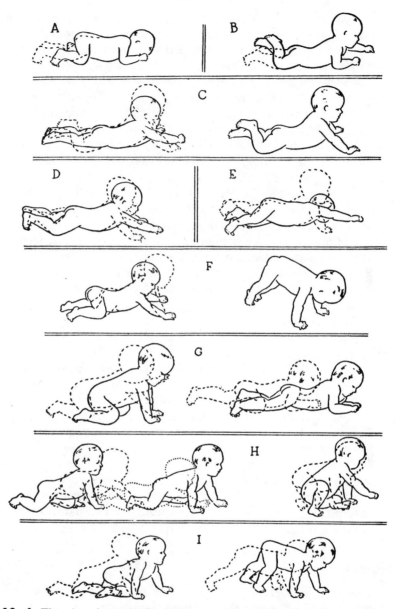

FIGURE 13–4. The nine phases (A–I) of the assumption of the all-fours position (crawling to creeping). (From McGraw MB. *The Neuromuscular Maturation of the Human Infant.* 1945, © Columbia University Press, New York. Reprinted with permission of the publisher.)

According to McGraw, the newborn phase of the prone progression (the first phase) describes the general posture of the infant, which is flexion. The weight is forward on the head, making head lifting in prone position difficult for the newborn. In *phase B, spinal extension,* the center of mass has moved inferiorly, and the extensor muscles actively promote head lifting in prone position. In *phase C, advanced spinal extension,* spinal extension is even more evident and the infant can maintain the head and trunk in an elevated position for some time. In *phase D, incipient propulsion in superior region,* the infant attempts to move the superior region of the body, but the inferior region of the body remains unorganized, and propulsion of the body is inhibited. In *phase E, incipient propulsion in inferior region,* the inferior region becomes organized but the two regions remain mostly unsynchronized, and the infant still cannot move the body as a unit. *Phase F, assumption of creeping posture,* represents some coordination between the regions of the body, but the infant does not make deliberate attempts to progress. Often in this phase, the infant lifts the abdomen from the surface but loses balance and falls. In this phase, the infant spends time rocking back and forth on hands and knees, but again without any progression. In *phase G, deliberate but unorganized progression,* the infant may raise one arm forward and then the other, but the legs move as a unit. The infant moves across the floor by pulling with the arms and pushing with the toes. In *phase H, organized progression,* the infant has a definite creeping pattern; abdomen up off the floor with contralateral movements of the extremities propelling the infant forward. McGraw describes the movement pattern as "staccato" and somewhat uncoordinated. In *phase I, integrated progression,* the progression is smoothly integrated.

Adult patterns of crawling and creeping have not been studied extensively. The literature indicates that the reciprocal pattern used in early childhood is the adult pattern of this movement behavior. How this pattern of locomotion evolves with aging has not yet been studied. One can assume, however, that the patterns of creeping and crawling for older adults remain very similar to the patterns that young adults display. The parameters that would change the progression of creeping in older adults most likely are biomechanical (e.g., muscle strength and joint flexibility).

Erect Walking

The erect ambulation pattern, walking, is defined as a two-phase pattern of movement in the upright position: the *stance phase,* which is approximately 60 per cent of a complete gait cycle, and the *swing phase,* which is approximately 40 per cent of a complete gait cycle. A *complete gait cycle* is defined as one complete stride of one limb: the time or distance from heel strike of one foot to heel strike of that same foot. In ambulation, the upper and lower extremities move in a reciprocal, contralateral pattern to propel the body forward or backward in space. In erect walking, a 50 per cent temporal and distance phasing relationship exists between the lower limbs. As stated earlier, 50 per cent phasing between the limbs indicates that when one limb is 50 per cent completed with its cycle, the contralateral limb starts its cycle. According to Clark and Whitall (1989), newly walking infants coordinate their limbs in a 50 per cent temporal phasing relationship, just like adults. These researchers revealed, however, that the young walkers exhibited significantly increased variability compared to older walkers (infants who had been walking 3 to 6 months).

McGraw defined seven phases for the development of erect locomotion, which are illustrated in Figure 13–5. In *phase A, the newborn* or *reflex stepping,* the infant is in a flexed posture when held upright, and attempts to step are the result of elicitation of the stepping reflex, a primitive reflex movement pattern. In *phase B, inhibition,* or the *static phase,* elicitation of the stepping reflex is not readily observed. As seen in the development of creeping, the infant can maintain a supported upright posture that includes active cervical and spinal extension. In *phase C, transition,* the infant moves the body up and down, holding the feet in position. The infant may stand in position and stamp the feet, but there is no progression forward. In *phase D, deliberate stepping,* the infant attempts to step when held upright. In *phase E, independent stepping,* the infant takes steps independently. During this phase, the early walker uses a wide base of support; feet are flat, and the upper extremities are maintained in a high regard position (arms held high with the shoulders in external rotation and abducted, with the elbows flexed and the wrist and fingers extended). The early walker maintains hips and knees in slight flexion, to bring the center of mass closer to the ground. At about 12 to 13 months of age, infants are learning to walk alone. The later, more mature walker ambulates with a narrower base of support. Feet are closer together and show a heel-toe progression. The upper extremities are in "low regard" (shoulders in more of a neutral position with the elbows in extension), and the hips and knees are extended more. McGraw called this pattern *phase F,* or *heel-toe progression. Phase G, integration,* or *maturity of erect locomotion,* finds the arms down and moving reciprocally, synchronous with the movements of the lower extremities; out-toeing has been reduced, and pelvic rotation is present, along with the double knee lock pattern. In the double knee lock pattern, there is knee extension just before heel contact, but at the moment of heel contact there is knee flexion to help absorb impact shock; then, as the body moves forward over the foot, the knee returns to extension for weight bearing during the stance cycle. These characteristics indicate a mature gait pattern, and usually have developed by age 3 or 4. According to Sutherland and co-workers (1988), 98 per cent of toddlers have mature gait pattern by age 4.

The gait parameters of time and distance—step length and width, stride length, cycle time, cadence, and walking velocity—all change as the physical characteristics of the child change. Step lengths grow as there is growth in leg length and stature. Walking velocity increases with age in a linear manner from 1 to 3 years of age. From 4 to 7, the rate of change diminishes, but the relationship remains linear (Sutherland et al, 1988).

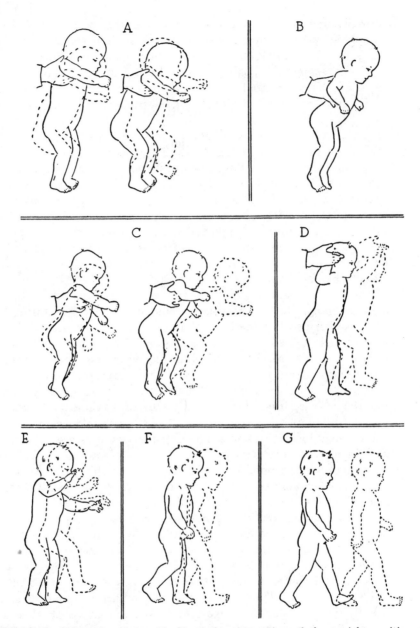

FIGURE 13–5. The seven phases (A–G) of the assumption of the upright position. (From McGraw MB. *The Neuromuscular Maturation of the Human Infant.* 1945, © Columbia University Press, New York. Reprinted with permission of the publisher.)

UPRIGHT LOCOMOTION IN THE OLDER ADULT

Attempts to clarify the relationship between aging and walking date back to at least the early 1940s and continue today. The literature provides conflicting information about exactly how the gait of elderly persons, particularly elderly women, changes with age. Murray and associates have provided much information concerning the characteristics of gait and the subsequent changes that accompany aging (Murray, 1967; Murray et al, 1964, 1966, 1970). In a 1970 study, Murray et al reported differences in the gaits of 30 women varying in age from 20 to 70 years. The six older women in this study had a slower walking velocity, shorter step length, longer stance, and shorter swing time than younger women. Murray's studies stated that women, compared to men, showed a slower walking velocity, shorter step length, and higher cadence that was not related to stature or body weight. Other researchers differed. Crowinshield and associates (1978) stated that female subjects are, on the average, shorter and lighter than male subjects. When the gait characteristics were normalized for subject height and weight, gender differences were nonsignificant.

Hageman and Blanke (1986) studied healthy women 20 to 35 years of age and 60 to 84 years of age. They found that the elderly women demonstrated significantly smaller values of step length, stride length, ankle range of motion, pelvic obliquity, and velocity when compared with the younger women. Stride width in this study was not found to be significantly different.

Elderly women prefer to walk more slowly than younger women. The temporal and kinematic variables of gait are speed-dependent (Crowinshield et al, 1978; Larish et al, 1988; Winter, 1983, 1984). If the younger women in many of these studies had walked at the slower speed chosen by the elderly women, the younger subjects might have shown a decrease in the ranges of motion used in the lower extremity, and possibly a decrease in the step length and, therefore, stride length.

Larish et al (1988) provided a most revealing study. This group used a wide range of younger and older subjects (for the 11 younger subjects, the mean age was 25.6; for the 17 older subjects, the mean age was 73.5 years). Gender information was not presented. The subjects walked at three different speeds, two controlled (0.81 m/second as the slow speed, 1.34 m/second as the fast speed) and one freely chosen speed. The authors found that the younger subjects took longer strides at the faster speeds. There was an age-related decrease in stride length for the 1.34 m/second (faster) condition, but not for the 0.81 m/second (slower) condition. In the freely chosen speed condition, the stride of the older adults was shorter than that of the younger adults. As a result of their shorter stride length in the 1.34 m/second condition, older adults compensated by increasing their stride frequency to a greater degree than younger adults. Of particular interest was the conclusion that the age-related decrease in stride length appeared only at faster walking speeds. In other words, certain age-related differences in gait may surface, but only when the functional capacity of the older adult becomes stressed. The full impact of the aging process on gait may be realized only when researchers begin to examine gait patterns across a variety of walking speeds and in a variety of environmental conditions.

In summary, much research is needed to identify more accurately the changes that occur in the gait of elderly women because of "normal" aging.

Running, Galloping, Hopping, and Skipping

The development of the locomotion patterns that evolve after upright walking are the patterns of running, galloping, hopping, and skipping (Clark & Whitall, 1989). Most literature on the development of these patterns has been descriptive research focusing on the head and neck, the trunk, and the extremities and on how these components relate to each other as a particular pattern evolves.

The contemporary theory of dynamic systems explains these subsequent patterns of locomotion as examples of different coordinative structures. A *coordinative structure* is defined as the coordination of the movement: how the muscles within a limb (intralimb) and between limbs (interlimb) are constrained to act as a unit. Dynamic action theory defines coordination of a movement pattern as the distance and temporal phasing relationships of the limbs, the stance swing relationships of the limbs, or some combination of time, distance, and velocity—collective variables that distinguish between different patterns of upright locomotion.

RUNNING

Running is defined as a pattern of movement that has a stance phase and a swing phase, but more importantly, a flight phase, a period of nonsupport. As with walking, the temporal phasing of running is such that halfway through the cycle of one limb, the other limb begins its cycle—50 per cent phasing (Clark & Whitall, 1989).

Many infants begin to run before they reach the mature level of walking. Footwork of the beginning runner recalls the early foot-flat pattern of walking. The early runner returns the arms to a high regard position. Initially there is no reciprocal arm swing or the forward-and-back driving swing of the arms. The arms are thought to be used more for balance. Stride length of the more advanced runner is longer because more force can be generated in the lower extremity during push-off. This ability to increase force also allows for a longer flight phase and heel strike. The more advanced runner demonstrates an increase in trunk rotation and arm swing. These patterns have been documented by descriptive studies of children aged 1.5 to 10 years (Woodward, 1986). The developmental levels of running are outlined below; these levels are adapted from the developmental levels of running defined by Roberton and Halverson (1984).

Level 1: *Upper extremities (UE)*—the arms are held in high regard to assist balance control, otherwise not active.

Lower extremities (LE)—the feet are flat; minimal flight; the swing leg is slightly abducted.

Level 2: *UE*—the arms begin to swing as spinal rotation counterbalances the rotation of the pelvis; the arms may give the appearance of "flailing."

LE—the feet may remain flat, may support knee flexes more during weight transfer; more flight time.

Level 3: *UE*—the arm swing increases because of the spinal rotation.

LE—heel contact is made at foot strike; the swing leg is in the sagittal plane; at toe-off, the support leg reaches full extension.

Level 4: *UE*—the arm swing becomes independent of spinal rotation; the arms move in opposition to each other and contralateral to the leg swing.

LE—similar to level 3.

The older adult form of running is defined according to the abilities of the adult being assessed. Many older adults who have remained active show no changes in their overall running patterns when compared to a younger group of adults. The assumption is that the qualities of the running pattern change when the characteristics of the individual (e.g., muscular strength, balance, range of motion) change. Although not substantiated, the logical conclusion is that as individual characteristics show the effects of aging, the running pattern returns to that of the early infant runner. Much research is needed to confirm or reject this notion, however.

GALLOPING

Galloping is defined as the first asymmetric gait mode in the young child, a walk on the leading leg followed by a running step on the rear leg. There is an asymmetric phasing of approximately 65/35 per cent (Whitall & Clark, 1986). Clark and Whitall (1989) state that galloping can be seen in young toddlers 20 months after first walking. The phasing modes are variable but predominantly consist of two distance phasing modes, 66/33 per cent and 75/25 per cent. The variability of temporal phasing was also found to be low across subjects who ranged in age from 2 to adulthood.

In early attempts at galloping, the arms are stiff and rarely become involved in projecting the body off the floor. They are usually held in the high regard position or out to the side to assist in balance, as was seen in the early form of running. During the early experiences of galloping, the stride is short, landings are flat-footed, and there is little trunk rotation. In addition, the tailing limb may land ahead of the lead limb. In contrast, the more advanced gallop appears more rhythmic and relaxed. The arms are no longer needed for balance and come into a low regard position or swing rhythmically in opposition to the movements of the lower extremities. These changes are accompanied by an increase in trunk rotation, which allows for more reciprocal arm movements. The literature appears to be void of any studies of older adults galloping.

HOPPING

Hopping (one-footed hopping) is an asymmetric pattern of locomotion. Halverson and Williams (1985) studied a group of children longitudinally and presented developmental levels for the upper and lower extremities for the hop. The developmental levels of hopping as defined by Roberton and Halverson (1984) are outlined below.

Level 1: *UE*—the arms are held in high regard, out to the side, not very active.
   LE—hip and knee quickly flex, pulling the body toward the floor more than lifting the body off the floor; the flight is momentary, only one or two hops; the swing leg is inactive.

Level 2: *UE*—the arms swing upward together, perhaps to assist in balance.
   LE—body lean allows extension of the knee and ankle to lift the body off the floor; there are repeated hops, but the swing leg is mostly inactive.

Level 3: *UE*—the arms are active together, pumping the body to help lift the body.
   LE—there is better coordination between the hip, knee, and ankle for functional takeoff and landing; the swing leg now assists in the movement by pumping up and down; the swing leg remains down and behind the support leg, however.

Level 4: *UE*—the arm in opposition to the swing leg is moving forward with the swing leg, assisting in the movement (to a minimal degree); the other arm is in the front or to the side.
   LE—the ball of the foot is now used for the landing; the support leg has good extension at takeoff; the swing leg helps in the upward and forward movement at takeoff; the increase in the swing leg's range of movement assists with the movement.

Level 5: *UE*—the arms work in coordination with the swing leg to assist the movement.
   LE—similar to level 4.

The swing leg is inactive in the earliest form of the one-leg hop. It is not until about 4 years of age that the swing leg begins to move in the hop, helping to propel the body forward. Ultimately, it is the swing leg that pumps up and down to assist in projection; the range of the swing leg increases so that it passes behind the support leg when viewed from the side. The arms follow a similar pattern. Initially, the arms are inactive, held in high regard.

As the pattern progresses, the arms become more active, swinging in opposition to the legs. Specifically, the arm opposite the swing leg moves forward and upward in a pumping action to assist the propulsion of the body forward; the other arm moves in the direction opposite the action of the swing leg. In the adult form of hopping, the arms and legs are active, swinging in opposition as just described. The interlimb phasing patterns are probably 50 per cent temporal and distance phasing. What should be remembered for this pattern of locomotion, as with all such patterns, is that children progress at different rates; the rate of progression can be attributed to many different parameters (e.g., muscle strength, balance).

No studies on the hopping patterns of older adults have been published. However, it might be appropriate to assume, as with the other patterns of locomotion, that the hopping patterns of older adults would resemble the patterns of the early hoppers; as muscle strength and balance decrease in the older adult hoppers, their hopping patterns resemble those of the young toddlers or children hopping at levels one, two, or three.

SKIPPING

Skipping is defined as an alternating gait, a step, then a hop on one leg, followed by a step, then a hop on the other leg. The developmental levels for skipping as defined by Roberton and Halverson are outlined below.

Level 1: *UE*—the arms move bilaterally to assist as the weight is transferred from foot to foot.

LE—one foot completes the step-and-hop sequence before weight is transferred to the other foot.

Level 2: *UE*—the arms begin to oppose each other, but they mostly work together.

LE—the child continues to complete one step-and-hop sequence before transferring the weight; the feet are flat during the movement.

Level 3: *UE*—the arms are in opposition to each other.

LE—action is completely on the ball of the foot; weight transfer is more smooth between the hop-and-step sequences.

The literature yields little information on skipping. The arms are initially held in high regard. The advanced pattern ultimately involves a swinging of the arms in opposition to the moving lower extremities. It has been suggested that interlimb phasing of this locomotion pattern is most likely 50 per cent (Clark & Whitall, 1989). Studies of older adults skipping were not found in a review of the literature. However, it is assumed that older adults demonstrate patterns similar to the early patterns of skipping, depending on the characteristics of the older population being studied.

INTERACTION OF SYSTEMS THAT PRODUCE THE BEHAVIORS OF LOCOMOTION

The transition from one form of locomotion to another form most likely depends on a number of factors: the interactions of the tasks to be accomplished, the bodily systems of the individual, and the environment in which the behavior is to be produced. Which system or combination of systems is ultimately responsible for producing the changes in a particular pattern of locomotion—that is, what are the system-sensitive scaling parameters that, when scaled (changed), create different gaits across the life span? In other words, what "causes" the older individual to walk slowly? Almost no research currently focuses on the identification of these parameters, especially for the later-developing locomotion skills of the older adult.

A review of the literature leads to the speculation that there are many body system parameters to consider, especially those that affect muscular strength, endurance, and postural control. In the transition from walking to running, the individual has to produce sufficient force to project the body into the air for the flight phase of running. The toddler, for instance, can run only when there are sufficient vertical ground reaction forces. These forces most likely result from increases in muscle mass, changes in anthropometric measurements, improved motoneuron recruitment, improved postural system, or some combination of these parameters and others not yet defined.

Older adults who maintain sufficient muscle strength, postural control, and other characteristics most likely maintain approximations of the most advanced form of a pattern of locomotion. Loss of function is common among the elderly. Muscle strength loss is one of the main causes of a decline in activities of daily living in the elderly population (Aniansson et al, 1978). As people get older, their physical activity patterns tend to change. It has been suggested that the changes observed in the locomotion patterns of aging adults are most likely the result of decreases in muscular strength. Wilder (1992) identified that 64% of the variation seen in the gait characteristics such as step length and time in double support of elderly adults was accounted for by the variable of muscle strength. This is one of only a few studies that have attempted to document exactly which system or combination of systems is responsible for the changes in motor pattern development across the life span. Most studies to date have not hypothesized the agent of change.

Continuous changes in body systems or environmental components can cause widespread reorganization of a particular pattern of locomotion. Systems are thought to be nonlinear and therefore able to respond to small changes with large effects. Wilder (1992) demonstrated that nonsignificant differences in ankle muscle strength and significant differences in hip muscle strength resulted in significant differences in certain gait pattern parameters of older adult women. Other studies have identified that older adults (over 70 years of age) sway more when standing erect, whether their eyes are open or closed (Horak et al, 1989; Maki et al, 1987). These studies have revealed that older adults with increased postural sway often are identified as the same individuals who frequently fall when moving from place to place. Thus, a relatively small change in postural sway appears to produce rather large effects in postural control.

Currently lacking in the literature are longitudinal studies (i.e., studies that follow one individual or a small group of individuals over a long period of time). What is available in the literature are cross-sectional research studies. To ultimately find out what forces a system or a combination of systems to change over time, we need studies that investigate the individual over time—the individual should be the unit of analysis.

SUMMARY

Descriptive studies have provided the bulk of our information on locomotion patterns: rolling, prone progression, walking, running, and galloping, skipping, and hopping. Some patterns have been validated only partially (galloping, hopping, and skipping), and then only by component analysis and for only one segment of the life span (the young child). Biomechanical studies have provided much information on the patterns of upright walking and running across the life span. The other patterns of locomotion await in-depth biomechanical analysis.

It is reasonable to assume that the evolution of a particular pattern of locomotion is ultimately the result of changes in the bodily systems that occur with aging.

References

Aniansson A, Grimby G, Hedberg M, L et al. Muscle function of old age. *Scand J Rehabil Med* 43(Suppl #6):43–49, 1978.

Clark JE, Whitall J. Changing patterns of locomotion: From walking to skipping. In Woollacott M, Shumway-Cook A (eds). *Development of Posture and Gait Across the Life Span*. Columbia, SC: University of South Carolina Press, 1989, pp 128–151.

Clark JE, Whitall J, Phillips SJ. Human inter-limb coordination and control: The first 6 months of independent walking. *Dev Psychobiol* 21:445–456, 1988.

Crowinshield RD, Brand RA, Johnston RC. The effects of walking velocity and age on hip kinematics and kinetics. *Clin Orthop* 132:140–144, 1978.

deVries JIP, Visser GHA, Prechtl HFR. *Fetal Motility in the First Half of Pregnancy*. In Prechtl HFR (ed). Continuity of Neural Functions Form Prenatal to Postnatal Life. *Clin Dev Med* 94, 1984. Philadelphia: JB Lippincott, pp 46–64.

Getchell N, Roberton MA: Whole body stiffness as a function of developmental level in children's hopping. *Dev Psychol* 25:920–928, 1989.

Hageman PA, Blanke DJ. Comparison of gait of young women and elderly women. *Phys Ther* 66:1382–1387, 1986.

Halverson LE, Williams K. Developmental sequences for hopping over distance: A prelongitudinal screening. *Res Q Exer Sport* 56:37–44, 1985.

Horak FB, Shupert CL, Mirka A. Components of postural dyscontrol in the elderly: A review. *Neurobiol Aging* 10:727–738, 1989.

Inman VT, Ralston HJ, Todd F. *Human Walking*. Baltimore: Williams & Wilkins, 1981.

Larish DD, Martin PE, Mungiole M. Characteristic patterns of gait in the healthy old. *Ann N Y Acad Sci* 515:18–33, 1988.

Larsson L. Aging in mammalian skeletal muscle. In Mortimer JA (ed). *The Aging Motor System.* New York: Praeger, 1982, pp 60–97.

Maki BE, Holiday PJ, Fernie GR. A postural control model and balance test for the prediction of relative postural stability. *IEEE Trans Biomed Eng* 34(10):797–810, 1987.

McGraw MB. *The Neuromuscular Maturation of the Human Infant.* New York: Hafner Press, 1945.

Murray MP. Gait as a total pattern of movement. *Am J Phys Med* 46:290–333, 1967.

Murray MP, Drought AB, Kory RC. Walking patterns of normal men. *J Bone Joint Surg [Am],* 46:335–360, 1964.

Murray MP, Kory RC, Clarkson BH, Sepic SB. Comparison of free and fast speed walking patterns of normal men. *Am J Phys Med* 45:8–24, 1966.

Murray MP, Kory RC, Sepic SB. Walking patterns of normal women. *Arch Phys Med Rehabil* 51:637–650, 1970.

Prechtl HFR. Prenatal motor development. In Wade MG, Whiting HTA (eds). *Motor Development in Children: Aspects of Coordination and Control.* Dordecht: Martinus Nijhoff, 1986.

Richter R, VanSant AF, Newton RA. Description of adult rolling movements and hypothesis of developmental sequences. *Phys Ther* 69:63–71, 1989.

Roberton MA, Halverson LE. *Developing Children—Their Changing Movement: A Guide for Teachers.* Philadelphia: Lea & Febiger, 1984.

Roberton MA, Halverson LE. The development of locomotor coordination: Longitudinal change and invariance. *J Motor Behav* 20:197–241, 1988.

Shirley MM. *The First Two Years: A Study of Twenty-Five Babies, vol 1: Postural and Locomotor Development.* Minneapolis: University of Minnesota Press, 1931.

Sutherland DH, Olshen RA, Biden EN, Wyatt MP. "The development of mature walking." *Clin Dev Med* 104/105, 1988.

Whitall J. A developmental study of the inter-limb coordination in running and galloping. *J Motor Behav* 21:409–428, 1989.

Whitall J, Clark JE. "The development of interlimb coordination in galloping: Theory and data." Paper presented at the North American Society for the Psychology of Sport and Physical Activity, June, 1986, Scottsdale, AZ.

Wilder PA. "Developmental changes in the gait patterns of women: A search for control parameters." PhD Thesis, University of Wisconsin, 1992.

Winter D. Biomechanical motor patterns in normal walking. *J Motor Behav* 15:302–330, 1983.

Winter DA. *The Biomechanics and Motor Control of Human Gait: Normal, Elderly, and Pathological,* 2nd ed. Waterloo, Canada: Waterloo Press, 1991.

Winter DA. Kinematic and kinetic patterns in human gait: Variability and compensating effects. *Hum Movement Sci* 3:51–76, 1984.

Woodward KM. In *Life Span Motor Development.* Champaign, IL: Human Kinetics, 1986.

Chapter 14

Prehension

by SUSAN V. DUFF

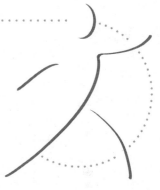

Objectives

AFTER STUDYING THIS CHAPTER, THE READER WILL BE ABLE TO:

1 Describe the components and systems involved in a prehensile task.
2 Describe the development of prehensile skills from the embryonic stage to adulthood.
3 Identify classic prehension patterns observed in the adult.
4 Describe the functional adaptations needed for prehension when underlying systems have been altered.

The human hand is a marvelous instrument. It enhances our life and serves to express not only our intelligence, but our emotions, through gestures. Dysfunction magnifies the remarkable capacity of prehensile skills. To understand dysfunction, it is important to review normal hand capabilities. This chapter explores prehensile skills and their importance at different phases of the life span.

COMPONENTS OF PREHENSION

Imagine yourself supported in a chair, looking at a cup of tea resting in front of you. Reach for the cup and secure the handle. As you drink the tea, adjust the handle within your hand. Now set the cup down on the table and let go of the handle. This simple task of drinking tea exemplifies the primary components of prehension: regard, approach, grasp, manipulation, and release. *Regard* is visual attention on the object, as when you observe the location of the cup of tea. *Approach,* or reaching, is the directing or adjusting of the hand toward an object, such as the handle of the cup. *Grasp* is the closing of the hand on the object, as when you secure the cup handle. *Manipulation* is the movement of the object while it is being held, as noted by your adjustment of the handle in your hand. *Release* is the method by which the object leaves the hand, as when you let go of the handle (Cliff, 1979). All of the components of

HANDS
by Melissa Goldstein

Some say the soul can be found
Pulsing in the heart
But I believe the soul resides
In our hands,
Flowing through the grasping, nimble fingers
Which separate us
From the kingdom of the beasts
Whose hearts beat like our own.
Towering pyramids,
Tapestries made of spun silver and gold—
All created by the work of our hands.

In the beginning
Before words,
We talked in fluid gesture.
Even now, though skilled artisans
In the craft of words,
We still use our hands to
Emphasize a point, grace our speech—
Saying "I love you" in a gentle caress,
Sometimes expressing our anger and hate
In a curled fist.
I look down at my own hands made
Stiff and clumsy by disease.
My fingers once spoke the language
Of music as they danced over the
Keys of the flute and piano.
Now they lie silent and still.
As I look at my hands
I realize that they are empty.
My soul took flight.
Traveled along the highways
Made of nerves and synapses
Until it finally came to rest
At the source of all expression.
Though my hands are mute.
My soul reaches out in these words.
The silence is broken.

—From Goldstein, Melissa. "Hands."
JAMA 269:1240, 1993. Copyright © 1993,
American Medical Association.

prehension are ideally accomplished from a point of stability and/or a stable base of support.

Stabilization

All movement is considered dynamic. It occurs from a point of stability, or a point from which there is a nonmoving part or a surface from which to move. When we rise to stand, we may push off with our arms from a static surface, the chair. If the chair were resting on wheels, the task would be much more difficult, because the surface would be dynamic, or movable. Our own body offers stabilization through skeletal structure and isometric muscle contraction.

TRUNK

Stabilization of the trunk during reaching tasks depends on the integrity of the bones of the trunk, including the spine, pelvis, ribs, and sternum. A stable trunk also involves recruitment or involvement of the slow-twitch muscle fibers present in large muscles such as the abdominals and hip extensors. These large muscles have large motor units; one axon may innervate 1000 muscle fibers (Lehmkuhl, 1983). The stabilizing contractions of these muscle groups prevent undesired movement and allow for adjustment in one's center of gravity when the upper limb moves in space. With the body stable proximally, one can engage in dynamic reaching and prehensile skill with less effort (Rood, 1962; Stockmeyer, 1967). For example, as you reach for a cup while sitting, the contractions of your trunk musculature act as synergistic stabilizers to maintain your center of gravity over your base of support. The muscle contractions prevent undesired trunk motion, such as lateral tilt to the same side as your reaching arm, which would result in a fall. If you are unable to reach for the cup without falling, external support, as from another individual, may provide a stable base. Stability of other joints is also needed during reaching tasks.

UPPER LIMB

Stabilization through muscle contraction occurs not only in the trunk, but also in the upper limb joints. The demands of the task determine which joints will be stabilized. If distal joint movement is desired, the proximal joints will stabilize, and vice versa. Consider the example of drinking tea: once the cup reaches your mouth and you sip the tea, your shoulder, elbow, and hand should remain in approximately the same position, while your forearm pronates to tilt the cup and allow the tea to flow into your mouth. (In other words, your forearm undergoes an isotonic contraction, and the other joints stabilize through isometric muscle contractions.) If the hand is undergoing sustained pinch or grasp through isometric contraction, this too is viewed as a form of stabilization. With the fingers and thumb providing the point of stability, the proximal joints are free to move. For example, when one holds a toothbrush, it is the wrist, forearm, and elbow that move while the fingers and thumb hold the toothbrush. In general, the joint to be stabilized will be determined by the activity and prehensile skills required.

Most prehensile skills are best performed with the wrist stabilized in approximately 20 to 30 degrees of extension and 10 degrees of ulnar deviation (O'Driscoll et al, 1992). With the wrist extended, the thumb can move into a plane of opposition in relation to the other digits, and the fingers can achieve full flexion (Kapandji, 1982). A sustained hold on the cup handle via finger flexion is an example. With the wrist positioned in extension, the long finger flexors can generate a strong contraction according to biomechanical concepts, including the *length-tension curve*. The length-tension curve, seen in Figure 14–1, correlates the tension produced or the strength of a muscle contraction with how close it lies to its resting length. Resting muscle length is defined as the length of a muscle when it is measured from attachment to attachment without a contraction. A strong muscle contraction can be generated when the muscle is within 70 to 105 per cent of its resting length, termed the *useful range* (Blix, 1895; Brand, 1985; Ramsey, 1940). Wrist extension keeps the finger flexors within this useful range, thus allowing for adequate strength during grip and pinch activities. When tasks are performed with the wrist

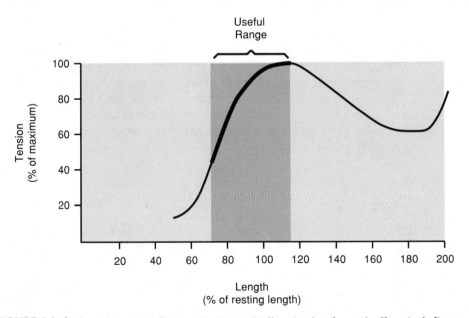

FIGURE 14–1. Length-tension diagram for isometrically stimulated muscle fiber, including extreme shortened and stretched states of fiber. (Redrawn from Lehmkuhl LD, Smith LK. *Brunnstrom's Clinical Kinesiology*. Philadelphia: FA Davis, 1983, p 132. Modified from Ramsey RW, Street SF. Isometric length-tension diagram of isolated muscle fibers of the frog. *J Cell Comp Physiol* 15:11, 1940.)

stabilized in flexion, the attachments of the finger flexors are close together. This may result in weaker grip and pinch, because the muscle-tendon unit may be at less than 70 per cent of its resting length (Blix, 1895; Brand, 1985; Ramsey, 1940; Kapandji, 1982). Some tasks are performed with the wrist in flexion, but tasks are more biomechanically efficient with the wrist in extension.

Visual Regard

Visual regard and perception play key roles in motivating an individual to reach for and grasp objects. Visual regard depends on the strength of one's attention, visual acuity, and ocular control, including accommodation and convergence. *Accommodation* involves adjusting the lens of the eye for distance. *Convergence* is the mechanism for maintaining single vision, by merging input from both eyes. Using our extraocular eye muscles, we can visually fix or sustain our gaze, track or follow moving targets, and scan from one object to the next (Bouska et al, 1985). Visual perception is the ability to use visual information to recognize, recall, discriminate, and understand what we see (Levine, 1991). As children gain experience through play involving various systems, perceptual constructs are developed. With exposure to and interaction with different environments, visual memory is laid down and complex processes develop, including visual sequencing and visuoconstructive abilities. Visual regard and perception guide our approach and manipulative skills in terms of accuracy and control, as noted when building a three-dimensional block design from a picture (Benbow et al, 1992; Bouska et al, 1985; Levine, 1991). For the purposes of this chapter, selected visual perceptual terms are defined in Table 14–1.

Approach

Reaching ability begins in infancy with random swiping and eventually is finely tuned to an accurate, continuous approach (Georgopoulos, 1986). Reaching integrates perceptual anticipation with motor preparation (Clifton, 1991). Visual-motor control, or eye-hand coordination, is the ability of an individual to utilize visual information for precise guidance of movement (Levine, 1991; Paillard, 1990). Sighted individuals use vision to guide reaching in many activities of daily living, such as retrieving a shirt hanging in the closet, or obtaining a carton of milk from the refrigerator. Practice plays a key role in terms of skill acquisition for specific tasks requiring visual-motor ability (Zernicke & Schneider, 1992). To function at a high level, eye-hand coordination requires collaboration between the visual and motor systems.

The motor preparation for reach and grasp may involve the entire upper limb. Movement of the shoulder can place the hand in space over a wide range. Elbow movements place the hand closer to or farther away from the body. The forearm and wrist make appropriate adjustments, in order to posi-

Table 14-1. VISUAL PERCEPTION TERMS

Visual Component	Definition	Functional Use
Depth perception	Ability to localize objects in space, estimate size and distance	Discriminating how far a cup is out of reach before retrieving it
Figure-ground	Ability to visually focus on selected details in the foreground by selectively screening out competing background stimuli	Locating an eraser in a desk drawer full of odds and ends or finding a geometric form embedded in a picture
Figure-closure	Ability to recognize a design or object despite incomplete information	Recognizing a toy half-covered in a blanket
Form constancy	Ability to recognize that an object may appear to change size or shape, depending on its position or location, yet remains the same	Recognizing a baby bottle anywhere, whether it's in the mother's hand or resting on the kitchen counter
Position in space	Ability to perceive the position of an object in relation to itself and the environment	Recognizing that a familiar stuffed animal is upside down versus upright, or recognizing letters or numbers in any position on a page
Spatial relationships	The relationship between two or more objects in terms of orientation in space	Recognizing that two objects are resting next to each other two inches apart or recognizing the relationship between letters, words, and sentences on a page
Visual memory	The reception, registration, and storing of information within the central nervous system	Retrieval of information stored, to confirm visual or nonvisual cues; recall of the shape and form of numbers
Visual sequencing	Ordering of visual patterns in time and space	Used when planning steps and anticipating the consequences of tasks that require ordering and step-by-step procedure
Visuoconstruction	Spatial planning involving building up and breaking down objects of two and three dimensions	Copying 2-D or 3-D designs, putting a puzzle together, wrapping gifts

Data from Bouska et al, 1985; Frostig, 1964; Levine, 1991.

tion the hand prior to grasp or receipt of a weight-bearing surface (Boehme, 1988). The hand itself adjusts for the object's perceived spatial properties, such as size and shape (Clifton, 1991). When reaching to grasp a cup visualized at chest level, the shoulder flexes to approximately 80 degrees, the scapula rotates up and protracts, and the elbow extends. As the cup handle is approached, the wrist extends and deviates in either an ulnar or a radial direction, while the forearm adjusts into neutral. As the handle is approximated, the fingers extend and the thumb abducts in preparation. The fingers complete the task by flexing, the thumb either adducts or opposes, and the proximal joints undergo sustained contractions to stabilize. When the activity demands greater than 90 degrees of shoulder flexion, the trunk and neck may need to flex laterally to the opposite side of the reaching arm, and the pelvis may elevate on the same side (Boehme, 1988). With maturity, our approach to objects during reaching is anything but random. Reaching involves precise timing and recruitment of needed muscle groups prior to grasping. Skilled adult reaching is typified by one smooth velocity peak that is followed by a small velocity change near the target (Absend, 1982). Visual regard in combination with precise motor preparation typically guides reaching behavior. Of course, we also can reach without vision, relying on alternative sensory cues and/or visual memory.

Grasp

Once an object is approached, one of various prehension patterns is used to secure it. Acquisition of reach and grasp is discussed in detail later in this chapter. For now, we will look at classic prehension patterns in the adult.

CLASSIFICATION OF ADULT PREHENSION

Adult prehension patterns have traditionally been classified according to Napier's work (1956) and Landsmeer's work (1962). Napier described two types of grip, power and precision. *Power grips* are defined as forcible activities of the fingers and thumb that act against the palm to transmit a force to an object (Long, 1970). Examples include the cylindric grip, spheric grip, and hook grip (Fig. 14–2). Muscular activity is generally isometric and involves sustained contraction of the extrinsic muscles of the hand with contributions from the intrinsic muscles. During *precision grip* and *pinch* activities, forces are directed between the thumb and fingers, not against the palm. Examples of precision grip or pinch include pad-to-pad prehension, tip-to-tip prehension, and pad-to-side, or lateral, prehension (Fig. 14–3). The muscular activity is generally isometric (Napier, 1956). Landsmeer kept the classification of power grip but used the term "precision handling" to describe the manipulative quality of precision functions. *Precision handling* requires a change in position of the handled object, either in space or about its own axes, as well as exact control of finger and thumb position. Movements are primarily isotonic. They involve a combination of patterns and are dynamic. For example, when using a lateral pattern to turn the stem of a watch, the dial is stabilized between the thumb and the index finger while the index finger undergoes isotonic movements of flexion and extension to turn the dial (Landsmeer, 1962). Grip and pinch patterns, along with the joints and muscles involved, are listed in Table 14–2. Despite their wide acceptance, the classic prehension patterns continue to be challenged.

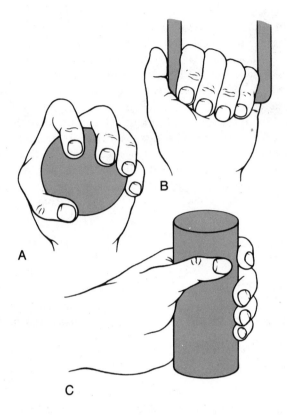

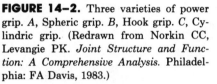

FIGURE 14–2. Three varieties of power grip. *A*, Spheric grip. *B*, Hook grip. *C*, Cylindric grip. (Redrawn from Norkin CC, Levangie PK. *Joint Structure and Function: A Comprehensive Analysis.* Philadelphia: FA Davis, 1983.)

Following an extensive survey of the literature, Casanova and Grunert (1989), introduced a new classification system based on anatomic nomenclature and contact surfaces. They proposed the use of the terms "static" and "dynamic" prehension. *Static prehension* refers to any form of prehension in which the object does not move within the hand, although proximal joint movement may occur. An example of static prehension is isometrically holding a key using a lateral pinch. *Dynamic prehension* refers to object manipulation within the hand. The positional changes of the object occur within the hand rather than at the proximal joints, as in rolling a needle between the fingers in order to clear the eye before threading the needle. Casanova and Grunert (1989) discuss how force sometimes is used during either static or dynamic prehension, and sometimes is used very little. For example, during precise static prehension, as in turning a key in a tough lock, force is used. However, it may not be needed when using a cylindric grasp on an empty soda can. We usually grade the force used during prehension. This ability to grade forces may be based on previous learning and memory of the weight and integrity of the object (Brooks, 1986). Despite the attempt to reclassify prehension, the classic patterns defined by Napier and Landsmeer continue to be widely ac-

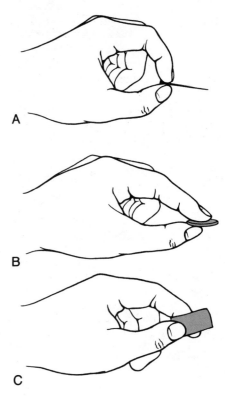

FIGURE 14–3. Three varieties of precision pinch and handling. *A*, Tip-to-tip. *B*, Pad-to-pad. *C*, Pad-to-side (lateral). (Redrawn from Norkin CC, Levangie PK. *Joint Structure and Function: A Comprehensive Analysis.* Philadelphia: FA Davis, 1983.)

cepted. In time, with more research, the alternative classification may gain more recognition and acceptance among professionals dealing with prehension.

SIGNIFICANCE OF OPPOSITION

Of all the digits, the thumb, because of its unique ability to oppose, is a common feature in all grasp classifications. Although prehension is evident in many forms of animal life, it attains maximum function in humans. The thumb contributes 40 to 70 per cent of total hand function (Beare, 1973; Flatt, 1977). What is the significance of thumb opposition?

The ability to oppose the thumb through a wide range of movements separate humans from the other primates. *Opposition* is the movement by which the pad surface of the thumb is placed diametrically opposite the terminal pad of one or all of the other digits of the hand, as seen in Figure 14–4. The primary digit, the thumb, opposes the index finger through rotation at the carpometacarpal joint (Napier, 1980). The comparative length of the index finger to the thumb is a major factor when attempting opposition or pad-to-pad contact. This comparison, called the *opposability index,* is represented by

Table 14-2. CLASSIFICATION OF PREHENSION PATTERNS

Patterns	Joint Motion	Muscles Used	Function
Cylindric grasp	Thumb opposition, finger adduction and flexion	FPL and thenar group, AdP, select interossei (task dependent), 4th lumbrical and FDP (FDS for more power)	Holding onto a cylindrically shaped object such as a soda can
Spheric grasp	Thumb opposition, finger flexion and abduction	FPL and thenar group, AdP, FDP (FDS for more power), 4th lumbrical interossei (except 2nd)	Holding onto a round object such as a baseball
Hook grasp	MCPs neutral; finger flexion at PIPs and DIPs; thumb extension	Finger FDS and FDP, thumb, EPL and EPB, EDC, 4th lumbrical and 4th dorsal interossei	Holding onto a briefcase handle
Pad-to-pad prehension	Thumb opposition and slight flexion of all thumb joints; finger flexion at MCP and PIP; flexion or extension of DIP of involved fingers	Thenar group, FPL, select interossei and FDS of involved fingers (FDP if DIP flexion is present)	Holding onto a coin
Tip-to-tip prehension	As above with greater thumb and finger flexion, including DIP flexion	As above with greater FDP force FDP secondary to DIP flexion, interossei of involved fingers	Holding a needle
Pad-to-side prehension (lateral)	Thumb adduction with IP flexion, index finger flexion, and abduction	Thumb, FPL, FPB and AdP, involved fingers, FDS and FDP, reduced interossei and lumbricals except 1st dorsal interossei	Holding a key

Data from Long et al, 1970; Landsmeer, 1962; Napier, 1956, 1980.

FPL = flexor pollicis longus, AdP = adductor pollicis, FDP = flexor digitorum profundus, FDS = flexor digitorum superficialis, MCP = metacarpophalangeal, PIP = proximal interphalangeal, DIP = distal interphalangeal, EPL = extensor pollicis longus, EPB = extensor pollicis brevis, EDC = extensor digitorum communis, IP = interphalangeal.

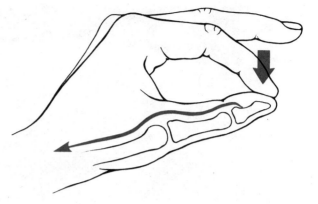

FIGURE 14–4. Opposition of the thumb to position its pad opposite the pad of one or all of the other digits.

the formula, total length of the thumb × 100 divided by the total length of the index finger. Humans have a high opposability index (65), and most primates have a lower index (40 to 45). The ape's opposability index lies closest to human's (Napier, 1980). A reduction in the opposability index can be noted in an individual whose distal phalanx of the thumb has been amputated, reducing its length and limiting the ability to fully rotate the thumb pad to the index pad, as pictured in Figure 14–5. Opposition of the thumb is significant in functional prehension, especially when used in combination with other joints (as when turning a doorknob or buttoning a shirt).

SIGNIFICANCE OF OTHER DIGITS

The index finger is considered the most important digit after the thumb because of its mobility and independent musculature attachments, such as the extensor indices. It accounts for 20 per cent of lateral pinch, 20 per cent of power grip from a supinated position of the forearm, and 50 per cent of power grip from a pronated forearm position (Tubiana, 1984). The long finger is the longest and strongest and thus has significant functional value. In some individuals, it replaces the index finger as the dominant finger and is used for pointing and manipulating small objects (Leatherwood & Skirven, 1987). The index and long fingers are considered the prehensile digits and the most stable anatomically. The small and ring fingers are recruited for power grip tasks. They are considered the most mobile anatomically, yet are the weakest digits (Tubiana, 1984). Both the index and small fingers can produce isolated extension. All of the digits are important in prehension, and the loss of any one of them will limit prehensile ability to some degree.

Manipulation

Once an individual obtains an object through grasp, he or she may either sustain a hold on the object or manipulate it with one or two hands to

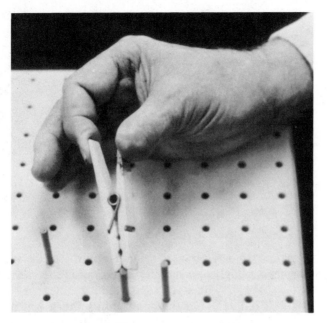

FIGURE 14–5. Opposition available given a partial amputation of thumb, representing a reduction in the opposability index.

accomplish a task. All forms of manipulation demand the use of the small intrinsic and extrinsic muscles of the fingers and/or thumb. These muscles have many fast-twitch fibers and small motor units, meaning that one axon may innervate approximately five muscle fibers (Lehmkuhl, 1983). These two features are important for precise movements such as manipulating a scalpel during surgical procedures and rolling dice with one hand. *Sustaining a grip or pinch* on an object or tool is done primarily with isometric contractions and intermittent isotonic contractions, as when writing with a pencil over a long period. The muscles used to sustain a hold will need to recruit many slow-twitch fibers in order to maintain the contraction.

The ability to move objects within one hand, called *in-hand manipulation,* is divided into three categories:

Shift: Movement of an object on the surface or among the fingers.

Rotation: Movement of an object around its axis using the fingers.

Translation: Movement of an object from fingers to palm or palm to fingers (Exner, 1990).

In-hand manipulation demands the use of fast-twitch muscle fibers in order to achieve quick movements. One example of in-hand manipulation is translation of a penny from the palm up to the fingertips, then shifting the penny across the finger pads to end with a hold between the index finger and the thumb. If you turned the coin over from heads to tails in your palm, that would be

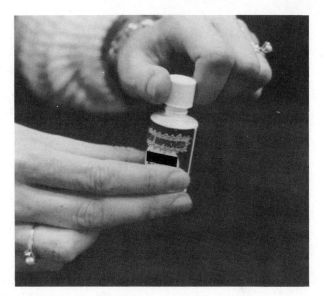

FIGURE 14-6. Bilateral hand use demonstrating two prehension patterns: three-fingered palmar pinch (three-jaw chuck) to hold the base, and dynamic lateral pinch to turn the top off.

considered a rotation. If two objects are held in the same hand, the ring and small (or "ulnar") fingers usually stabilize one object while the index and long (or "radial") fingers manipulate the other object.

Bilateral hand use, or using both hands to perform a task simultaneously, is practiced and refined in early childhood. Skill for complex tasks advances with development. Eventually each hand can perform a separate role to accomplish a task with success, which is called *differentiation* or *asymmetry.* Activities such as opening a small bottle demonstrate differentiation. Note in Figure 14–6 how two different prehensile patterns are used for each part of the bilateral task. One hand is holding the base with a three-fingered palmar pinch, and the other is demonstrating a dynamic lateral pinch to turn the cap off. In summary, manipulation is demonstrated by sustained holding activities, one-handed manipulation, or tasks requiring two hands simultaneously.

STEREOGNOSIS

Stereognosis, or *haptic perceptual exploration,* is the ability to recognize objects by name without vision. The rich number of receptors in our fingertips, muscles, and joints provide the tactile, proprioceptive, and kinesthetic cues used to identify characteristics of an object (Royeen & Lane, 1991). Sensory nerve endings in the fat pads and ridges of our fingers supply the varied tactile information (Riordan, 1978). Muscle spindles, along with tactile input, detect the sense of position (Clark, 1985). Joint receptors, in the joint capsule, detect the sense of movement (Proske, 1988). Golgi tendon organs, located at the musculotendinous junction, and other receptors including the muscle spindle, detect the sense of force (Schmidt, 1981). Our kinesthetic sense, needed for fine-motor skills, is strengthened as our skin is stretched over joints and muscles of the hand and forearm (Moberg, 1983). We use our manipulation abilities as well as our sensory systems to foster object identification, yet it is the memory of the object that serves to make it recognizable. Reach into your purse or pocket and retrieve a quarter. How did you know it was a quarter and not a nickel? You probably used tactile cues and proprioceptive-kinesthetic input to judge the size and weight of the coin, based on memory of a previous visual or other sensory experience. Although visual memory is a strong component, individuals without sight can develop strong stereognosis ability once they are taught, demonstrating that memory from various types of sensory input must play a significant role in recognition.

Release

Release is the process of letting go of a held object or taking pressure away. Release can be crude, as when one drops the hot handle of a frying pan, or it can be graded and controlled, as when setting a crystal glass onto a counter. Graded release is mastered and refined individually through practice of specific tasks. Playing a musical instrument is a beautiful demonstration of how graded release is achieved. A master jazz pianist is able to hold pressure on the keys and release the pressure in such a controlled and graded fashion that the end result is a varied sound combination of loud or soft, sustained or quick tones. A novice player may not exhibit the same degree and finesse with regard to hold and release of the pressure on the piano keys, perhaps making all the tones loud and sustained. Tool use also demonstrates graded release. In the process of using a screwdriver to drive in screws, a series of quick, graded gross grasps and releases occurs, in order to turn the handle effectively and not involve the whole shoulder girdle. If you could imagine a 5-year-old performing the same task, he or she would probably display an alternating lateral trunk tilt and/or involve the shoulder girdle. This may be secondary to weakness, reduced ability to supinate the forearm, and/or insufficiently graded gross grasp and release. As control of release is gained, one's repertoire of prehension activities enlarges.

Summary

In summary, the components of prehension begin ideally from a stable base of support, such as is provided by the trunk. The amount of stabilization required by joints of the upper limb varies depending on the demands of the prehensile task. Primarily, a point of stability is needed from which to move. All components of prehension are important: visual regard, approach or reach, grasp, manipulation, and release. The development of the components requires various, interdependent systems. Dysfunction arises when a related system is underdeveloped or not operating to full capacity, eventually affecting some aspect of fine motor function.

PROGRESSION OF PREHENSILE TASKS ACROSS THE LIFE SPAN

The time frame for acquisition of prehensile skills has been researched from conception to old age. The periods outlined in Chapter 2 will be used as a guide as we consider meaningful tasks encountered at different phases in the life span.

Prenatal Period

The upper limb buds, which represent the earliest form of the upper limb, begin to appear around the 26th to 27th day of gestation, as seen in Figure 14–7. By the end of the 7th week, the fingers are defined and the upper limb has rotated medially to its typical position at birth. Table 14–3 describes and illustrates upper limb development up until the 7th week. The dermatomes of the skin, which represent the tactile system, begin to develop as early as 7 weeks of gestation. Our proprioceptive system develops in utero with the differentiation of the articular skeleton and muscle system, beginning around the 7th week of gestation (Moore, 1982). The prenatal period ends with full development of the upper limbs. Incomplete development of the central ner-

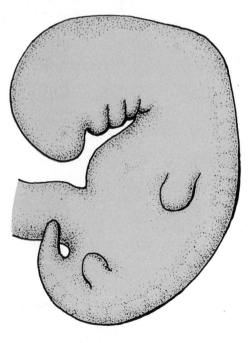

FIGURE 14–7. Limb bud appearance in embryo at about 28 days of gestation. (From Moore KL. *The Developing Human: Clinically Oriented Embryology*, 4th ed. Philadelphia: WB Saunders, 1988.)

Table 14–3. DEVELOPMENT OF THE UPPER LIMB IN THE EMBRYONIC PERIOD

Age of Embryo	Upper Limb Development	Illustration
28–30 days	Upper limb buds "flipper-like" Lower limb buds appear	
31–32 days	Upper limb buds "paddle-like"	
33–36 days	Hard plates formed	
41–43 days	Digital or finger rays appear	
44–46 days	Elbow region visible, notches appear between finger rays	
47–48 days	All limb buds extend ventrally	
49–51 days	Upper limb longer and bent at elbow Fingers distinct but webbed	
52–53 days	Hands and feet approach each other Fingers are free and longer	
7th week	Upper limb rotates 90° laterally in longitudinal axis (elbows face posterior) Lower limb rotates 90° medially (knees face anterior) Tissue breaks down between digits from the circumference inward, producing fingers and toes	

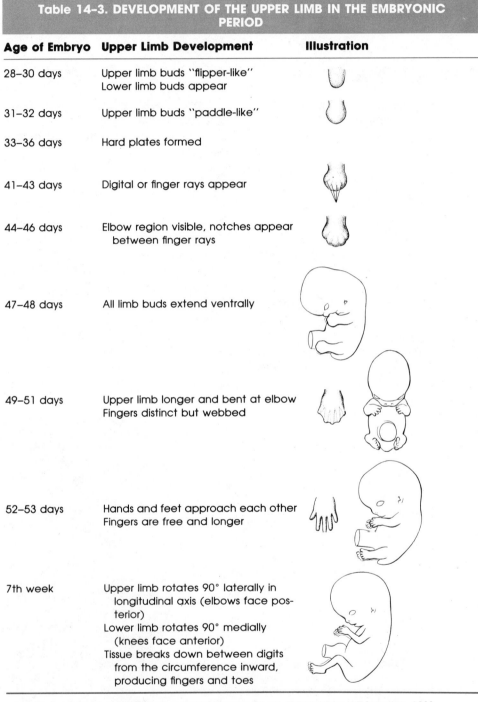

Adapted from Moore KL. *The Developing Human,* 4th ed. Philadelphia: WB Saunders, 1988.

vous system and lack of nerve myelinization prevent full upper limb control at birth.

Infancy

REFLEXES

The newborn infant is dominated by primitive reflexes that provide most of the initial response to stimuli from the external world. Tactile and proprioceptive stimuli elicit the reflexes that most influence early hand function (Gesell, 1947). These reflexes are listed in Table 14–4. The early development of the tactile and proprioceptive systems allows for the elicitation of these reflexes at birth (Ayres, 1972). As the newborn enters infancy, the hand reflexes are gradually integrated, and voluntary prehensile function develops.

GROSS MOTOR SKILLS

Early gross motor skills contribute to the development of prehension skills. When making transitions from one position to another, the infant stretches various muscle groups that are used in later prehensile and stabilization tasks.

Prone Position. In the prone position, propping on forearms, the 4-month-old infant may attempt to shift weight to reach. If the infant is successful, one arm is freed to allow reaching toward a toy, while the weight-bearing forearm supinates and the weight-bearing shoulder externally rotates. The child may end up in a roll, but the weight shift will help stretch shoulder girdle musculature and the pronator muscles of the forearm. Weight bearing on the upper limbs recruits muscles to stabilize, which will be used later for reaching tasks. Weight bearing on the elbows or forearms recruits the pectorals; weight bearing on extended arms recruits the pectorals, triceps, and scapular muscles. As strength increases, the infant is able to horizontally adduct the arms to position the hands directly beneath the shoulders during extended arm weight bearing (Bly, 1983). Once an infant can move into quadruped position and rock, greater weight shifting through the hands alternates pressure from the ulnar to the radial side, stretching out the intrinsics of the hand, as seen in Figure 14–8. Boehme (1988) entitled this open-palm weight bearing *expansion of the hand* and considers it a prerequisite to manipulation. Later in life, we use expansion of the hand to push off from supporting surfaces when standing from a sitting position and when using objects such as a stapler, as seen in Figure 14–9 (Boehme, 1988).

Supine Position. In the supine position, the infant gains abdominal strength and, with full hand-to-foot play, stretches out the elbow flexors in preparation for full arm weight bearing. Control of the pectorals and other muscles gained in prone weight bearing strengthens full reaching against gravity and object play above chest height for sustained periods. This may include hand-to-

Table 14-4. HAND REFLEXES				
Reflex	**Appears**	**Disappears**	**Stimulus**	**Response**
Grasp	2 weeks	4–5 months	Tactile stimulus initially; later, proprioceptive input also is needed to elicit grasp	Flexion of fingers, adduction and flexion of the thumb
Traction response	28 weeks' gestation	2–5 months	Stretch to shoulder flexors and adductors with traction	Flexion of the wrist and fingers with synergistic flexion of elbow and shoulder
Avoidance response	Neonatal period	5–6 months; fully integrated by 6–7 years	Light tactile stimulus along dorsum of hand to fingertips	Extension and abduction of fingers and wrist (withdraw from stimulus)
Instinctive grasp reaction	4–5 months	Remnants persist into adult life	Stationary or moving light touch; radial palm contact; ulnar palm contact	Orienting reaction Slight supination Slight pronation
	6–7 months		Ulnar or radial palm contact	Orienting and groping to find the object
	8–10 months		Moving stimulus withdrawn from any part of the palm	Orienting, groping, and grasping of stimulus
Asymmetric tonic neck reflex (ATNR)	28 weeks' gestation	4–5 months	Passive rotation of head	Elbow flexion on skull side, with elbow extension on face side

Data from Twitchell, 1970; Ammon & Etzel, 1974; Fiorentino, 1972; Gesell, 1947; Illingsworth, 1987; Dargassies, 1977.

mouth play or hand-to-hand transfer (Boehme, 1988; Erhardt, 1982). Abdominal strength, used to bring the knees up, will be needed to help stabilize the trunk for future upper limb activities. By 6 months, the infant has enough abdominal and back control to sit upright during upper limb reaching and grasping activities. Once strength through the trunk and upper limb is

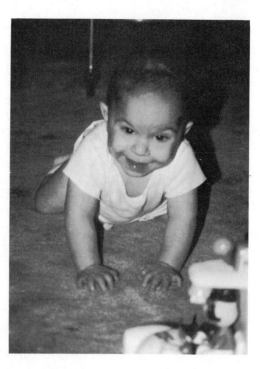

FIGURE 14–8. Expansion of the hand during weightbearing in quadruped.

achieved, the infant is able to demonstrate reaching both unilaterally and bilaterally. Reaching becomes more accurate as the infant gains control in the middle ranges of shoulder movement. With increasing proximal stability, the infant can focus on distal control and begin to acquire greater prehensile skill.

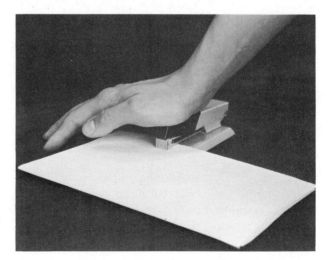

FIGURE 14–9. Expansion of the hand during functional tasks — in this case, using a stapler.

ACQUISITION OF PREHENSION

As an infant matures in intelligence, physical development, and neuromuscular abilities, all components of prehension develop. *Regard* demands the use of vision. The visual system in newborns is more advanced than the manual system. In early infancy, the asymmetric tonic neck reflex (ATNR) position channels the infant's gaze toward the hand. Although the neonate seems obligated by reflexes and will not gain control of hand movements until months later, he or she can visually fixate or sustain gaze for brief periods and track or follow a moving target through a small range (Bushnell, 1985). By 2 to 3 months of age, convergence and accommodation are advancing. This enables the infant to fixate on objects for sustained periods and to follow a moving target through a wider range (Bouska et al, 1985; Hatwell, 1990). By 4 to 5 months, the child will reach for objects in his or her visual field. As visual memory develops, between 6 and 7 months, the infant begins to realize that an object still exists even if it falls out of the visual field, and by 8 months will search for it. Binocular vision (or two eyes working together), accommodation, and acuity progress over a child's second year of life, strengthening eye-hand coordination.

Early approach, also termed *visually elicited reaching,* begins in the neo-natal period and ends at approximately 7 weeks. This early form of reaching is described as a "fling or thrust" and is considered a ballistic, preprogrammed, and inaccurate movement (Bower, 1974; Bushnell, 1985; von Hofsten, 1984). The connection between the eye and the hand is strengthened, in part, through the presence of the ATNR. As the ATNR is integrated and symmetry is gained, *visually guided reaching* emerges (Bower, 1974; Halverson, 1931). This occurs around 4 months and is differentiated from visually elicited reaching because it is guided, accurate, and based on matching the seen target with the seen hand (Bushnell, 1985). Infants at 5 to 6 months can reach toward a target and make hand and arm adjustments to accommodate an object's shape and size before it is encountered (Hofsten, 1984; Clifton, 1991). Clifton (1991) found that infants with previous visual experience demonstrated this hand and arm orientation even when reaching to grasp objects in the dark, if cued by a sound. By the time an infant reaches 9 months, practically all reaches are unilateral and directed straight at the target (Halverson, 1931). The nerves to the proximal joint musculature myelinate approximately 1 month ahead of the small hand muscles (McBryde & Ziviani, 1990). This accounts for the fact that proximal muscle control develops first, contributing to proximal stability and accurate reach to objects.

Grasp and manipulation progress as we gain control of our small hand muscles, the intrinsics (McBryde & Ziviani, 1990). Initial grasp patterns primarily involve the fingers only, leaving the thumb passive. Thumb function, including opposition, develops between 3 and 12 months and is responsible for the progression in prehensile patterns. By 11 months, the infant demonstrates pad-to-pad opposition of the thumb to the index. Index isolation begins around 10 months, and by the end of the first year, the infant is able to isolate the index finger as a dominant pointer (Erhardt, 1974; Knobloch, 1987; Hohlstein, 1982). In his study of reach and grasp patterns, Halverson (1931) found very little improvement in 60-week-old infants in comparison to adults in terms of the neatness and quickness of the grasp, or the balanced placement of the digits in holding activities. Gradation of pressure while holding objects is initially exaggerated, but by the end of the infant's first year, subtle adjustments are possible, allowing for only necessary pressure to be exerted when holding objects (Halverson, 1932). Stereognosis develops gradually after birth. According to *sensory integrative theory,* our tactile system is the foundation for form and space perception, as well as eye-hand coordination. Disruptions or alterations in the tactile system may result in functional deficits and interfere with the acquisition of all components of prehension, including tool use (Ayres, 1972; Fischer & Murray, 1991). Hirschel and colleagues (1990) studied performance and environmental support during execution of grasp and specific prehension patterns in infants 7 to 14 months old. They found that external support was required in the absence of internal stability in order to execute patterns off an unstable surface. As infants mature, internal stability develops, allowing exhibition of higher-level prehensile patterns with less support.

Release progresses in early infancy, as voluntary control over wrist, finger, and thumb extensors emerges. Boehme (1988) suggests that release develops off a point of stability. For example, mutual fingering in mid-line by the 4-month-old and transferring of objects from hand to hand in the 5- to 6-month-old is possible because one hand can release off the stability provided by the other hand. Voluntary release emerges around 7 to 9 months. It is initially achieved through stabilization provided by an external surface, such as the tray of a highchair or from the stable hand offered by someone attempting to take an object from the infant. Once a child is able to accurately release an object into a container, without external support, he or she is on the way to developing mature control and graded release patterns. Typically, an infant can release a block into a small container by 12 months (1 year) and release a pellet into a small container by 15 months (Boehme, 1988; Erhardt, 1982; Hirschel, 1990; Knobloch, 1987). Ball throwing is an example of release that improves in control and accuracy as the infant moves into childhood (Cliff, 1979).

Table 14–5 outlines sequential development of prehension. Although this outline is adapted from the work of major authors, there is still room for refinement. Hohlstein (1982) challenges previous approaches to classify prehension. She feels that a high degree of inconsistency in the prehensile responses of normal infants makes it difficult to accurately label patterns. Instead, she groups all prehensile responses into three phases. During *phase one,* infants use their whole hands in a gross or unspecialized manner. In *phase two,* infants use parts of their hands as they begin to develop specialization. By *phase three,* infants use the pads of their distal phalanges in a precise, specialized manner. Hohlstein is just one of the many researchers to question

Table 14–5. SEQUENTIAL ACQUISITION OF PREHENSION FROM BIRTH TO 1 YEAR

Description	Age	Illustration	Stimulation
Recognizes hands	8 wks (2 mos)		Hand enters visual field assisted by the ATNR
Reflexive ulnar grasp	12 wks (3 mos)		Ulnar placement of objects encourages grasp; hanging toys may promote visual tracking
Retains objects placed in hand: Midline fingering; mouthing of fingers; swiping in visual field	16 wks (4 mos)		Placing objects anywhere in hand will encourage grasp; hanging toys will encourage swiping if they are within visual field and reach
Primitive squeeze grasp (wrist flexed); raking	20 wks (5 mos)		Introduction of toys of varied textures, sizes, and shapes will promote voluntary grasp and raking
Palmar grasp (no thumb participation, wrist moving into neutral)	24 wks (6 mos)		Placing toys in different positions will encourage eyes and hands to search prior to reach and grasp
Radial palmar grasp (thumb adduction begins); mouthing of objects	28 wks (7 mos)		Ideal toys are washable and those that can be picked up and transferred easily from one hand to the other

currently accepted methods of prehension classification. Further revisions are expected in the future.

BILATERAL ARM AND HAND USE

Bilateral arm and hand use, or bimanual coordination, combines the components of prehensile function previously outlined. However, it is unique in terms of development. Some components of bilateral hand use are included in Table 14–5. Infants progress through stages of asymmetry to symmetry to differentiation. Initially, asymmetry predominates, as seen in the 2-month-old, and antigravity control is limited. The 3-month-old demonstrates greater symmetry as noted during bilateral hand play on their chest in mid-line. If an

Table 14-5. *Continued*			
Description	**Age**	**Illustration**	**Stimulation**
Scissors grasp (thumb adduction stronger)	32 wks (8 mos)		Introduction of toys with a thin circumference will strengthen thumb adductor
Radial-digital grasp (beginning opposition)	36 wks (9 mos)		Pliable materials such as clay or finger food will encourage opposition of thumb
Inferior pincer grasp (volar hold vs. pad to pad; hand supported prior to grasping); isolated index pointing	36–52 wks (9–12 mos)		Small objects varied in shape will promote exploration via poking, feeling, and manipulation
Pincer grasp—pad to pad (some support before grasping)	38–52 wks (10–12 mos)		Tiny objects, such as raisins, to pick up and drop will encourage development
Superior pincer grasp — tip to tip (hand unsupported prior to grasping)	52–56 wks (1 yr)		Thin yet safe objects the size of a pin will encourage development
Three-jaw chuck (wrist extended and ulnarly deviated); maturing release	52–56 wks (1 yr)		Toys requiring a strong radial finger hold and blocks and containers providing repeated motions will encourage strong grasp and release

object is placed near the infant's hand, he or she may swipe the object with a fisted hand. The 4-month-old often displays a bilateral, or two-handed, approach to reach objects visible in mid-line. After 5 months, object presentation and size determines whether the reach will be unilateral or bilateral (Fagard, 1990). The 5-month-old is able to crudely transfer objects from one hand to the other. Mid-line hand play away from the chest becomes more extensive as shoulder girdle strength improves. At this age, the infant can hold the bottle with two hands and displays more active object manipulation, as in banging and shaking toys. The 6- to 7-month-old displays unilateral reach and a mature hand-to-hand transfer. By 8 to 10 months, the infant demonstrates initial differentiated movements; this is when the two hands begin to have different roles or functions. For instance, one hand can hold the bottle while the other reaches to grasp a new toy. The 12- to 18-month-old demonstrates advancing differentiated movements; each hand assumes either the active role or the stabilizing role. For example, the active hand may operate the dial of a toy phone with the index finger, and the stabilizing hand may hold the edge of the toy phone. After 2 years of age, the complexity of bimanual, or two-handed, tasks, increases significantly (Ammon & Etzel, 1977; Bly, 1983; Conner, 1978; Exner, 1989; Fagard, 1990). Basic prehensile patterns and bilateral hand use progress over time and are refined into complex patterns through childhood.

Preschool Child

REFINEMENT AND PRACTICE

During childhood, early prehensile patterns and eye-hand coordination skills are refined and practiced. Learning prehensile tasks through trial and error and rehearsal from a model are hallmarks of early childhood (McCullagh et al, 1989). Often a young child is unable to demonstrate a particular skill independently, yet can do so in the presence of an adult or more capable peer. Vygotsky (1978) defined this distance between actual and potential problem solving ability as the *zone of proximal development*. A 3-year-old child may be unable to cut paper with scissors independently, yet may be successful in the presence of other capable 3-year-olds, by internalizing the perceptual and problem-solving strategies provided (Exner, 1990; Lyons, 1984; Vygotsky, 1978). Skilled hand function and implement use develops rapidly during this period.

MANIPULATION

Early use of implements begins as the toddler becomes socialized. Implements commonly used at this age, as defined by Coley (1978), include the following:

Utensils: Eating devices, banging instruments.

Tools: Scissors, writing implements.

Self-Care Items: Fasteners, shoelaces, hairbrush.

Implement use requires all three forms of manipulation: sustained pinch, in-hand manipulations, and bimanual coordination or bilateral hand use. It is possible to use all three forms within the same task. As strength of the intrinsics develops, the child is able to *sustain a hold* on objects, such as when holding onto a crayon for a prolonged period. As distal control improves, abilities in terms of crayon and pencil grip advance. The sequence of pencil grip is outlined in Table 14–6. Initially, the child must adjust the crayon position with the opposite hand (Erhardt, 1982; Rosenbloom & Horton, 1971). As the coordination of the fingers improves, the child demonstrates *in-hand manipulation* as needed to translate the crayon from the palm to the fingertips without assistance from the opposite hand. *Bimanual coordination* expands in the preschool years as coordinated, asymmetric roles are assumed by each hand. Initially, the child may need to stabilize with both elbows the paper he

Table 14-6. SEQUENTIAL ACQUISITION OF PENCIL GRIP			
Pencil Grip	**Age**	**Description**	**Illustration**
Palmar-supinate	1–2 yrs	Pencil or crayon is held by fisted hand; forearm slightly supinated; wrist slightly flexed; shoulder motion produces movement of pencil	
Digital-pronate	2–3 yrs	Pencil or crayon is held by fingers and thumb; forearm pronated, wrist ulnarly deviated; pencil controlled by shoulder movement	
Static-tripod	3+ yrs	Pencil held proximally between thumb and radial two fingers; minimal wrist mobility; pencil controlled by shoulder movement	
Dynamic-tripod	4+ yrs	Pencil is held distally through thumb opposition to the index and long fingers, with the ring and small fingers stabilizing in flexion; small movements at the metacarpolphalangeal and interphalangeal joints control the pencil; stabilization occurs at the shoulder, elbow, forearm, and wrist	

Data from Erhardt, 1982; Rosenbloom and Horton, 1971; Knoblock, 1987.

or she is coloring on, until eventually just the opposite hand is needed. Other examples of bilateral skill are when the preschooler cuts paper with scissors, buttons clothing, zips a zipper, and ties shoelaces. Motor planning, or the ability to execute novel motor acts, plays a significant role in the acquisition of new fine-motor tasks such as those described above. Both the tactile and proprioceptive systems combine with cognitive processes to execute good motor planning (Cermack, 1991; Fischer & Bundy, 1991). Modeling of novel tasks with immediate rehearsal is another mode of learning (McCullagh et al, 1989). Through modeling and practice, the preschool child expands and refines sustained pinch strength, in-hand manipulation, and bilateral hand use. By the end of this period, a hand preference for specific tasks such as coloring is demonstrated.

HAND PREFERENCE

Hand preference and hand dominance are often confused in definition. Preference refers to a *tendency* to use one hand for prehension instead of the other.

(Hand dominance is the *consistent use* of one hand over the other for such tasks as throwing a ball, writing with a pencil, and eating with a fork.) Although some researchers report that hand preference for swiping objects can be noted within days after birth, it remains controversial (Korczyn et al, 1978). The preschool child develops a hand preference as he or she practices skilled tasks such as eating with utensils, coloring, and throwing a ball. By 4 to 6 years, hand preference is well established (Levine, 1987, p. 472). Lateralization of the brain, or the process in which the hemispheres become specialized for particular functions, is generally thought to be the driving force behind hand dominance. By 6 to 7 years, laterality is demonstrated by consistent and superior use of one hand over the other to hold a pencil during writing tasks (Ayres, 1972; Murray, 1991).

School-Aged Child

MASTERY

This period brings mastery of many components of prehension. Mastery of specific prehensile skills depends on the amount of time spent practicing and the strength of the supporting systems. A child's knowledge and abilities for an activity are considered domain- or task-specific, which allows for rapid encoding and response to certain fine-motor situations (Starkes, 1990). School-aged children often spend much of their time involved in task-specific practice. The demands for written work increase by the fourth grade, necessitating skill in holding and sustaining a pencil grip while completing the complex task of handwriting (Levine et al, 1981). Writing requires selective attention and is affected by the state of arousal (Benbow et al, 1992). By the time a child reaches school age, his or her systems are ready to engage in higher-level prehensile tasks such as writing.

HANDWRITING

Most of the components of prehension play a role in handwriting. Visual regard of the paper and pencil and an accurate perception of the workspace are needed. When copying from a chalkboard, one is required to shift visual gaze from the board to the paper without losing one's place. The spatial relationships between the desk, the paper, and the blackboard need to be accurately perceived, as do the spatial relationships between the letters, words, and sentences on a page. Position in space and form constancy will guide recognition of letters and numbers. Grasp and manipulation, sustained grip and pinch, in-hand manipulation, and bimanual coordination are strong factors and can be analyzed separately for clarity. Pencil grip is an example of sustained pinch. Examples are pictured by order of frequency in Figure 14–10.

The most frequently occurring example is the dynamic tripod, which is

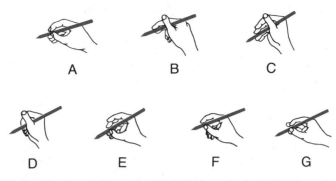

FIGURE 14–10. Pencil grips. *A,* Dynamic tripod. *B,* Lateral tripod. *C,* Transpalmar interdigital. *D,* Cross-thumb. *E,* Dynamic bipod. *F,* Dynamic bipod with omitted third digit. *G,* Static tripod. (Redrawn from Bergmann KP. Incidence of atypical pencil grasps among nondysfunctional adults. *Am J Occup Ther* 44[8]:736–740, 1990.)

demonstrated when a pencil is held between the pads of the index and thumb while it rests against the long finger (Jaffe, 1990). This position is considered the most efficient in terms of speed and dexterity, because pencil movement is controlled distally by the fingers and thumb. Alternative pencil grips are considered efficient if the thumb and index form a circle or open web space, allowing for skillful distal manipulation. Inefficient alternative grips limit the range, speed, and fluidity of distal movement. In other words, there is a greater need to incorporate proximal movements of the wrist and elbow to control the pencil, reducing precision (Benbow et al, 1992; Bergmann, 1990; Schneck, 1991; Schneck & Henderson, 1990). The lateral tripod, considered a functional yet inefficient grip, because the web space is closed, is used by up to 25 per cent of nondysfunctional children and up to 10 per cent of adults (Bergmann, 1990; Schneck & Henderson, 1990). With adequate strength and somatosensory feedback, a child can sustain a hold on a pencil without the need for excess pressure (Benbow, 1991; Erhardt, 1982). Endurance for sustained pinch required during prolonged handwriting tasks is gained with practice. Gains in grip and pinch strength contribute to all prehensile abilities, including sustained activities. Mathiowetz and colleagues (1986) collected normative data on grip and pinch strength for children and adolescents 6 to 19 years of age, comparing males to females. Figure 14–11 graphs the upward strength progression in the three-fingered palmar pinch or three-jaw chuck, and Figure 14–12 depicts the trend with key pinch. Pencil grip strength may be inferred from palmar pinch and key pinch strength. Figure 14–13 demonstrates the upward trend with regard to grip strength for the same age group. In-hand manipulation is frequently used for pencil writing (Levine et al, 1981). If a demand is made for writing and erasing quickly, a child learns to adjust the pencil in one hand through translation or shift and rotate it longitudinally to use the eraser, without laying it down or obtaining assistance from the other hand. Bimanual coordination is required for writing because one hand

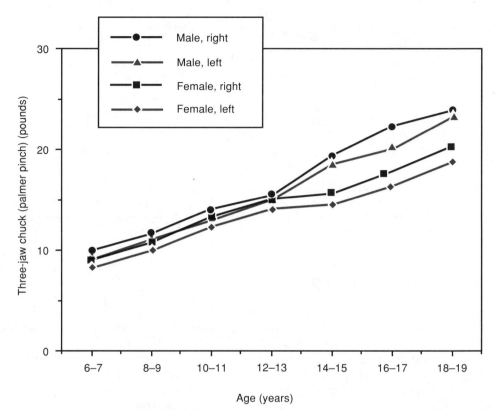

FIGURE 14–11. Three-jaw chuck (palmar pinch) of males and females from 6 to 19 years of age. Graph depicts the upward trend in strength. (Data from Mathiowetz V, Wiemer DM, Federman SM. Grip and pinch norms for 6 to 19 year olds. *Am J Occup Ther* 40[10]:705–711, 1986.)

must stabilize the writing surface and the other hand must actively use the pencil. Complex bimanual coordination progresses during school age. One complex task is that of building model airplanes, which requires one hand to stabilize the base and the other to place small parts. As the child matures into adolescence, interest will further guide the refinement of prehensile skills.

Adolescence

PREREADINESS SKILLS

During this phase of development an individual's primary occupations include schoolwork, socialization, part-time employment, and prereadiness for later employment and/or career. The prehensile demands resemble those of the school-age child, except that the skill level is often higher, with less time spent in trial and error and more time spent in task-specific practice. Skills performed with the dominant hand continue to advance beyond those of the nondominant hand. However, bilateral hand skills, including use of a computer

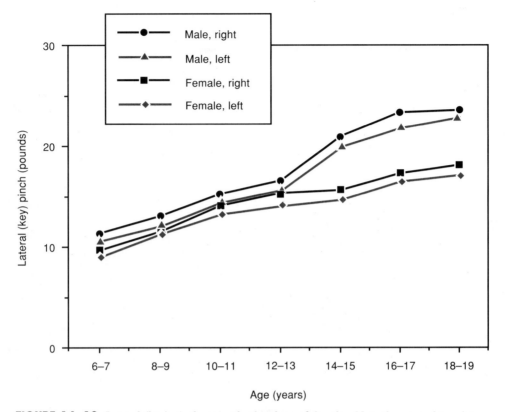

FIGURE 14–12. Lateral (key) pinch strength of males and females. Note the upward trend from 6 to 19 years of age. (Data from Mathiowetz V, Wiemer DM, Federman SM. Grip and pinch norms for 6 to 19 years olds. *Am J Occup Ther* 40[10]:705–711, 1986.)

keyboard or sports-related activities, do play a strong role at this stage of development. Adolescents often are cognitively aware of their strengths and weaknesses in terms of coordination and skill with manipulative tasks. Success heightens interest and helps boost self-esteem; thus, motivation for a task and practice are strongly correlated. A comparison between male and female adolescents, in terms of grip and pinch strength, is made in Figures 14–11 through 14–13. Young adults demonstrate a significant increase in grip and pinch strength, which may translate into functional gains for prehensile tasks in terms of force generated and endurance.

Adulthood

OCCUPATIONAL CHOICES

Early in adulthood, most career choices are made. Some occupations require fine dexterity and skilled hand use. Dental hygiene, surgery, and stained glass

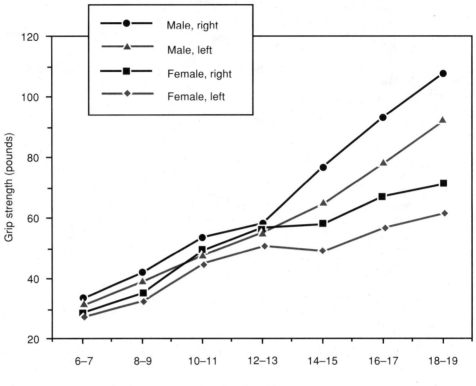

FIGURE 14–13. Grip strength of males and females from 6 to 19 years of age. (Data from Mathiowetz V, Wiemer DM, Federman SM. Grip and pinch norms for 6 to 19 year olds. *Am J Occup Ther* 40[10]:705–711, 1986.)

artistry all require skill in precision handling and a strong pinch for sustained tool use. Pickelman and Schueneman (1987) devised a rating form for testing proficiency in surgery and a neuropsychologic test battery for assessing psychomotor, perceptual, and perceptual-motor abilities in surgical residents. They found that technical proficiency did improve over time, which probably correlates with task-specific practice. In addition, they found that those with demonstrated strength in the area of complex visuospatial problem-solving and manual dexterity displayed superior surgical technique. Although not measured, other components enter the equation, such as endurance, efficiency, and accuracy. As one enters early adulthood with strong prehensile skill, those other components may require nurturing prior to achievement of true mastery. With motivation, patience, and task-specific practice, most prehensile skills improve. If they do not, the individual may choose a profession in which strong prehensile skills are not required.

MAINTENANCE OF PREHENSILE SKILL AND FUNCTION

In middle adulthood, most of the systems involved with prehension continue to function well, as long as they are well maintained and not overextended. Performance in most activities of daily living (ADL) is maintained easily because such activities are practiced repeatedly over the years and are generally nonstrenuous. What differentiates this period from early adulthood in terms of performance is the amount of domain-specific practice, motivation, and efficiency of performance. As interest in and motivation for activities drop, so does practice time. One may have been an expert at the piano at the age of 25 years, but by age 50 may spend too little time at the keyboard to maintain and preserve one's former skill. Conversely, concert pianists, who continue to demonstrate fine technique well into their elder years, may be able to maintain their skills because of continued practice. Sustained practice time promotes greater endurance, yet it is demanding. It requires one to maintain a high tolerance of aerobic work in order to avoid fatigue of associated structures. Musculoskeletal disorders such as carpal tunnel syndrome and tendinitis, called *cumulative trauma disorders (CTDs)* result from sustained pinch or prehensile activity without adequate endurance and thus adequate rest to refuel energies. CTDs are the most frequent cause of lost work and worker's compensation claims in certain industries. For example, as many as 30 per cent of professional musicians will develop CTDs (Armstrong, 1987; Markson, 1990). For adults, the best methods for maintaining prehensile skill without causing undue harm require one to maintain correct alignment for tasks, take frequent breaks during sustained pinch or grip tasks, use tools to simplify tasks, and redesign the tools and musical instruments used to prevent undue stress on anatomic structures (Blair & Bear-Lehman, 1987; Dortch, 1990; Markson, 1990; Meagher, 1967).

STRENGTH

Mathiowetz and colleagues (1985) outlined normative data on persons older than 20 years in terms of grip strength, as illustrated in Figure 14–14. There may or may not be a difference between dominant and nondominant hands in terms of grip strength. Evaluation using the Jamar dynamometer suggests that if the right hand is dominant, strength of the right hand is usually 10 per cent higher in comparison to the left; if the left hand is dominant, the strength of the two hands are usually equal (Crosby & Wehbe, 1992; Peterson et al, 1989). This can be important when reporting relative strength and during the rehabilitation phase following injury to the hand or upper limb.

Older Adulthood

SYSTEM CHANGES

Functional adaptation to system changes seems to be the biggest challenge for older adults. Many changes vary with regard to age of onset, and they occur in

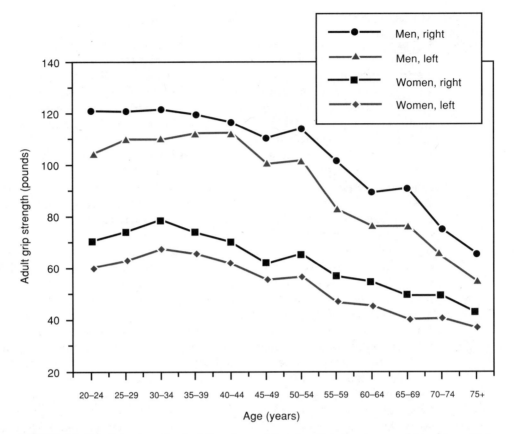

FIGURE 14–14. Grip strength of adult males and females. Note the downward trend from 20 to 75 years of age. (Data from Mathiowetz V, Kashman N, Volland G, Dowe M, Rogers S. Grip and pinch strength: Normative data for adults. *Arch Phys Med Rehabil* 66:16–21, 1985.)

those systems directly involved in object manipulation and eye-hand coordination. These systems include the visual and somatosensory system, the nervous system, and the musculoskeletal system. Visual acuity, imaging power of the retina, and the transparency of the lens are all reduced during the elder years. It takes older individuals 33 per cent longer to process visual information than younger individuals (Kline, 1983; Sekuler & Hutman, 1980). Also, there is a sharp decrease in depth perception from 60 to 75 years (Williams, 1990). Changes in the nervous system predominantly involve the brain. There is a loss of brain weight secondary to death of neurons and synapses. Neuronal changes also include a decrease in motor and sensory nerve conduction. Secondary to changes in the neural end organs of joints and muscles, there may be a greater dependency on muscular feedback to maximize proprioception, or awareness of joint position and movements. Despite the proprioceptive alterations, Williams and colleagues (1987) reported that few changes in kinesthetic sense occur with age. There is an increased threshold to touch pressure input and a decreased sensitivity to vibration sense. In terms of neuromuscular status, there is a general decrease in the number of muscle fibers, which affects strength and mass. Functionally, there is a decrease in the speed of muscle contraction and in the ability to sustain a contraction (Williams, 1990). Common changes in the skeletal system occur as one ages; osteoarthritis may damage articulations by destroying cartilage, and osteoporosis weakens bone by reducing the amount of calcium. The system changes that occur in elderly individuals affect hand function, yet somehow most persons manage to adapt and remain functional.

ADAPTATIONS

What are some adaptations that elderly individuals make in response to system changes, and what are the resultant alterations in hand function? Shiffman (1992) found that hand strength, performance time, and the frequency with which prehension patterns are used are affected by age. Other factors, such as reduction in sensory feedback, can also influence function. We count on a sustained grip to hold onto such items as a hairbrush, a toothbrush, and eating utensils. If somatosensory feedback is reduced, a tighter grip will be used to provide the needed sensory input. This tighter grip may not only strain joints, but also may recruit more muscle fibers to secure a sustained contraction. This extra effort may put the muscle at even greater risk for fatigue, because the muscles already have a reported reduction in strength and speed of contraction.

Quick dexterous function will be reduced if the speed of a contraction is reduced. Thus, when elderly persons have to count out change at the checkout line, they may require extra time, because their in-hand manipulation skills used to count coins may be slower. Reaction time has been used to measure the capacity of the central nervous system to plan and initiate movement. Williams and colleagues (1987), in their study of normal individuals free of impairment, found that the time needed to plan for precise movements of the distal extremities increased linearly from 50 years to 90 years of age. Variability in terms of planning simple movements was considerable. During complex hand movements, an increase in planning time in elderly persons was most frequently noted (Williams, 1990). However, many other studies indicate that, with significant practice, elderly persons can decrease their overall response time (Conrad & Longman, 1965; Falduto & Baron, 1985; Fleishman & Fruchter, 1960; Provins, 1956, 1958). Thus, despite the system changes that occur with aging, overall eye-hand coordination and manipulative skills may be relatively maintained in elderly persons as long as task-specific practice is continued and the systems involved remain generally intact.

ADAPTATIONS TO ALTERATIONS IN PREHENSION

Adaptive Strategies

Earlier in this chapter, it was mentioned that the presence of a thumb and even the length of the thumb separates humans from other primates in terms of prehensile skill. The complexity of approach was also reviewed in terms of the forearm and wrist motion required to make adjustments prior to grasp of an object. One would expect difficulties given either the absence of a thumb for opposition tasks or the inability to make adjustments in the forearm and wrist during approach. However, one only has to observe a 25-month-old child with bilateral congenital absence of the thumb and radius to confirm the creative and adaptive capacity of humans. The child in Figure 14–15 can be observed picking up pegs with a modified small spheric grasp, demonstrating a wider abduction approach to make up for the lack of thumb opposition. She can also engage in two-handed tasks, such as bringing a large cookie to her mouth, as seen in Figure 14–16. In the picture she demonstrates a modified scissors grasp with the right hand, and with the left hand she counterbalances forces by placing the ulnar fingers on top and the index and long fingers on the bottom side of the cookie. Because her radius is absent, this child lacks forearm rotation. Thus, as pictured, she abducts and internally rotates her right shoulder to successfully bring the cookie to her mouth. Typically for this activity, the forearm supinates and the shoulder needs only to flex. Most adaptive acts occur naturally, as the child described above illustrates. It is interesting to note, however, that even following surgical replacement of the thumb, these children retain and often use the ingrained adaptive patterns previously displayed.

Adaptive Devices

Most individuals adapt to subtle deficits in prehension. If the deficits make it difficult to perform simple tasks, one may require the use of adaptive devices. Self-care items commonly used to maximize abilities include universal cuffs to

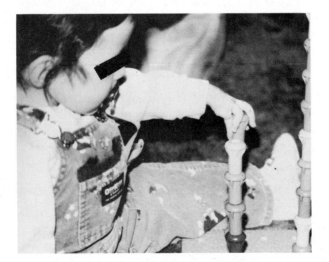

FIGURE 14–15. Adaptive spheric grasp demonstrated by a 25-month-old child born with absent radius and thumb.

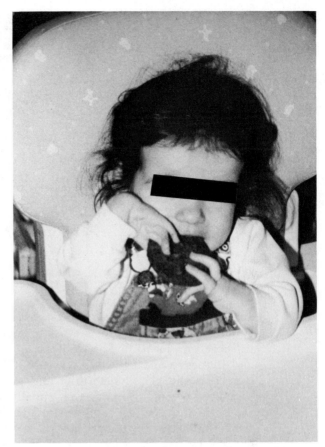

FIGURE 14–16. Bilateral hand use in same child seen in Figure 14–15, demonstrating adaptive scissors grasp with one hand and an interdigitating grip with the other.

hold various implements (e.g., a toothbrush or an eating utensil) and button-hooks used to button clothing with one hand. For those without full active motion, writing devices that place the fingers and thumb in a position resembling the tripod hold are available (Fig. 14–17). If accepted, adaptive devices can increase independent function in daily activities for an individual with prehension deficits.

Intervention

Surgical reconstruction and prosthetic devices provide an alternative means of prehension to those with reduced function or nonfunctional hands. A common goal for both interventions is to provide an opposing digit and a pad to oppose to. If *surgery* is elected, the small child discussed previously will first undergo an operation to centralize the right ulna or place it in the center of the carpal bones. Following that procedure, she will undergo further surgery to rotate the second metacarpal and its adjacent index. The rotated metacarpal and index

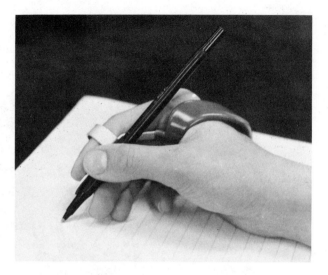

FIGURE 14–17. Adaptive writing tool used to promote tripod hold on writing utensil.

will serve as the opposing digit or new thumb (Bora, 1986; Muniz & Dell, 1989). *Prostheses* are available to those who opt against surgery or who are not surgical candidates. Various types of prosthetic devices are currently available to those who lack full or partial use of one or both hands. Conventional hook and harness units are body powered. The aluminum or stainless-steel hooks can open and close voluntarily and provide a strong pinch force. They are supported through a harness proximally and driven by a cable that runs from the harness to the terminal device. As proximal muscles move, the cable drives the terminal device. Electrically powered prostheses, termed *myoelectric units,* operate by battery. Electrodes are placed over proximal muscle bellies, and distal motion is activated by conscious control of specific muscle contraction. The most frequently issued terminal device for myoelectric units resembles a hand, and like the hook provides a strong pinch force. Finally, there are cosmetic prostheses without moving parts. These passive prostheses are often flesh-colored gloves covering an amputated body part. Because they are made to resemble the missing part, they can greatly improve one's self-image. Functionally, they can be used to assist with tasks demanding bilateral hand and arm use. As with adaptive devices, prostheses are not always accepted. Prior to purchase of a costly prosthesis or surgical intervention, it is important to evaluate the needs and long-range plans of the individual, given his or her current functional level.

SUMMARY

Normal prehensile abilities are a remarkable demonstration of human adaptation to the demands of everyday life. Many systems work cooperatively to form the components of normal hand skills. When we explore prehension through the life span, with its many facets, we can only marvel at the highly developed features. Even more amazing are the prehensile abilities of a person of any age who has deficits in hand function. Simple tasks become outstanding acts of adaptation with a touch of creativity.

References

Absend W, Bizzi E, Morasso P. Human arm trajectory formation. *Brain* 105:331–348, 1982.

Ammon JE, Etzel ME. Sensorimotor organization in reach and prehension: A developmental model. *Phys Ther* 57(1):7–14, 1977.

Armstrong TJ, Fine LJ, Goldstein SA, Lifshitsz YR, Silverstein BA. Ergonomic considerations in hand and wrist tendonitis. *J Hand Surg [Am]* 12:830–837, 1987.

Ayres AJ. *Sensory Integration and Learning Disorders.* Los Angeles: Western Psychological Services, 1972, pp 25–234.

Beare RLB. Upper limb abnormalities. *Proc R Soc Med* 66:634–638, 1973.

Benbow M. *Loops and Other Groups: A Kinesthetic Writing System, Instructor's Edition.* Randolph, NJ: OT Ideas Inc., Appendix v–viii, 1991.

Benbow M, Hanft B, Marsh D. Handwriting in the classroom: Improving written communication. In Royeen CB (ed). *AOTA Self Study Series: Classroom Applications for School-Based Practice.* Rockville, MD: American Occupational Therapist's Association, 1992, pp 5–41.

Bergmann KP. Incidence of atypical pencil grasps among nondysfunctional adults. *Am J Occup Ther* 44(8):736–740, 1990.

Blair SJ, Bear-Lehman J. Editorial comment: Prevention of upper extremity occupational disorders. *J Hand Surg [Am]* 12(5):821–822, 1987.

Blix M. Die Lange und die Spannung des Muskes. *Scand Arch Physiol* 3:295, 1891; 4:399, 1892–1893; 5:150, 175, 1895. In Lehmkuhl LD, Smith LK. *Brunnstrom's Clinical Kinesiology,* 4th ed. Philadelphia: FA Davis, 1983, pp 129–132.

Bly L. *The Components of Normal Development During the First Year of Life and Abnormal Motor Development.* Birmingham, AL: Pittinger, 1983.

Boehme R. *Improving Upper Body Control.* Tucson: Therapy Skill Builders, 1988, pp 19–127.

Bora FW. Congenital anomalies of the upper extremity. In Boyd S (ed). *Pediatric Upper Extremity Diagnoses and Management.* Philadelphia: WB Saunders, 1986, pp 28–32.

Bower TGR, Broughton JM, Moore MK. The coordination of visual and tactual inputs in infants. *Percept Psychophys* 8:51–53, 1970.

Bouska MJ, Kauffman NA, Marcus SE. Disorders of the visual perceptual system. In Umpred D (ed). *Neurological Rehabilitation.* Princeton: CV Mosby, 1985, pp 555–585.

Brand PW. *Drag in Clinical Mechanics of the Hand.* St. Louis: CV Mosby, 1985, pp 166–191.

Brooks VB. *The Neural Signs of Motor Control.* Oxford: Oxford Press, 1986.

Bushnell EW. The decline of visually guided reaching during infancy. *Infant Behav Dev* 8:139–155, 1985.

Casanova JS, Grunert BK. Adult prehension: Patterns and nomenclature for pinches. *J Hand Ther* 2(4):231–244, 1989.

Cermack SA. Somatodyspraxia. In Fisher AG, Murray EA, Bundy A (eds). *Sensory Integration: Theory and Practice.* Philadelphia: FA Davis, 1991, pp 137–170.

Clark FJ, Burgess RC, Chapin JW. Role of intramuscular receptors in the awareness of limb position. *J Neurophysiol* 54:1529–1540, 1985.

Cliff S. *The Development of Reach and Grasp.* El Paso, TX: Guynes Printing, 1979.

Clifton RK, Tochat P, Litovsky RY, Perris EE. Object representation guides infants reaching in the dark. *J Exp Psychol Hum Percept Perform* 17(2):323–329, 1991.

Coley IL. *Pediatric Assessment of Self-Care Activities.* St. Louis: CV Mosby, 1978.

Cooney WP, An Kai-Nan, Daube JR, Askew LJ. Electromyographic analysis of the thumb: A study of isometric forces in pinch and grasp. *J Hand Surg [Am]* 10:202–210, 1985.

Conner FP, Williamson GG, Siepp JM (eds). *Movement in Program Guide for Infants and Toddlers with Neuromotor and Other Developmental Disabilities.* New York: Teachers College Press, 1978, pp 99–128.

Conrad R, Longmann D. Standard typewriter versus chord keyboard—An experimental comparison. *Ergonomics* 8:77–88, 1965.

Crosby C, Wehbe MA. "Normative values for hand strength." Paper presented at The American Society of Hand Therapists 15th Annual Conference, Phoenix, November 6, 1992.

Dargassies S. *Neurological Development in the Full-Term and Premature Neonate.* New York: Excerpta Medica, 1977.

Dortch HL, Trombly CA. The effects of education on hand use with industrial workers in repetitive jobs. *Am J Occup Ther* 44(9):777–782, 1990.

Exner C. Development of hand functions. In Pratt P, Allen A (eds). *Occupational Therapy for Children,* 2nd ed. St. Louis: CV Mosby, 1989, pp 235–259.

Exner C. The zone of proximal development in in-hand manipulation skills of nondysfunctional 3 and 4 year old children. *Am J Occup Ther* 44(10):884–891, 1990.

Erhardt RP. *Developmental Hand Dysfunction: Theory, Assessment, and Treatment.* Laurel, MD: RAMSCO, 1982, pp 9–43.

Erhardt RP. Sequential levels in the development of prehension. *Am J Occup Ther* 28:592–596, 1974.

Fagard J. Development of bi-manual coordination. In Bard C, Fleury M, Hay L (eds). *Development of Eye-Hand Coordination Across the Life Span.* Columbia, SC: University of South Carolina Press, 1990, pp 262–282.

Falduto L, Baron A. Age-related changes and effects of practice and task complexity on card sorting. *J Gerontol* 41(5):659–661, 1960.

Fischer AG, Murray EA. Introduction to sensory integration. In Fisher AG, Murray EA, Bundy AC (eds). *Sensory Integration: Theory and Practice.* Philadelphia: FA Davis, 1991, pp 3–26.

Fiorentino MR. *Normal and Abnormal Development: The Influence of Primitive Reflexes on Motor Development.* Springfield, IL: Charles C Thomas, 1972.

Flatt A. The absent thumb. In Flatt A (ed). *The Care of Congenital Hand Anomalies.* St. Louis: CV Mosby, 1977.

Fleishman E, Fruchter B. Factor structure and predictability of successive stage of learning Morse code. *J Appl Psychol* 44:97–101, 1960.

Frostig M. *Frostig Developmental Test of Visual Perception.* Palo Alto, CA: Consulting Psychologists Press, 1964.

Georgopoulos AP. On reaching. *Annu Rev Neurosci* 9:147–170, 1986.

Gesell AL, Amatruda CS. *Developmental Diagnosis: Normal and Abnormal Child Development, Clinical Methods and Pediatric Applications,* 2nd ed. New York: Paul Hoeber, 1947.

Goldstein M. Hands. *JAMA* 269:1240, 1993.

Halverson HM. An experimental study of prehension in infants by means of systematic cinema recording. *Genet Psychol Monogr* 19:107–285, 1931.

Halverson HM. A further study of grasping. *J Gen Psychol* 7:34–64, 1932.

Hatwell Y. Spatial perception by eyes and hand: Comparison and intermodal integration. In Bard C, Fleury M, Hay L (eds). *Development of Eye-Hand Coordination Throughout the Life Span.* Columbia, SC: University of South Carolina Press, 1990, pp 99–132.

Hirschel A, Pehoski C, Coryell J. Environmental support and the development of grasp in infants. *Am J Occup Ther* 44(8):721–727, 1990.

Hohlstein RR. The development of prehension in normal infants. *Am J Occup Ther* 36(3):170–175, 1982.

Illingworth RS. *The Development of the Infant and Young Child: Normal and Abnormal,* 9th ed. New York: Churchill Livingstone, 1987.

Jaffe L. "Influence of grip on legibility, speed, and fatigue in adult handwriting." PhD Thesis, Boston University. In Bergmann KP. Incidence of atypical pencil grasps among nondysfunctional adults. *Am J Occup Ther* 44(8):736, 1990.

Kapandji IA. *The Physiology of the Joints, vol. 1: Upper Limb,* 5th ed. New York: Churchill Livingstone, 1982, pp 162, 248–271.

Kline D, Schieber F, Coyne A. Aging, the eye and visual channels: Contrast sensitivity and response speed. *J Gerontol* 33:211–216, 1983.

Knobloch H, Stevens F, Malone AF. *Manual of Developmental Diagnosis: The Administration and Interpretation of the Revised Gesell and Amatruda's Developmental and Neurological Exam.* Houston: Developmental Evaluation Materials, 1987, pp 24–260.

Korczyn AD, Sage JI, Karplus M. Lack of limb motor asymmetry in the neonate. *J Neurobiol* 9:483–488, 1978.

Landsmeer JMF. Power grip and precision handling. *Ann Rheum Dis* 21:164–169, 1962.

Leatherwood D, Skirven T. "Dominance of the long finger." Paper presented at The American Society of Hand Therapists 10th Annual Meeting, San Antonio, TX, 1987.

Lehmkuhl LD, Smith LK. *Brunnstrom's Clinical Kinesiology.* Philadelphia: FA Davis, 1983, pp 85–88, 121–136, 147–258.

Levine KJ. *Fine Motor Dysfunction: Therapeutic Strategies in the Classroom.* Tucson: Therapy Skill Builders, 1991, pp 333–379, 505.

Levine MD. *Developmental Variation and Learning Disorders.* Toronto: Educators Publishing Service, 1987, pp 68–136, 208–345, 472.

Levine M, Oberlaid F, Meltzer L. Developmental output failure: A study of low productivity in school-aged children. *Pediatrics* 67:18–25, 1981.

Long C, Conrad PW, Hall EA, Furler SL. Intrinsic-extrinsic muscle control of the hand in power grip and precision handling. *J Bone Joint Surg [Am]* 52(5):853–867, 1970.

Lyons BG. Defining a child's zone of proximal development: Evaluation process for treatment planning. *Am J Occup Ther* 38(7):446–451, 1984.

Markison RE. Treatment of musical hands: Redesign the interface in hand injuries. *Sports Performing Arts Hand Clin* 6(3):525–544, August, 1990.

Mathiowetz V, Wiemer DM, Federman SM. Grip and pinch strength norms for 6 to 19 year olds. *Am J Occup Ther* 40(10):705–711, 1986.

Mathiowetz V, Kashman N, Volland G, Weber K, Dowe M, Rogers S. Grip and pinch strength: Normative data for adults. *Arch Phys Med Rehabil* 66:16–21, 1985.

McBryde C, Zivani J. Proximal and distal upper limb motor development in 24 week old infants. *Can J Occup Ther* 57(3):147–154, 1990.

McCullagh P, Weiss MR, Ross D. Modeling considerations in motor skill acquisition and performance: An integrated approach. In Randolph KB (ed). *Exercise and Sport Sciences Reviews, vol. 79.* Baltimore: Williams & Wilkins, 1989.

Meagher SW. Tool design for prevention of hand and wrist injuries. *J Hand Surg [Am]* 12(5):855–857, 1987.

Moberg E. The unsolved problem—How to test the functional value of hand sensibility. *J Hand Ther* 4(3):105–110, 1991.

Moore KL. *The Developing Human,* 4th ed. Philadelphia: WB Saunders, 1988, pp 70–110, 366–374.

Muniz RE, Dell PC. Rehabilitation following surgical reconstruction of the hypoplastic thumb. *J Hand Ther* 2(1):29–34, 1989.

Murray EA. Hemispheric specialization. In Fisher A, Murray EA, Bundy AC (eds). *Sensory Integration Theory and Practice.* Philadelphia: FA Davis, 1991.

Napier JR. Function of the hand. In Napier J (ed). *Hands.* New York: Pantheon Books, 1980, pp 68–83.

Napier JR. The prehensile movement of the human hand. *J Bone Joint Surg [Br]* 38:902–913, 1956.

Norkin CC, Levangie PK. *Joint Structure and Function: A Comprehensive Analysis.* Philadelphia: FA Davis, 1983, pp 157–253.

O'Driscoll SW, Horil E, Ness R, Richards RR. The relationship between wrist position, grasp size, and grip strength. *J Hand Surg [Am]* 17(10):169–177, 1992.

Paillard J. Basic neurophysiological structures of eye-hand coordination. In Bard C, Fleury M, Hay L (eds). *Development of Eye-Hand Coordination Across the Life Span.* Columbia, SC: University of South Carolina Press, 1990, pp 26–74.

Peterson P, Petrick M, Connor H, Conklin D. Grip strength and hand dominance: Challenging the 10% rule. *Am J Occup Ther* 43(7):444–447, 1989.

Pickleman J, Schueneman AL. The use and abuse of neuropsychological tests to predict operative performance. *Am Coll Surg Bull* 72(2):7–10, 1987.

Proske U, Schaible HG, Schmidt RF. Joint receptors and kinaesthesia. *Exp Brain Res* 72:219–224, 1988.

Provins K. The effect of training and handedness on the performance of two simple motor tasks. *J Exp Psychol* 10:29–39, 1958.

Ramsey RW, Street SF. Isometric length-tension diagram of isolated skeletal muscle fibers of frog. *J Cell Comp Physiol* 15:11, 1940. In Lehmkuhl LD, Smith LK. *Brunnstrom's Clinical Kinesiology,* 4th ed. Philadelphia: FA Davis, 1983, pp 130–132.

Riordan DC. Functional anatomy of the hand and forearm. *Orthop Clin North Am* 5(2):199–203, 1974.

Rosenbloom L, Horton ME. The maturation of fine prehension in young children. *Dev Med Child Neurol* 13:3–8, 1971.

Royeen CB, Lane SJ. Tactile processing and sensory defensiveness. In Fisher AG, Murray EA, Bundy AC (eds). *Sensory Integration: Theory and Practice.* Philadelphia: FA Davis, 1991, pp 108–131.

Salthouse T, Somberg B. Skilled performance: Effects of adult age and experience on elementary processes. *J Exp Psychol* 111(2):176–207, 1982.

Schmidt RF. Somatovisceral sensibility. In Schmidt RF (ed). *Fundamentals of Sensory Physiology,* 2nd ed. New York: Springer-Verlag, 1981, pp 81–101.

Schneck CM. Comparison of pencil-grip patterns in first graders with good and poor writing skills. *Am J Occup Ther* 45(8):701–706, 1991.

Schneck CM, Henderson A. Descriptive analysis of the developmental progression of grip position for pencil and crayon control in nondysfunctional children. *Am J Occup Ther* 44:893–900, 1990.

Sekuler R, Hutman C. Human aging and spatial vision. *Science* 209:1255–1256, 1980.

Shiffman LM. Effects of aging on adult hand function. *Am J Occup Ther* 46(9):785–792, 1992.

Starkes JL. Eye-hand coordination in experts: From athletes to microsurgeons. In Bard C, Fleury M, Hays L (eds). *Development of Eye-Hand Coordination Across the Life Span.* Columbia, SC: University of South Carolina Press, 1990, pp 312–323.

Stockmeyer SA. An interpretation of the approach of Rood to the treatment of neurological dysfunction. *Am J Phys Med* 46:900–956, 1967.

Tubiana R. Architecture and functions of the hand. In Tubiana R, Thomine JM, Mackin EJ (eds). *Examination of the Hand and Upper Limb.* Philadelphia: WB Saunders, 1984, pp 1–98.

Twitchell TE. Reflex mechanisms and the development of prehension. In Connelly K (ed). *Mechanisms of Motor Skill Development.* London: Academic Press, 1970, pp 25–59.

von Hofsten C, Ronnqvist L. Preparation for grasping an object: A developmental study. *J Exp Psychol Hum Percept Perform* 14(4):610–621, 1988.

Vygotsky LS. *Mind in Society: The Development of Higher Psychological Processes.* Cambridge, MA: Harvard University Press, 1978.

Williams HG. Aging and eye-hand coordination. In Bard C, Fleury M, Hay L (eds). *Development of Eye-Hand Coordination Across the Life Span.* Columbia, SC: University of South Carolina Press, 1990, pp 327–357.

Williams H, Keith J, Richter D, Clancy M, Carter J. "Aging, CNS processes and movement planning." Paper Presented at North American Society of the Psychology of Sport and Physical Activity, University of British Columbia, 1987. In Bard C, Fleury M, Hay L (eds). *Development of Eye-Hand Coordination Across the Life Span.* Columbia, SC: University of South Carolina Press, 1990, pp 343–345.

Williams WN, Hanson CS, Crary MA, Wharton PW. Human pinch-force discrimination. *Percept Motor Skills* 73:663–672, 1991.

Zernicke RF, Schneider K. Biomechanics and developmental neuromotor control in child development. In Thelen E, Lockman J (eds). *Developmental Biodynamics: Brain, Body, and Behavior Connections.* Calgary, Alberta, Canada: University of Calgary, 1992.

SUGGESTED READINGS

Ager CL, Olivett BL, Johnson CL. Grasp and pinch strength in children 5 to 12 years old. *Am J Occup Ther* 38(2):107–113, 1984.

Atkins D, Meier R (eds). *Comprehensive Management of the Upper Limb Amputee.* New York: Springer-Verlag, 1989.

Beasley RW. Amputations and prosthetic considerations. In *Hand Injuries.* Philadelphia: WB Saunders, 1981.

Bower TGR. *The Perceptual World of the Child.* Cambridge, MA: Harvard University Press, 1977.

Brand PW, Hollister A. *Clinical Mechanics of the Hand,* 2nd ed. St. Louis: CV Mosby, 1993.

Bruner JS. The growth and structure of skill. In Connelly K (ed). *Mechanisms of Motor Skill Development.* London: Academic Press, 1970, pp 63–91.

Casanova JS (ed). *Clinical Assessment Recommendations,* 2nd ed. Chicago, IL: American Society of Hand Therapists, 1992.

Clancy H, Clark MJ. *Occupational Therapy with Children.* New York: Churchill Livingstone, 1990, pp 21, 261–300.

Galley PM, Forster AL. *The Function of the Upper Extremity with Special Reference to the Hand in Human Movement: An Introductory Text for Physiotherapy Students,* 2nd ed. New York: Churchill Livingstone, 1987, pp 211–226.

Kamm K, Thelen E, Jensen JL. A dynamic systems approach to motor development. *Phys Ther* 70(12):763–775, 1990.

Kopp CB. Fine motor abilities of infants. *Dev Med Child Neurol* 16:629–636, 1974.

Levine MD. *Developmental Variations and Learning Disorders.* Toronto: Educators Publishing Service, 1987.

Schmidt RA. *Motor Control and Learning: A Behavioral Emphasis,* 2nd ed. Champaign, IL: Human Kinetics, 1988.

Schneck CM. Joint position changes in the dynamic tripod grip in children aged three to seven years. *Phys Occup Ther Pediatr* 10(4):85–103, 1990.

ACKNOWLEDGMENTS

I would like to thank the following individuals for reviewing the content of this chapter: Lisa Kurtz, MEd, OTR/L; Wendy Davis, MEd, OTR/L; and Ruth Levine, EdD, OTR/L.

Chapter 15

Health and Fitness

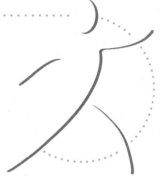

Objectives

AFTER STUDYING THIS CHAPTER, THE READER WILL BE ABLE TO:

1 Discuss the relationships among health, fitness, and physical activity.
2 Understand the integrated role of all body systems in the development and maintenance of fitness.
3 Identify the effects of exercise and training on the body systems.
4 Appreciate age-related considerations in developing exercise and training programs.

The preceding chapters of this book discuss the role of different body systems in functional physical activity. The ability to function at one's best in all activities throughout the life span is a goal shared by everyone. What is "functioning at one's best"? Is it health? What role does fitness play? More importantly, how can one be proactive and ensure an optimal level of functioning throughout the life span? This chapter discusses these issues and encourages readers to incorporate concepts of health and fitness into their own life plans. As health care providers, we are uniquely qualified to assist clients in reaching the goal of lifelong fitness.

HEALTH AND FITNESS

Health

General definitions of health describe a state of physical, mental, and social well-being (McArdle et al, 1991). These definitions discuss freedom from defect, pain, and disease, while emphasizing that health is not merely the absence of these entities. In reality, health is a condition of the human body and mind. As a condition, health is represented on a continuum from good health to poor health.

Bouchard and colleagues (1990) define health as a human condition with physical, social, and psychologic dimensions on a continuum with positive and

355

negative poles. Positive health reflects the ability to enjoy life and withstand challenges, not merely the absence of disease. It has also been referred to as the highest level of functional capability (McArdle et al, 1991). Negative health reflects morbidity and ultimately mortality. Currently the term *wellness,* which comprises biologic and psychologic well-being, is also used to denote a state of positive health (Bouchard et al, 1990). This term reflects a holistic concept of health.

Fitness

There is no universally accepted definition of fitness (O'Toole & Douglas, 1988). Some general definitions describe fitness as a state of optimal well-being and the capacity to successfully meet the present and potential physical challenges of life. To be fit is to be adapted, adjusted, qualified, or suited to some purpose, function, or aim. "Fit" also describes a person in good physical condition, or "healthy." Physical fitness allows one to carry out daily tasks with vigor and alertness, without undue fatigue, and with ample energy to enjoy leisure and to meet unusual circumstances and unforeseen emergencies (Biegel, 1984).

More specifically, from an exercise perspective, physical fitness is related to a person's ability to perform physical activity (McArdle et al, 1991). The World Health Organization defines physical fitness as the ability to perform muscular work satisfactorily. Cardiovascular and respiratory endurance, muscular strength, and flexibility contribute to fitness. Physical fitness is determined by habitual activity level, diet, and heredity (Bouchard et al, 1990). Therefore, fitness is determined by one's physical work capacity and varies with activity level (O'Toole & Douglas, 1988). Exercise scientists differentiate physical from physiologic fitness. *Physiologic fitness* is the fitness of the biologic systems and also is influenced by physical activity. Blood pressure, glucose tolerance, blood lipid level, and body composition are markers of physiologic fitness (Bouchard et al, 1990).

COMPONENTS

The components of fitness are cardiovascular and respiratory endurance, muscular strength and endurance, flexibility, and body composition. They contribute to one's agility, power, balance, coordination, and speed during physical activity.

Cardiovascular and respiratory endurance reflects the ability of the heart, vasculature, and lungs to provide oxygen to working muscle during physical activity (Payne & Isaacs, 1972). *Muscular strength* is the force that can be generated in a muscle, whereas *muscular endurance* reflects the ability of the muscle to complete many repetitions of muscle contraction before fatiguing. *Flexibility,* the ability to move without restriction, depends on adequate muscle length and appropriate mobility within the joints of the body. Good flexibility improves efficiency of movement and decreases the potential for injury. *Body*

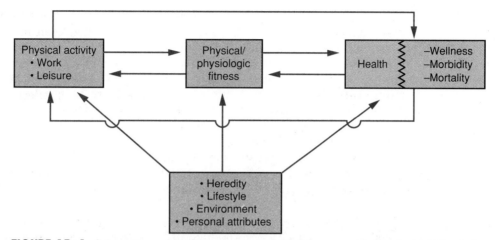

FIGURE 15–1. Schematic model of the complex relationships among habitual physical activity, fitness, and health. (Redrawn from Bouchard C, Shepard RJ, Stephens T, Sutton JR, McPherson BD. *Exercise, Fitness and Health: A Consensus of Current Knowledge.* Champaign, IL: Human Kinetics. Copyright © 1990 by Human Kinetics Publishers, Inc. Reprinted by permission.)

composition refers to the amount of lean body mass and fat mass. Lean body mass includes muscle, bone, other nonfat substances (e.g., water, minerals), and a small amount of fat stored in the nervous system and bone marrow (McArdle et al, 1991). Because, in most physical activity, one must support and carry the body weight, it is preferred that active lean body mass be greater than nonactive fat mass (O'Toole & Douglas, 1988).

Factors Influencing Health and Fitness

Individual factors such as heredity, age, sex, physical activity, lifestyle, and environment contribute to one's level of physical and physiologic fitness. A model of the interactions among exercise, health, and fitness, as developed by Bouchard and colleagues (1990), is shown in Figure 15–1. Personal attributes as defined for this diagram are age, sex, socioeconomic status, personality, and motivation.

PHYSICAL FACTORS

Age, growth, and gender can influence fitness. The ability to perform physical activities with physiologic efficiency improves through childhood, adolescence, and young adulthood, but then declines. Some of this decline may be related to physical changes, but social and environmental factors also are influential. Recent studies indicate that the functional "losses" in physical fitness may be due not to aging but to decreased activity level. An active lifestyle appears to minimize physical changes within the various body systems (Frontera &

Evans, 1986; McArdle et al, 1991). Physiologic improvements through training occur at a similar rate and magnitude in all individuals, regardless of age (McArdle et al, 1991).

Growth leads to changes in height and weight. The developmental pattern of aerobic capacity, muscular strength and endurance, and power is similar to that of growth (Malina, 1990). Increase in stature gradually slows and ceases after adolescence, whereas weight increases into the middle twenties (Malina, 1990). After age 35, body weight continues to slowly increase, reflecting an increase in body fat. After age 60, the percentage of lean body mass decreases further because of age-related decreases in muscle and bone mass (McArdle et al, 1991). McArdle and colleagues (1991) discuss several studies in which physical activity appeared to minimize increases in fat mass of older individuals.

Before puberty, gender does not appear to significantly affect fitness. Maximal aerobic capacity per kilogram of body weight is the same in boys and girls. After puberty, maximal aerobic capacity is greater in men than in women. This change reflects the increased percentage of body fat, lower oxygen carrying capacity, and smaller muscle fiber area in women as compared to men (O'Toole & Douglas, 1988). Training responses in men and women are equivalent (Katch & Katch, 1988; O'Toole & Douglas, 1988).

HEREDITY

Heredity influences several factors that contribute to fitness, such as body size and muscle fiber composition. Whether someone is tall or short is determined by heredity. The percentage of slow-twitch muscle fibers and fast-twitch muscle fibers found in skeletal muscle also is determined genetically (Faulkner & White, 1990; McArdle et al, 1991). Twin studies have shown genetics to be a factor in determining maximal aerobic capacity and heart rate (Cunningham et al, 1984). Inherited factors may influence an individual's selection of physical activities (e.g., choosing to be a sprinter rather than a marathon runner). They may also impose limits on the possible level of fitness one may achieve.

ENVIRONMENTAL FACTORS

Environmental factors such as climate, oxygen pressure, and air quality can affect exercise performance. Extreme hot or cold climates stress the exercising individual trying to maintain internal body temperature. People who live and exercise in regions of high altitude must adjust to low oxygen pressures. Indoor air contaminants such as cigarette smoke, radon, and wood smoke may diminish air quality. Environmental air quality is compromised by byproducts of industry and engine exhaust. Specific pollutants such as ozone and sulfur dioxide affect lung function (Folinsbee, 1990).

SOCIAL FACTORS

Social factors play a role in determining an individual's involvement in physical activity and fitness. Toddlers and preschoolers are very active. Their "job" is to learn new skills and explore their environment through movement. Parents may influence this level of activity by guiding the child's choice of movement experiences. By school age, children become more competitive, and achieving an adequate level of skill is important for the child's social acceptance. Children who function well motorically are encouraged to continue with physical activities, while children who are less skilled may become frustrated and less active. Successful motor performance is a positive reinforcer. In adolescence, societal modeling and peer pressure often discourage vigorous physical activity for girls (Porter, 1989). Physical activity decreases for both boys and girls in late adolescence. This reduction may be influenced by social models and the need to enter the work force (Malina, 1990). Adults report that job and family demands frequently do not allow time for exercise programs (Buskirk, 1990). Other lifestyle changes, such as smoking, alcohol consumption, and use of contraceptives, may affect fitness in adolescence and adulthood (Malina, 1990).

Society is beginning to influence awareness of and participation in fitness programs. With increased public awareness of the benefits of fitness, fitness centers and aerobic exercise programs have become more available in the United States. Fitness has become an industry. Corporations also provide fitness programs for their employees, seeking to improve health and productivity.

How Fit Are We?

Fitness has been associated with increased health and well-being. Improved quality of life and preventive health maintenance are valuable benefits of fitness. In recognition of these benefits, the U.S. Department of Health and Human Services included physical fitness and exercise objectives in their Year 2000 objectives for the nation (Public Health Service, 1990). These fitness and exercise objectives strive to increase public awareness of appropriate levels of exercise, promote cardiovascular fitness, and increase participation in physical activity programs (Table 15–1).

Public awareness of the importance of fitness may be increasing, but surveys conducted in the 1980s found only a small percentage of Americans participating in sufficient physical activity to maintain health and fitness (Brooks, 1987; Caspersen et al, 1986). Buskirk (1990) reviewed several studies of regular participation in physical activity by adults in the United States and found some evidence that it had increased slightly in recent years. Most studies reflect that only 10 to 20 per cent of adults in the United States exercise regularly and vigorously enough to benefit health and fitness.

A progressive and predictable decline in participation with age has been

Table 15-1. OBJECTIVES TO INCREASE PHYSICAL ACTIVITY AND FITNESS: YEAR 2000 OBJECTIVES FOR THE NATION

BY THE YEAR 2000 . . .

RISK REDUCTION

1. Increase to at least 60 per cent the proportion of people age 6 and older who participate in moderate physical activities 3 or more days per week for 20 or more minutes per occasion (baseline: 50 per cent in 1985).
2. Increase to at least 30 per cent the proportion of people age 6 and older who participate in vigorous physical activities that promote the development and maintenance of cardiorespiratory fitness 3 or more days per week for 20 or more minutes per occasion (baseline: 25 per cent in 1985).
3. Increase to at least 50 per cent the proportion of people age 6 and older who regularly perform physical activities that maintain muscular strength, muscular endurance, and flexibility (baseline data not available).
4. Reduce overweight among people ages 20 through 74 to a prevalence of no more than 20 per cent (baseline: 25.7 per cent in 1976–1980, 24.2 per cent for men and 27.1 per cent for women).
5. Reduce overweight among adolescents ages 12 through 17 to a prevalence of less than 15 per cent (baseline: 15 per cent in 1976–1980).
6. Increase to 75 per cent the proportion of overweight people age 12 and older who have adopted sound dietary practices combined with physical activity to achieve weight reduction (baseline: 25 per cent of overweight men and 30 per cent of overweight women for people age 18 and older in 1985).

PUBLIC AWARENESS

7. Increase to at least 80 per cent the proportion of people age 6 and older who know that regular exercise reduces the risk of heart disease, helps maintain appropriate body weight, reduces the symptoms of depression and anxiety, and enhances self--esteem (baseline data unavailable).
8. Increase to at least 40 per cent the proportion of people age 6 and older who know that cardiorespiratory fitness, muscular strength, muscular endurance, flexibility, and body composition (percentage of body fat) are important to health (baseline data unavailable).
9. Increase to at least 25 per cent the proportion of people age 6 and older who can identify correctly the frequency and duration of exercise thought to most effectively promote cardiorespiratory fitness (baseline: 10 per cent in 1985).

reported (Brooks, 1987; Buskirk, 1990; Caspersen et al, 1986; Katch & Katch, 1988; McArdle et al, 1991). A 1985 National Health Interview Survey showed that only 7 percent of adults over the age of 65 participate in regular physical activity. Regular physical activity by adults also has been reported to decrease as education and income levels decrease (Caspersen et al, 1986).

Physical fitness of the nation's children is also a concern: 20 per cent of children fail one or more standards on fitness tests (Pate & Shepard, 1989). Malina (1988) reviewed studies of the activity level of adolescent girls and reported that they do not get enough regular exercise to maintain high aerobic fitness.

Table 15-1. *Continued*

PROFESSIONAL EDUCATION AND AWARENESS

10. Increase to at least 65 per cent the proportion of primary care providers who assess and counsel their patients regarding the frequency, duration, type, and intensity of each patient's physical activity practices as part of a thorough evaluation and treatment program (baseline: an estimated 47 per cent routinely "inquired" in 1985).

SERVICES AND PROTECTION

11. Increase to at least 45 per cent the proportion of children and adolescents in grades 1 through 12 who participate in daily school physical education programs (baseline: 36 per cent in 1984–1986).
12. Increase to at least 70 per cent the proportion of teachers who teach physical education who spend 30 per cent or more of class time on skills and activities that promote lifetime physical activity participation (baseline data unavailable).
13. Increase the proportion of worksites offering employer-sponsored fitness programs as follow:
    ● Worksites with 50–99 employees: 25 per cent (baseline 14 per cent in 1985).
    ● Worksites with 100–249 employees: 35 per cent (baseline 23 per cent in 1985).
    ● Worksites with 250–749 employees: 45 per cent (baseline 32 per cent in 1985).
    ● Worksites with 750 or more employees: 65 per cent (baseline: 54 per cent in 1985).
14. Increase to at least 40 per cent the proportion of people age 6 and older who participated in the physical activity program of at least one community organization within the past year (baseline data unavailable).
15. Increase community swimming pools; hiking, biking and fitness trail miles; and park and recreation open space to at least one pool per 25,000 people, one trail per 10,000 people, and 4 acres of developed open space per 1000 people, respectively (baseline: estimated at one pool per 53,000 people; one trail mile per 60,000 people; and 1.8 acres of developed open space per 1000 people in 1986).
16. Increase to at least 30 per cent the proportion of life insurers that offer lower individual premiums to people who exercise regularly and maintain a regular physically active lifestyle (baseline: one life insurance company offered lower premiums in 1988).

From U.S. Department of Health and Human Services. "Promoting health, preventing disease: Year 2000 objectives for the nation." Washington, DC: Public Health Services, NIH, 1990.

SYSTEMS INVOLVED IN FITNESS

Fitness results when several body systems—the cardiovascular, pulmonary, musculoskeletal, nervous, and endocrine systems—interact optimally and efficiently. In the course of development, changes in these systems affect the way in which the body delivers fuel and produces energy for movement. Levels of fitness and capacity for physical activity may vary throughout development as a result.

Exercise and training have been found to improve body system function and levels of fitness. *Exercise* is defined as leisure-time physical activity (Bouchard, 1991) that is planned, repetitive, and purposeful (McArdle, 1991). *Training* is regular and repeated exercise, carried out over several weeks or months, with the intention of developing physical and/or physiologic fitness

(Bouchard et al, 1990). *Trainability* reflects the ability of different body systems to adapt to repeated exercise stimuli (Bar-Or, 1988).

This section will determine

1. How each body system contributes to fitness and physical activity.
2. The effects of exercise and training on the systems.
3. The developmental changes that affect fitness.

Cardiovascular System

ROLE IN FITNESS

The role of the cardiovascular system is to deliver nutrients to the muscles and remove waste products. The structure, function, and development of this system are presented in Chapter 8. During exercise, the cardiovascular system must carry large amounts of oxygen to the muscle tissue and remove waste products associated with energy production.

The functional capacity of the heart is expressed as cardiac output (CO) and reflects the amount of blood pumped from the heart per minute. Cardiac output is affected by the heart rate, amount of cardiac filling, vascular resistance, heart muscle performance, and neurohormonal regulation (Wei, 1986). It is the product of the heart rate and the stroke volume ($CO = HR \times SV$). *Stroke volume* is the amount of blood pumped from the heart with each beat. The heart size, contractile force of the heart muscle, vascular resistance, and venous return determine the stroke volume (Payne & Isaacs, 1987).

EFFECTS OF EXERCISE AND TRAINING

Cardiovascular responses to exercise and training are summarized in Table 15–2.

Table 15-2. CARDIOVASCULAR ADAPTATION TO EXERCISE AND TRAINING	
Exercise	**Training**
↑ CO	↑ Heart weight
↑ HR	↑ Heart volume
↑ Blood flow to working muscles	↑ Plasma volume
↑ Systolic blood pressure	↑ Hemoglobin
↑ Cardiac contractility	↓ Resting heart rate
↓ Peripheral resistance	↑ Max. CO and SV
↑ Venous return	↑ a-vO$_2$ difference
	↓ Systolic and diastolic BP

Short-Term Adaptation. During aerobic exercise, skeletal muscle demand for oxygen increases, resulting in increased cardiac output. Heart rate increases in proportion to the intensity of the exercise for 3 to 5 minutes. A steady state is then attained and maintained for short periods of exercise. After 15 to 30 minutes, heart rate again begins to rise because of fatigue and increased body temperature. Vasodilation occurs, helping shunt blood flow away from the viscera to the working skeletal and heart muscles. Muscle contraction squeezes nearby veins, facilitating venous return. Systolic blood pressure increases in proportion to exercise intensity and theoretically is related to the increased cardiac output. Diastolic blood pressure increases only slightly. In general, dynamic, aerobic exercise results in increased cardiac contractility, decreased peripheral resistance, and increased venous return (Noble, 1986).

Long-Term Adaptation. Heart weight and volume, plasma volume, and hemoglobin levels increase with training (Green, 1990; McArdle et al, 1991; Zernicke et al, 1991). Ventricular filling, stroke volume, and cardiac output increase (Saltin, 1990). Therefore, more blood can be pumped per heart beat, and necessary circulation is delivered to body tissues at a lower heart rate. Increased blood volume improves removal of waste products and heat, dilution of hormones, and perfusion of the kidneys while decreasing resistance to capillary flow.

Resting heart rate decreases, an effect that appears to be related to decreased sympathetic input. Maximum heart rate remains relatively stable, whereas maximum cardiac output and stroke volume increase (Noble, 1986). Stroke volume increases because of greater end-diastolic volume of the left ventricle and more forceful contraction of strengthened cardiac muscle (McArdle et al, 1991; Noble, 1986).

Both systolic and diastolic blood pressure decrease with training (McArdle et al, 1991; Noble, 1986; Zernicke et al, 1991). Decreases in blood pressure may be related to reduced sympathetic input, which decreases peripheral resistance to blood flow (McArdle et al, 1991).

The trained individual is better able to extract oxygen from the blood, as reflected by the arterial to venous oxygen difference (a-vO_2 difference) (McArdle et al, 1991; Noble, 1986). The a-vO_2 difference compares the oxygen concentration of the arterial and venous blood, reflecting the amount of oxygen extracted from the capillaries at the tissue level. Increased capillarization and mitochondrial capacity are seen in working muscle, improving the muscle's ability to extract oxygen from the capillaries (Noble, 1986; Zernicke et al, 1991).

DEVELOPMENTAL CHANGES

Childhood. Body size and especially body height are predictive of cardiovascular system capacity in childhood (Cunningham et al, 1984). Heart rate changes with age, decreasing as body size increases. Because of the smaller size and functional ability of the cardiovascular system, the stroke volume of children is smaller than that of adults. It begins to increase significantly when the adolescent is undergoing maximal growth in height. The child's higher heart rate does not appear to totally compensate for decreased stroke volume, because the cardiac output of children is smaller than that of adults (Haywood, 1986; Payne & Isaacs, 1984).

Other differences in the cardiovascular system of children as compared to adults are seen. Children have less hemoglobin than adults and therefore less oxygen carrying capacity. The a-vO_2 difference is smaller in children than in adults, reflecting less efficiency in extracting oxygen from the blood. The a-vO_2 difference increases slightly with age, especially after puberty, and reaches adult levels by late adolescence. This change may be related to the growing child's increased muscle mass, changes in muscle enzyme perfusion, and changes in the ratio of capillary to muscle fiber (Cunningham et al, 1984).

Training effects, specifically improvements in maximal aerobic power, in prepubescent children have not been conclusively demonstrated. High levels of habitual activity, mechanical inefficiency in performing physical activity, and body size limitations affect the maximal aerobic capacity of children (Bar-Or, 1983). Hollman and colleagues (1988) report significant effects of endurance training on aerobic capacity and "athlete's heart" (increased heart volume, increased left ventricular wall diameter, increased end diastolic diameter) in prepubescent swimmers. Cunningham et al (1984) report that physical activity can help improve cardiorespiratory function in the year before peak height increases and thereafter. Other reviews of the effectiveness of training with adolescents report inconsistent results (Bailey & Mirwald, 1988; Malina, 1988).

Adulthood. Once adult levels of cardiovascular performance have been reached, some sex-related differences surface. The stroke volume of women is approximately 25 per cent less than that of men. Men have 15 to 16 g Hb/100 ml blood, whereas women have 14 g Hb/100 ml blood; this gives men a greater oxygen carrying capacity. Teenage and adult women have a 5 to 10 per cent higher cardiac output during submaximal exercise than men, possibly to compensate for their decreased oxygen carrying capacity (McArdle et al, 1991).

Older Adulthood. Structural changes are seen in the heart, valves, and vasculature with aging. Elastic tissue, fat, and collagen increase in the endocardium and myocardium of the heart, resulting in a stiffer, less compliant ventricle (Kitzman & Edwards, 1990; Peel, 1990). After the age of 60, the number of pacemaker cells in the sinoatrial node decreases. This may contribute to the increased incidence of electrocardiographic abnormalities in older adults (Peel, 1990). Valves thicken and calcify, affecting the closure and efficiency of the cardiac valves (Kitzman & Edwards, 1990; Peel, 1990). Blood vessels, especially proximal arteries, dilate with age. The vascular walls become thicker because of increased connective tissue and lipid deposition. Calcification and atrophy of the elastic fibers in the vasculature also are seen. These factors increase vascular stiffness and reduce vascular compliance (Peel, 1990; Wei, 1986).

Functional changes also are seen with aging in the cardiovascular system, but most are not apparent at rest. Minimal or no change occurs in resting heart rate (Shepard, 1987; Wei, 1986). Resting systolic and diastolic blood pressures increase secondary to increased stiffness of the vascular system and decreased size of the peripheral vascular bed. These blood pressure changes are not seen in all populations and so may not be a natural effect of aging (Peel, 1990). Blood pressure increases also are seen in older adults during submaximal and maximal exercise and are due to decreased arterial compliance (Noble, 1986).

Oxygen consumption and heart rate changes with submaximal exercise in older adults are similar to those seen in young adults. During maximal exercise, the older adult's cardiac output, cardiac contractility, and a-vO$_2$ difference are decreased. Diminished cardiac compliance, valvular thickening, higher vascular resistance, poor myocardial perfusion, and poor contractility contribute to reduced stroke volume. Decreased pacemaker activity and sensitivity to catecholamines may contribute to decreased peak heart rate (Peel, 1990). Lower arterial oxygen saturation, less hemoglobin, and poor peripheral vascular distribution may decrease maximal a-vO$_2$ difference (Shepard, 1987; Wei, 1986).

Pulmonary System

ROLE IN FITNESS

The pulmonary system allows oxygenated air to be taken in from the environment and delivered to the tissues. It also removes carbon dioxide waste products from the body. During exercise, greater airflow is required to meet the demands of the body. This is accomplished by taking deeper breaths and increasing the respiratory rate.

EFFECTS OF EXERCISE AND TRAINING

Adaptations of the pulmonary system to exercise and training are summarized in Table 15–3.

Table 15-3. PULMONARY ADAPTATION TO EXERCISE AND TRAINING	
Exercise	**Training**
↑ Minute ventilation	↑ Vital capacity
↑ Tidal volume	↑ Tidal volume
↑ Breathing frequency	↓ Respiratory rate at submaximal exercise
↓ Inspiratory/expiratory reserve	

Short-Term Adaptation. At the onset of exercise, ventilation increases rapidly and reaches a steady state within 3 to 4 minutes (Noble, 1986). The amount of air exchanged with the atmosphere per minute (minute ventilation) is increased as more air is moved in each breath (tidal volume) and as breathing frequency increases. At low-intensity exercise, changes in tidal volume are sufficient to maintain adequate minute ventilation. Greater tidal volume allows inspired air to perfuse more lung tissue, opening more alveoli and maximizing the ability for gas exchange between the capillaries and the alveoli (Shepard, 1987). As exercise intensity becomes greater and tidal volume is 50 to 60 per cent of vital capacity, breathing rate increases (Frontera & Evans, 1986).

Breathing rate at rest is approximately 14 breaths per minute. During exercise, the respiratory rate may rise up to 40 breaths per minute. Even at these higher rates, there is enough time for alveolar gas exchange to occur because alveolar ventilation increases more than pulmonary capillary blood flow. This process works until fatigue or cardiac function limit the exercise (Noble, 1986).

In light to moderate exercise, ventilation increases linearly with levels of oxygen consumption and carbon dioxide production. At higher exercise levels, ventilation increases in relation to increased carbon dioxide concentrations produced by anaerobic metabolism. For example, blood lactate levels increase during anaerobic metabolism and must be buffered to prevent acidosis. The end product of this buffering is carbon dioxide. As the carbon dioxide levels in the blood increase, chemoreceptors in the aortic and carotid bodies, as well as in the medulla, cue the system to increase ventilation (McArdle et al, 1991; Noble, 1986).

Long-Term Adaptation. With training, the efficiency of the ventilatory system increases in adolescents, young adults, and older adults (McArdle et al, 1991). Conclusive studies of the effects of training on children have not been done (Mahon & Vaccaro, 1989).

Following training, resting lung volumes show little change. Slight increases in vital capacity may occur as respiratory muscle strength is improved (Shepard, 1987). During submaximal exercise, respiratory rate decreases and tidal volume increases. Air stays in the lungs longer, allowing more oxygen to be extracted (McArdle et al, 1991; Shepard, 1987). The amount of air that must be breathed in to deliver adequate oxygen to the tissues is decreased, requiring less work by the respiratory system. Studies of endurance athletes have demonstrated increased vital capacity and increased total lung capacity (Nobel, 1986).

DEVELOPMENTAL CHANGES

Childhood. As with other systems, the growth of the lungs parallels the general growth of the child. Under 10 years of age, children have not yet developed the number of alveoli they will have as adults (Tecklin, 1989). Their airways are small in diameter, resulting in higher resistance to airflow and increased work of breathing. Because children demonstrate poorer ventilatory efficiency than adults in both submaximal and maximal exercise, they must maintain a higher breathing frequency when performing similar tasks (Porter, 1989).

Older Adulthood. Structural changes in older adults affect the compliance and elastic recoil of the pulmonary system, making it harder for respiratory muscles to move air into the system. Some of these changes are increased stiffness of the chest wall, thoracic ankylosis and kyphosis, increased anterior-posterior diameter of the thorax, increased rigidity of the bronchioles, thickening of the mucous layer of the lungs, and structural changes of the elastic fibers of the lungs. As a result, residual volume increases, because more air is retained in the lungs. Inspiratory reserve, expiratory reserve, and vital capacity decrease in both resting and dynamic states.

The surface area available for gas exchange also is decreased because of changes within the alveoli and a decrease in the number of pulmonary capillaries (Irwin & Zadai, 1990; Peel, 1990; Shepard, 1987). Ventilatory responses to increased CO_2 or decreased O_2 levels in the blood also decrease with age, possibly because of receptor, neuronal, or muscular changes (Peel, 1990).

Older adults require increased ventilation during activity compared to young adults, but they may not be able to breathe fast enough. For this reason, the pulmonary system, rather than the cardiovascular system, of older adults often limits the amount of exercise performed (Peel, 1990; Shepard, 1987). Some evidence shows that training can counter the changes in lung function attributed to age (McArdle et al, 1991).

Musculoskeletal System

ROLE IN FITNESS

The muscular and skeletal systems are the mechanical basis for human movement. Muscle cells also contain energy stores necessary for movement. Oxygen provided during respiration activates metabolic pathways that convert carbohydrates, fats, and proteins into stored energy sources in muscle.

At the onset of exercise, energy is produced anaerobically as the high-energy phosphate bonds of adenosine triphosphate (ATP) and creatinine phosphate (CP) stored within the muscle are broken. Only small amounts of these substances are stored; this source of energy can be used only for short periods. ATP stores in muscle can be replenished through anaerobic and aerobic pathways utilizing carbohydrates, fats, and proteins. In light to moderate exercise, oxidative pathways can successfully meet the energy demands. In more strenuous exercise, carbohydrate stores in the form of glycogen can be broken down anaerobically to release energy. Lactic acid is formed as an end product and is transferred from muscle to the blood. As blood levels of lactic acid increase, fatigue results. This may be due to the increased acidity produced as attempts are made to buffer the lactic acid. Anaerobic threshold is reached when the lactate buildup limits continued activity (McArdle et al, 1991).

Table 15-4. MUSCULOSKELETAL ADAPTATION TO EXERCISE AND TRAINING	
Exercise	**Training**
↑ Blood flow to working muscle	↑ Bone density
	↑ Strength, flexibility, and thickness of ligaments
	↑ Thickness of articular cartilage
	↑ Muscle strength
	↑ Oxidative capacity: onset of blood lactate accumulation at higher max VO$_2$

Skeletal muscle is made up of two main types of muscle fibers. Slow-twitch muscle fibers, also called type I muscle fibers, work during long-term endurance activity. They have many mitochondria and high myoglobin levels, which enable them to utilize oxygen. They also are rich in capillaries, making oxygen readily available. Fast-twitch muscle fibers, also called type II muscle fibers, work during short-burst, maximal strength actions. They utilize anaerobic glycogen metabolism to produce energy. There are two groups of fast twitch muscles: type IIa, which can work aerobically or anaerobically, and type IIb, which operate only anaerobically. It is unclear whether one fiber type can be converted to another with training. It appears that some type IIb fibers can switch to type IIa fibers, improving oxidative capacity, but conversion of type II to type I fibers has not been demonstrated (Faulkner & White, 1990; McArdle et al, 1991; Shepard, 1987; Zernicke et al, 1991). McArdle and colleagues (1991) reviewed studies that appear to show a conversion of type I to type II fibers. This is definitely an area of current and future research.

EFFECTS OF EXERCISE AND TRAINING

Adaptations of the musculoskeletal system to exercise and training are summarized in Table 15-4.

Short-Term Adaptation. At the onset of exercise, blood flow to exercising muscle increases. Increased blood flow delivers more oxygen to the muscle and helps to dissipate heat, which results from the muscle work. With exercise at less than 60 to 70 per cent of maximum aerobic power, first type I and then type IIa muscle fibers are recruited.

Long-Term Adaptation. Training affects all components of the musculoskeletal system. Exercise increases the bone density and strengthens the bone architecture. Ligaments become stronger, thicker, and more flexible. Articular cartilage also becomes thicker and more resistant to compression (Shepard, 1987). Muscle tissue undergoes significant change, which varies with the type of exercise performed.

Resistance training increases muscle strength via hypertrophy of muscle fibers and/or neural recruitment of motor units. Children and older adults increase strength primarily via increased neural recruitment. In older adults, increases in strength also have been related to reversal of fast-twitch fiber atrophy (Knortz, 1987). Muscle hypertrophy is seen in adults when high levels of resistance are used. Anaerobic metabolic pathways are used primarily, resulting in increased anaerobic enzyme levels in type II muscle fibers.

With endurance training, oxidative capacity of the muscle is maximized. Levels of enzymes used by oxidative metabolic pathways increase, especially in oxidative type I and type IIa muscle fibers. The size and number of mitochondria increase with training (Knortz, 1987; Zernicke et al, 1991), as does capillarization (Green, 1990; Noble, 1986; Shepard, 1987) and myoglobin content (Zernicke et al, 1991).

Anaerobic threshold increases during submaximal exercise as a result of increased mechanical efficiency and muscle strengthening (Shepard, 1987). Blood lactate accumulation begins at 55 to 65 per cent of maximal oxygen uptake in the untrained individual, and at approximately 80 per cent of maximal oxygen uptake in the trained individual (McArdle et al, 1991).

DEVELOPMENTAL CHANGES

Childhood. The potential for aerobic and anaerobic muscle metabolism is smaller in children as compared to adults. Aerobic capacity is related to the available muscle mass and increases with growth. Children have smaller muscles and therefore less aerobic capacity. Anaerobic capacity is also limited in children becasue of lower glycogen concentration, rate of glycogen utilization, lactic acid concentration, level of enzymes necessary to break down glycogen, and tolerance of acidosis. Anaerobic capacity improves in adolescence and appears to be related to sexual maturity (Bailey & Mirwald, 1988; Bar-Or, 1984).

Older Adulthood. Muscle changes with aging are reported. Decreases in strength, which appear to be related to decreased muscle mass, are reported after the age of 30. Muscle fibers are lost through denervation and selective atrophy of type II muscle fibers. Type I fibers are used in activities of daily living and remain stable (Knortz, 1987). It is difficult to determine whether these changes are due to inactivity or to aging (McArdle et al, 1991). Increases in strength with training have been demonstrated regardless of age.

Endocrine System

The endocrine system is composed of several glands and organs that secrete hormones. These hormones help integrate and control all body functions. They regulate growth, development, reproduction, and the ability to deal with physical and psychologic stress. Hormones also adjust electrolyte levels and acid/base balance within the body. Hormonal levels are determined by stimulation

Table 15-5. HORMONAL ACTIVITY RELATED TO PHYSICAL ACTIVITY

Hormone	Secreted by	During Exercise
Growth hormone	Anterior pituitary gland	↓ Carbohydrate utilization ↑ Fat utilization
ACTH	Anterior pituitary gland	↑ Fat utilization; ↑ Protein utilization; stimulates secretion of cortisol
ADH	Posterior pituitary gland	↑ Water retention
Norepinephrine/ epinephrine	Adrenal medulla	Affects cardiac contractability and distribution of blood in vascular system; Fat⟶fatty acid, glycogen⟶glucose
Cortisol	Adrenal cortex	Protein⟶glucose; fatty acid⟶glucose
Insulin	Pancreas	↓ Secretion during exercise; inhibits epinephrine and glucagon
Glucagon	Pancreas	↑ Secretion during exercise; forms glucose from liver, glycogen, and amino acids; breaks down fat

from other hormones, blood levels of ions or nutrients, and neural input (McArdle et al, 1991).

ROLE IN FITNESS

The endocrine system allows the body to adapt to vigorous physical activity and ensures that fuel is delivered to working muscles (Shepard, 1987). Several endocrine organs are activated during exercise. The hormones they secrete play a role in utilization of carbohydrates and fatty acids, maintenance of fluid volume, contractility of the heart, and distribution of blood within the vascular system. The hormonal activity related to increased physical activity is summarized in Table 15–5.

GROWTH HORMONE

Growth hormone is secreted by the anterior pituitary gland. It decreases the use of carbohydrates and increases the use of fat metabolism for energy production. By maintaining glucose levels, growth hormone increases endurance. Growth hormone also promotes protein synthesis, cartilage formation, and skeletal growth. Intensity and duration of exercise affect the secretion of growth hormone. The mechanism for control of growth hormone secretion during exercise is not known, but it is probably related to neural mechanisms (McArdle et al, 1991).

CORTICOTROPIN (ACTH)

ACTH also is secreted by the anterior pituitary gland. It improves the mobilization of fat as an energy source, increases the rate of glucose formation, and stimulates the breakdown of proteins. ACTH also controls the secretion of hormones from the adrenal cortex, including cortisol, which is important during intense exercise (McArdle et al, 1991).

ANTIDIURETIC HORMONE (ADH)

The secretion of ADH is controlled by the posterior pituitary gland. During exercise, this gland increases water retention by the kidneys, maintaining fluid volume (McCardle et al, 1991).

NOREPINEPHRINE AND EPINEPHRINE

Secretion of these hormones by the adrenal medulla is stimulated by exercise and increases as the intensity of the exercise increases. A greater response to exercise is seen in older than in younger individuals, and in men than in women. Also known as catecholamines, these hormones are related to activity of the sympathetic branch of the autonomic nervous system. They increase cardiac contractility, heart rate, distribution of blood within the vascular system, and so forth. They are also active in the breakdown of stored fat into free fatty acids and of glycogen into glucose (McArdle et al, 1991; Noble, 1986).

CORTISOL

Cortisol is secreted by the adrenal cortex. It promotes the formation of glucose from proteins and fatty acids during intense exercise. ACTH stimulates the release of cortisol.

INSULIN

Insulin is secreted by the pancreas when blood glucose levels are too high. It inhibits the effects of epinephrine and glucagon on fat metabolism and facilitates glucose uptake by the muscle cells. Insulin secretion is usually decreased during prolonged exercise (McArdle et al, 1991; Noble, 1986; Sutton et al, 1990).

GLUCAGON

Glucagon also is secreted by the pancreas when blood glucose falls below a threshold. It stimulates the formation of glucose from liver glycogen stores and amino acids. It can also stimulate the breakdown of fat stores. Glucagon acts in opposition to insulin; its secretion is increased during exercise (McArdle et al, 1991; Noble, 1986).

LONG-TERM EFFECTS OF TRAINING

With training, insulin and glucagon are maintained at closer to resting levels during exercise (McArdle et al, 1991). Levels of epinephrine and norepinephrine at rest and during submaximal work are decreased. Cortisol and ACTH levels are slightly elevated during exercise. Training does not appear to have an effect on the resting levels of growth hormone in adults (McArdle et al, 1991). In older adults, insulin receptors become more active following training (Shepard, 1987).

Integration of All Systems

All of the systems discussed above work together to allow the body to efficiently utilize its energy stores and produce the mechanical work necessary for physical activity. A measure of how efficiently the body can perform this task is the *maximal aerobic capacity,* or *maximal oxygen uptake.* Maximal aerobic capacity, which measures the maximum level of work an individual can perform, is a major determinant of overall functional ability. This measure improves as an individual's level of fitness improves and decreases with inactivity. McArdle and colleagues (1991) surveyed several research studies and reported that regular vigorous physical activity can result in physiologic improvements, regardless of age. One's habitual level of physical activity is thought to be more of a determinant of aerobic capacity than chronologic age.

Maximal oxygen consumption refers to the largest amount of oxygen that can be consumed at the tissue level. This value decreases with age (Payne & Isaacs, 1987). Oxygen consumption can be increased two ways. The first is to increase blood flow to the muscles by increasing cardiac output. The second is to extract more oxygen at the tissue level by increasing the capillarization of the trained muscle tissue, number of mitochondria, and levels of enzymes necessary for aerobic metabolism (Knortz, 1987; McCardle et al, 1991; Noble, 1986; Shepard, 1987; Zernicke et al, 1991).

Age affects maximal aerobic capacity. Maximal aerobic capacity appears to be lower in children than in adults, but it increases through childhood as size increases. Effectiveness of training on the maximal aerobic capacity of children has been inconclusive (Bar-Or, 1983; Cunningham et al, 1984; Porter, 1989). As discussed by McArdle and colleagues (1991), after age 25, maximal aerobic capacity decreases by approximately 1 per cent per year. In the elderly, maximal oxygen uptake is limited by the inability to increase cardiac output (O'Toole & Douglas, 1988; Saltin, 1990), but older adults in exercise programs demonstrate improved maximal aerobic power (Cunningham et al, 1987).

EXERCISE AND TRAINING CONSIDERATIONS ACROSS THE LIFE SPAN

As discussed throughout this book, exercise and training programs can improve one's health and fitness. Quality of life is improved as one feels better, does more, and develops a positive self-image. Exercise helps one attain and maintain body efficiency, allowing one to function optimally within the environment. This is why health promotion and fitness activities are increasingly important in today's health care arena. Exercise planning and programming is a complex process. Detailed assessment of a person's ability to participate in an exercise program is necessary. Exercise programs differ according to a person's age, health, level of fitness, and interests. The following discussion focuses on special considerations in the development of exercise programs for children and older adults.

Childhood

The child's response to exercise or aerobic training is not well understood (Bar-Or, 1984; Porter, 1989). It is difficult to separate effects of growth and maturation from the effects of the conditioning program. Many of the changes in cardiovascular, pulmonary, and muscle function that result from conditioning also are seen as a result of normal growth and maturation (Bar-Or, 1983). Children also maintain naturally high levels of physical activity, but this activity is mechanically inefficient. A running child must move her short legs more frequently and faster than an adult, who can sprint with a long stride. This inefficient pattern results in high energy cost. As the child grows, mechanical efficiency increases and endurance improves (Bar-Or, 1983; Porter, 1989; Smith, 1988).

In general, younger children have more difficulty in maintaining aerobic or anaerobic work than do adolescents. Determinants of aerobic capacity such as muscle mass, stroke volume, cardiac output, and vital capacity are directly proportional to size (Gandy, 1987). Anaerobic capacity of children is limited by their diminished ability to process glycogen.

The thermoregulatory capacity of children is different from that of adults. Children have a high ratio of surface area to body weight, allowing a greater rate of heat exchange with the environment. For this reason, children may have more difficulty exercising in extremely hot or cold weather. Children also sweat less then adults, making them less able to dissipate heat (Bar-Or, 1984).

It is difficult to define optimal intensity, duration, and frequency of endurance training for children. Regular physical activity should be encouraged to promote optimal physiologic fitness and to establish health behavior patterns for the child to carry into adulthood. Children are learning and perfecting motor skills that promote agility, balance, coordination, speed, and power. Fitness evaluations and programs for children should include a motor skills component (Malina, 1990). Endurance activities that require anaerobic metabolism should be thoroughly evaluated for appropriateness. Events such as long distance running for prepubescent children may be inappropriate (Smith, 1988).

Older Adulthood

Older adults are generally happy with their level of fitness but underestimate their ability to exercise (Buskirk, 1990). As maximal exercise capacity decreases with age, it begins to affect the intensity of exercise that can be considered submaximal work. For example, activities of daily living are considered submaximal work. The energy required to perform these activities remains constant, but the percentage of maximal capacity they require increases as the maximal exercise capacity decreases. These activities then become more stressful. If the individual can no longer complete activities of daily living because of the level of physiologic stress, functional independence is decreased (Peel, 1990). Studies have shown that regular exercise, even in the 7th decade of life, can increase maximal aerobic capacity and submaximal work capacity (Cunningham & Patterson, 1990).

Exercise programming for the older adult should emphasize the functional needs of the individual. A person's level of fitness and interests must be kept in mind (Thomas & Rutlege, 1985). Both aerobic exercise (to strengthen the cardiovascular system) and low-intensity exercise (to control weight and loss of bone mineral, to improve flexibility, and to retain muscle endurance) should be included. Additional time should be allowed for warm-up and cool-down (Peel, 1990). Use of large muscle groups in continuous rhythmic movements is also recommended (O'Toole & Douglas, 1988).

SUMMARY

One's level of health and physical fitness is related to one's level of physical activity. Many body systems work together to produce efficient, effective physical activity. Each of these systems develops uniquely; this development can be positively influenced by participation in physical fitness programs.

Because optimal health and fitness reflect the ability to maintain a physically active and independent lifestyle, fitness programming is an important focus of health care. Health care providers should familiarize themselves with the age-related aspects of exercise and training programs to help themselves and their clients attain lifelong fitness.

References

Bailey DA, Mirwald RL. The effects of training on the growth and development of the child. In Malina RM (ed). *Young Athlete's Biological, Psychological and Educational Perspectives.* Springfield, IL: Human Kinetics Press, 1988, pp 33–47.

Bar-Or O. *Pediatric Sports Medicine for the Practitioner.* New York: Springer Verlag, 1983.

Bar-Or O. The growth and development of children's physiologic and perceptional responses to exercise. In Ilmannen J, Valimaki I (eds.). *Children and Sport—Pediatric Work Physiology.* New York: Springer Verlag, 1984, pp 3–17.

Bar-Or O. The prepubescent female. In Shangold MM, Mirken G (eds). *Women and Exercise: Physiology and Sports Medicine.* Philadelphia: FA Davis, 1988, pp 109–119.

Biegel L. *Physical Fitness and the Older Person: A Guide to Exercise for Health Care Professionals.* Rockville, MD: Aspen Publishing, 1984.

Bouchard C, Shepard RJ, Stephens T, Sutton JR, McPherson BD. *Exercise Fitness and Health: A Consensus of Current Knowledge.* Champaign, IL: Human Kinetics Books, 1990.

Brooks CM. Leisure time physical activity assessment of American adults through an analysis of time diaries collected in 1981. *Am J Public Health* 77:455–460, 1987.

Buskirk ER. Exercise, fitness and aging. In Bouchard C, et al (eds). *Exercise, Fitness and Health: A Consensus of Current Knowledge.* Champaign, IL: Human Kinetics Publishers, 1990, pp 687–697.

Caspersen CJ, Christenson GM, Pollard RA. Status of the 1990 physical fitness and exercise objectives—evidence from NHIS 1985. *Public Health Rep* 101:587–592, 1986.

Cunningham DA, Paterson DH. Discussion: Exercise, fitness and aging. In Bouchard C, et al (eds). *Exercise, Fitness and Health: A Consensus of Current Knowledge.* Champaign, IL: Human Kinetics Books, 1990, pp 699–704.

Cunningham DA, Paterson DH, Blimke CJR. The development of the cardiorespiratory system with growth and physical activity. In Bouleau RA (ed). *Advances in Pediatric Sport Science, vol. 1: Biological Issues.* Champaign, IL: Human Kinetics Publishers, 1984, pp 85–116.

Cunningham DA, Rechnitzer PA, Howard JH, Donner AP. Exercise training of men at retirement — A clinical trial. *J Gerontol* 42:17–23, 1987.

Faulkner JA, White TP. Adaptation of skeletal muscle to physical activity. In Bouchard C, et al (eds). *Exercise, Fitness and Health: A Consensus of Current Knowledge.* Champaign, IL: Human Kinetics Books, 1990, pp 256–279.

Folinsbee LJ. Discussion: Exercise and environment. In Bouchard C, et al (eds). *Exercise, Fitness and Health: A Consensus of Current Knowledge.* Champaign, IL: Human Kinetics Books, 1990, pp 179–183.

Frontera WR, Evans WJ. Exercise performance and endurance training in the elderly. *Top Geriatr Rehabil* 2:17–32, 1986.

Gandy J. Adolescent sports injury. In Tecklin JS (ed). *Pediatric Physical Therapy.* Philadelphia: JB Lippincott, 1989, pp 318–341.

Green HJ. Discussion: Adaptation of skeletal muscle to physical activity. In Bouchard C, et al (eds). *Exercise, Fitness and Health: A Consensus of Current Knowledge.* Champaign, IL: Human Kinetics Publishers, 1990, pp 281–291.

Haskell WL. Cardiovascular benefits and risks of exercise: The scientific evidence. In Straus RH (ed). *Sports Medicine.* Philadelphia: WB Saunders, 1984, pp 57–76.

Haywood KM. *Lifespan Motor Development.* Champaign, IL: Human Kinetics Books, 1986.

Holman W, Klemt F, Rost R, Liesen H, Heck H. Comparative studies of physical work capacity of children in 1964 & 1984 and adaptations during competitive training. In Malina RM (ed). *Young Athlete's Biological, Psychological and Educational Perspectives.* Springfield, IL: Human Kinetics Publishers, 1988, pp 49–59.

Irwin SC, Zadai CC. Cardiopulmonary rehabilitation of the geriatric patient. In Lewis CB (ed). *Aging: The Health Care Challenge,* 2nd ed. Philadelphia: FA Davis, 1990, pp 181–211.

Katch FI, Katch VL. Optimal health and body composition. In Shangold MM, Mirkin G (eds). *Women and Exercise: Physiology and Sports Medicine.* Philadelphia: FA Davis, 1988, pp 23–39.

Kitzman DW, Edwards WD. Minireview: Age-related changes in the anatomy of the normal human heart. *J Geriatr Med Sci* 45(2):33–39, 1990.

Knortz KA. Muscle physiology applied to geriatric rehabilitation. *Top Geriatr Rehabil* 2(4):1–12, 1987.

Leeson TS, Leeson CR, Paparo AA. *Test/Atlas of Histology.* Philadelphia: WB Saunders, 1988.

Mahon AD, Vaccaro T. Ventilatory threshhold and Vo_2 max changes in children following endurance training. *Med Sci Sports Exerc* 21(4):425–431, 1989.

Malina RM. Growth, performance, activity and training during adolescence. In Shangold MM, Mirken G (eds). *Women and Exercise: Physiology and Sports Medicine.* Philadelphia: FA Davis, 1988, pp 120–128.

Malina RM. Growth, exercise fitness and later outcomes. In Bouchard C, et al (eds). *Exercise, Fitness and Health: A Consensus of Current Knowledge.* Champaign, IL: Human Kinetics Publishers, 1990, pp 637–653.

McArdle WD, Katch FI, Katch VL. *Exercise Physiology: Energy, Nutrition and Human Performance,* 3rd. ed. Philadelphia: Lea & Febiger, 1991.

Noble BJ. *Physiology of Exercise and Sport.* St Louis: Times Mirror/Mosby College Publishing, 1986.

O'Toole ML, Douglas PS. Fitness: Definition and development. In Shangold MN, Mirkin G (eds). *Women and Exercise: Physiology and Sports Medicine.* Philadelphia: FA Davis, 1988, pp 3–19.

Pate RR, Shepard RJ. Characteristics of physical fitness in youth. In Grisolfi CV, Lamb DR (eds). *Perspectives in Exercise Science and Sports Medicine: Youth Exercise and Sport,* Vol 2. Indianapolis: Benchmark Press, 1989, pp 1–45.

Payne VG, Isaacs LD. *Human Motor Development: A Life Span Approach.* Mountain View, CA: Mayfield Publishing, 1987.

Peel C. Cardiopulmonary changes with aging. In Irwin S, Tecklin JS (eds). *Cardiopulmonary Physical Therapy,* 2nd ed. St. Louis: CV Mosby, 1990, pp 477–489.

Porter RE. Normal development of movement and function: Child and adolescent. In Scully RM, Barnes MR (eds). *Physical Therapy.* Philadelphia: JB Lippincott, 1989, pp 83–98.

Saltin B. Cardiovascular and pulmonary adaptation to physical activity. In Bouchard C, et al (eds). *Exercise, Fitness and Health: A Consensus of Current Knowledge.* Champaign, IL: Human Kinetics Books, 1990, pp 187–203.

Shepard RJ. *Exercise Physiology.* Toronto: BC Decker, 1987.

Sinclair D. *Human Growth After Birth,* 3rd ed. London: Oxford University Press, 1978.

Smith AD. Children and sport. In Scoles P (ed). *Pediatric Orthopedics in Clinical Practice,* 2nd ed. Chicago: Year Book, 1988, pp 269–285.

Sutton JR, Farrell PA, Harber VJ. Hormonal adaptation to physical activity. In Bouchard C, et al (eds). *Exercise, Fitness and Health: A Consensus of Current Knowledge.* Champaign, IL: Human Kinetics Books, 1990, pp 217–257.

Tecklin JS. Pulmonary disorders in infants and children and their physical therapy management. In Tecklin JS (ed). *Pediatric Physical Therapy.* Philadelphia: JB Lippincott, 1989, pp 141–172.

Thomas GS, Rutledge JH. Fitness and exercise for the elderly. In Dychtwald K (ed). *Wellness and Health Promotion for the Elderly.* Rockville, MD: Aspen Publishing, 1985, pp 165–177.

U.S. Department of Health and Human Services. "Promoting health–Preventing disease; Year 2000 objectives for the nation." Washington, DC: Public Health Services, NIH, 1990.

Wei JY. Cardiovascular anatomic and physiologic changes with age. *Top Geriatr Rehabil* 2(1):10–16, 1986.

Zernicke RF, Salem GJ, Alejo RK. Endurance training. In Reider B (ed). *Sports Medicine: The School Age Athlete.* Philadelphia: WB Saunders, 1991, pp 3–17.

Index

. . . .

Note: Page numbers in *italics* refer to illustrations; page numbers followed by t refer to tables.